P9-DVJ-034

Adult Leukemia

A Comprehensive Guide for Patients and Families

Barbara Lackritz

O'REILLY®

Beijing • Cambridge • Farnham • Köln • Paris • Sebastopol • Taipei • Tokyo

Library of Congress Cataloging-in-Publication Data:

Lackritz, Barb (Barbara B.)
    Adult leukemia : a comprehensive guide for patients and families / Barb Lackritz.
        p. cm.—(Patient-centered guides)
    Includes bibliographical references and index.
    ISBN: 0-596-50001-7 (pbk.)
        1. Leukemia—Popular Works. I. Title. II. Series.

RC643 L33 2001
616.99'419—dc21   00-046478

[M]

This book is dedicated to my family.

I wouldn't be here now if it weren't for my husband, Irv,
who was with me all the way, and my children Hilary and
Tony Ticknor, Pamela and Bill Kuehling, and Neal
and Marjorie Lackritz.

Neal and his lovely wife took amazing care of me
when I had my transplant; I shall never forget their kindness.
My brother Michael Bank and his incredible wife, Nancy,
were always there for me.

Grandchildren Benjamin and Lauren Moehle, and
Randall Ticknor are three of the most wonderful reasons
to celebrate life and to live it to the fullest.

Table of Contents

Foreword

FEW MORE DEVASTATING WORDS CAN BE HEARD THAN "You have leukemia." After hearing this you enter a bewildering world full of totally foreign words—the world of someone battling leukemia. The good news is that over the past few decades, tremendous advances have been made in the treatment of acute and chronic leukemias, and new treatment approaches are constantly offering more hope that these once invariably fatal diseases will soon be conquered.

Along with advances in the medical treatment of leukemias have come new methods for disseminating information (most notably, the Internet). Patients arrive in clinics vastly more informed about their diseases than seemed possible only a few years ago. Making this information more freely available to all patients is a goal for us all. Thanks to user groups and information sites on the Internet, information can be found and digested in the patient's own time in a way that a visit to the doctor's office could never provide. Barb Lackritz—or "GrannyBarb," as she is known to her legions of fans on GrannyBarb and Art's Leukemia Links and the CLL Internet support group—has not only fought her own battles with leukemia, but also arms patients with the information needed to fight their own battles. Recently, exciting results have emerged regarding a new drug treatment for chronic myelogenous leukemia that will likely revolutionize the way we treat this disease. Hopefully this pattern will be repeated for the other leukemias. How does a person with leukemia and their family find the information about these new treatments and understand it in the context of his or her own specific disease? The answer lies in using the information in this book to help ask the right questions and having frank discussions with caregivers.

This book is a tremendous resource. Barb Lackritz goes further than providing the type of information now available on the Internet. She provides a comprehensive guide to patients and families to help them navigate through the world of battling leukemia. This is deliberately written not as a standard medical textbook, but as a compendium of terms, explanations, and perhaps most importantly, descriptions from patients who have experience battling leukemia. Some of their stories are good, some bad, but all provide the benefit of experience, of someone else who has been there before. I was particularly struck by one individual's response to diagnosis. After hearing the words "You have leukemia," every other word in the meeting with their physician was lost in a flurry of emotion. A number of stories describe physicians passing on such news in such an uncaring manner that you wince when you read them. But, of course, there is no easy way to tell someone such devastating news. The important thing is how to get to "cure." Clearly, complex treatments for leukemia require working closely with the caregiver team led by your oncologist. Understanding fully what is happening and why will help you win the battle!

GrannyBarb's book offers valuable help to those fighting leukemia, and her continued commitment to others is indeed an inspiration to all of us in the community who are resolved to treat and cure leukemia. Hopefully *Adult Leukemia* will motivate others to become more involved in patient resources.

— Dr. John Gribben
Dana-Farber Cancer Institute
Associate Professor of Medicine
Harvard Medical School, Boston

Preface

IF YOU ARE READING THIS BOOK IT IS LIKELY that you or someone close to you has been diagnosed with leukemia. A cancer diagnosis is shocking and frightening. It changes your life in many ways and affects every member of your family. It brings you face to face with your own mortality. Your friends will be concerned and many won't know how to deal with you. You will be afraid of pain and possible dependence on others, and you will fear dying. Nevertheless, do not despair!

This book offers facts about the disease and contains stories from people who have been through what you face. It offers hope and helps you to deal with and to understand things you are likely to experience. It even suggests ways to make yourself a very well informed patient so that you regain some control over your life.

Why I wrote this book

Everyone in life has to face a dragon or two. I met my dragon in 1988 shortly after my 50th birthday. I awakened that morning thinking that I liked my life. My children were delightful, good friends. My husband was doing well and had his health. I loved my profession and thoroughly enjoyed going to work each day. Life was good.

I've been taught from childhood never to tempt fate. Perhaps I should have known better than to have counted blessings that morning. After work, I stopped off at the doctor's office to have my cholesterol checked. I left the blood sample, and drove home singing despite the traffic. The next morning the call came, "Barb, the blood work looks strange. Come in and we'll do it again." I came in, blithe and unaware. That time the doctor did the pathology himself. He told me:

> *Your white blood count is high. There are some strange smudge cells*
> *in the blood sample. I hate to say it, but I want you to see a hematologist*

because I think you have chronic lymphocytic leukemia. Oh yes, one thing more. Your cholesterol is within normal limits.

So began my first encounter with this dragon. My cholesterol was fine. That was why I had the blood test done. The dragon swooped down like a lightning bolt. There was no warning, no symptoms, nothing to give me any idea that I was fighting for my life.

It was a quiet, patient dragon. It didn't give me any trouble for almost four years (after we were introduced), but then it roared into battle. My counts had been climbing slowly during those years, but they were nothing to worry about. Suddenly I was fatigued and had a hard time getting out of bed. Bruises on my arms stayed black and blue for weeks. Sinus infections moved in to stay.

The time had come to meet the dragon in battle. Six months of fludarabine monophosphate chemotherapy administered intravenously gave me a temporary victory. More battles followed with shorter spaces between, until I was in a last ditch battle for my life. An autologous bone marrow transplant using my own purged cells gave me the latest victory and I've been cancer free since June 1997. The dragon is sleeping, and I hope it has finally conceded victory to me. If not, I shall battle again.

The battles were not easy. I had great help all along the way. Family, friends, and health professionals provided strong support, good choices, and the best of medical care. My colleagues fought with me right to the last dragon roar and since then we have celebrated life, each day, every day. May my dragon never wake!

When I was diagnosed with chronic lymphocytic leukemia I had no idea that it was a hematological malignancy. I knew nothing about the disease. My mother's sister had died in the 1920s of Hodgkin's disease, but all I knew was that it was a blood disease. I had lots to learn, but there were few resources.

I started at the public library looking for books on leukemia. There was almost nothing there. I called the Leukemia Society of America and (800) 4 CANCER, but they had little to offer an information-starved patient. I tried the Internet, but in those days there was little information online and finding it was not an easy task. As I gained knowledge, I promised myself that I would never let anyone else go through the frustration I encountered alone as I tried to research my disease.

In an attempt to make the information more accessible to the public, I wrote GrannyBarb's chronic lymphocytic leukemia (CLL) story (*http://www.acor.org/ leukemia/storydir/barb.html*) and posted it on the World Wide Web. It is used now as a teaching tool for young doctors studying at the National Institutes of Health. I also created a web site called "GrannyBarb's Leukemia Links," which subsequently was joined with another leukemia links site run by Arthur Flatau, PhD, an acute myelogenous leukemia survivor, to become GrannyBarb and Art's Leukemia Links (*http://www.acor.org/leukemia*).

I joined Internet support lists to help myself, and ended up helping to found the Hem-Onc List, supporting those with hematological malignancies. Hem-Onc is the grandmother of the hematological cancer lists. Presently I work with support lists for every kind of leukemia, and with many non-leukemia lists as well. I sit on the board of directors of ACOR, the Association of Cancer Online Resources, and the CLL Foundation to increase visibility and to educate people about leukemia. The CLL Foundation raises funds for research into CLL. I speak at forums throughout the country and, with top CLL specialists in the US, have participated in online web casts that are promoted by the Leukemia and Lymphoma Society (available at *http://www. healthtalk.com*). Now I'm writing this book to try to bring information to people who are dealing with this disease but who may not yet be online.

I strongly believe that an informed patient is the best kind of patient. We make today's healthcare institutions give us the quality of care we need. We know what questions to ask and what treatment options we have. I sincerely hope this book will provide you with as much information about leukemia as you feel you want to learn.

My quest is to enable others to walk the paths I've walked with less fear and trepidation. Yes, it is a quest! Those of us who battle the leukemia dragon know we must ensure that the dragon does not defeat anyone due to a lack of information, support, education, or medical choices.

Organization of the book

The book is organized to take you along the path of a patient's experiences from symptoms, to understanding the nature of the disease, to testing and diagnosis. You'll learn what leukemia is and what it isn't. We survivors will share the questions we wish we had known to ask our doctors. We'll discuss tests and procedures so that you will know what to expect before you have to deal with them, or so that you understand what you have experienced and why.

In Chapter 6, we look at risks and possible causes for and predispositions to leukemia. Chapters 7 and 8 discuss staging and standard treatments for each leukemia. We'll not only talk about what possible treatments might be, but about how the treatments are given. The information is complex and I've tried to make it understandable. If you are only interested in one type of leukemia, feel free to read only the sections that deal with it.

Many leukemias are treated with bone marrow or stem cell transplants, so in Chapter 9, *Transplantation,* we'll cover the topic in depth. Because new treatments arrive frequently, we'll discuss what clinical trials can and can't do for you in Chapter 10, *Clinical Trials and Beyond.* Clinical trials move rapidly and something really exciting may happen between the writing and publishing of this material. While we've tried to be as current as possible, new ideas and research results will invariably change the landscape of leukemia therapy as it exists today.

With all the treatment options available, choices become most confusing for patients. Families and caregivers are often called upon for help, so we'll cover ways to make the best treatment decision. Working with your doctor and his team is a key issue, so we've devoted Chapter 11, *Communicating with Your Medical Team,* to ways to make this important relationship effective.

Treatment helps, but sometimes there are side effects. In Chapter 12, *Side Effects of Treatment,* topics of discussion include what to expect and how to deal with unexpected side effects. In Chapter 13, *Stress and the Immune System,* we'll talk about stress and what it does to the immune system, and we'll discuss ways of getting support when you need it in Chapter 14, *Getting Support.* Treatment takes over our world at times, but how do we deal with life when treatment is over and we're back in real-time again? Chapter 16, *After Treatment* deals with ways to face that problem.

Sooner or later that hard-won remission may deteriorate and we may face a recurrence of leukemia. We'll consider ways to deal with that situation head on. At some point we may have used all the available options and all treatments may have failed. That's when we'll talk about end of life issues and how to deal with what comes next (see Chapter 18, *If All Treatments Have Failed*).

Chapter 19, the final chapter of this book, is dear to my heart, for it talks about how you can research your leukemia. We've put many references in the chapter and given you addresses for web sites where you will find still more information.

Appendix A includes general resources for assistance. Appendix B provides blood and marrow test values so blood work reports make sense to you. Appendix C provides charts for calculating body surface area; Appendix D explains acute leukemia staging; Appendix E provides genetic explanations of the different leukemias; Appendix F explains the progression of cell development; and Appendix G provides charts of common chemotherapies used for leukemia treatments. Yes, there is a Glossary of terms, because we need to become conversant with the language we're exposed to during leukemia battles. The book ends with a blood and marrow donor card for those who care about others who have leukemia and wish to give a gift of life.

Who this book is written for

If you've recently been diagnosed with leukemia, you're likely feeling panic and pain. Your whole world has fallen apart and you've been left in the rubble. No matter who is there to help you, the ultimate decisions are yours. How do you pick up the pieces and weave them back into your life again? How do you help your family and friends accept and understand the situation? How do you step back from the worry and accept the help that others are offering?

The information in this book was assembled with you in mind. It has been gathered over a long period and includes the experiences of hundreds of cancer patients, their children and families, and their caregivers. We hope that when you're finished reading this, you feel that you have met friends who have been there and done that and are sharing their experiences so that you know what to expect down the line.

For those of you who have been dealing with this dragon for a while now, you know what a canny old beast it is. You've had first-hand some of the experiences we relate. We hope you'll be reading and shaking your head thinking, "Oh yes! That was quite an experience, and mine was similar." There is as much new information in this text as could be found to share. Leukemia research is moving very rapidly and new information is coming weekly from the human genome project, which is impacting every facet of cancer research. The treatment options of the future may make current practices look barbaric. We may even achieve that wonderful dream—a cure for leukemia!

You may be a spouse, a child, a family member, a good friend, or a medical professional. In all those cases the information in this book should be of help to you in understanding what the patient is undergoing and how those experiences are being perceived. We hope that you will find suggestions that will enable you to help your patient deal with this illness. We also hope that whatever your relationship, you will find information here that will ease the load of worry you carry as you watch the battle with the dragon, knowing that all you can do is wait for the outcome. Many patients say that they think the watching and waiting is harder for the caregiver and family members. Patients are being treated. Something is being done for them. All the others can do is watch and worry.

What this book provides

This book is written by a patient, not a doctor. It provides information that is based upon patient experiences and perceptions. Scientific terminology has been kept to a minimum, but common terms that the patient needs to understand are explained. Patients communicate with medical professionals who use special jargon. Some of their language simply needs to be translated; other bits and pieces need to be restated in ways the patient can understand.

As patients, we need to know some basic medical information so that things that happen and continue to happen in our lives can be put into a frame of reference that makes sense to us. We have to know the basic tests and information from the results of tests so that we can put them into a logical context. Treatment options need to be explained in ways that show us how we benefit. We will try to provide that frame of reference in these chapters.

Acknowledgments

This book wouldn't have been written without immeasurable help from Lorraine Johnston, who lent me material that she had already researched and organized. Thanks too go to the editor, Linda Lamb, for her unfailing good nature, organizational skills with material, and uncanny ability to help me see how to make my words say what I thought they were saying originally. Linda, I consider you a gift! Thanks to Shawnde Paull who clarified, streamlined, and made the sections of this book go together as seamlessly as they could. Thanks also for her technical expertise in creating the tables that make things so clear.

Special thanks to David Olliver, friend and mentor, who has kept me informed of the latest developments in leukemia treatments and so, saved my sanity. Another mentor is friend and neighbor Dr. Scott Martin, who clarified when the science became too complex and helped me make sense of the pathology information. Professor Susan Leclair was always willing to answer questions about blood work and tests and contributed the content of Appendix F, *Progression of Cell Development*. Dr. Gerald Marti of the FDA was another unfailing mentor who spent hours working with me. They have my great appreciation. Dr. Alex Denes, Dr. John Gribben, and Dr. Maria Sgambatti all donated their time to make this book as correct as they could.

None of these people can be held responsible for any errors you find here: those must be blamed on me.

Research assistance came from the Dana-Farber Cancer Institute's Katherine F. Stephans, RN; Susan Woods, RN, of Dr. Kipps's and Dr. Wierda's office at UCSD; Linda Mercer of the M. D. Anderson Information Line; Sue Laurent, RN and Medical Case Manager for Strategic Health Development Corp.; and Michelle Keating, RN, and Michelle Nobs, RN, of the St. John's Mercy Resource Center. Thanks to Mary Fox-Geiman, PharmD, BCOP who helped with information about drugs and other treatment substances.

Susan K. Stewart of the BMT News Information Network was most helpful with the transplant chapter. Michael Keating, MB, BS; Andrew Bosanquet, BSc, PhD; and Michael Andreef, MD, provided specific background information. Thousands of thanks to most generous technical reviewers including Hector Bensimon, MD, FACS; Bruce Chesson, MD; Costas Giannakenas, MD, PhD; and John Gribben, MD, PhD.

Many members of the ALL-L, AML, CLL, CML, Hairy cell, Hem-Onc, MPD-Net, and other online cancer support lists clarified the topics, found URLs, and generally provided me with what they do best—support and encouragement. Very special appreciation, acknowledgment, and many thanks to Hazel Silverstein, who went through chapter after chapter dealing with all the nitty-gritty details. Thanks also to Charlene Prost, and David Covell for their time and review.

This book is greatly enhanced by the many leukemia survivors' stories that bring its pages to life. My thanks and cheers to these marvelous individuals. Some people asked that their names not be used, and that confidence has been honored, but their stories make this book all the more readable. Story contributions were made by Stephen Addison, Sally Armour, Neeraj Arora, Linda Bier, Rosemary Bradford, Bettina A. Brumbaugh, Danielle Chaikin, Rand Costich, David Covell, Lynn Crawford, Nell Day, Ellen Diamond, Arthur Flatau, Sharon Foster, Mark Freymiller, Pat Gardiner, Merrill Hayes, Elizabeth Hawes, Paul Hoffman, Antoine Ioannides, Michael Keener, E. Hubbard Kennady III, Dr. Monta Kennady, Karin Laakso, Kathy Lebedun, Kim Murphy, J. F. S. Le Noury, Judit Luger, Tom McCune, Gary Moon, Jenny O'Brien, David Palmer, Dan Peiser, Daryl Rutherford, Trudy Rhynsburger, Ed Sakal, Hazel Silverstein, Danielle Simmons, Michele Stevens, Merlyn L. Stock, Tom Storer, Janet Upchurch, Suzanne Wohl, and John Wood.

CHAPTER 1

What Leukemia Is

IT'S A SHOCK TO HEAR that you have been diagnosed with leukemia, that tests on your blood are suspicious and you might have leukemia, or that you have a condition that might later lead to leukemia (a preleukemic condition). It's difficult to know what this disease is or what it might mean to you. For many people, leukemia is a childhood disease that is more curable today than ever before. Adult leukemia is less publicized and most people know little about it.

Leukemia is a cancer of the blood-forming cells. Specifically, it usually involves white blood cells that may not mature fully and that reproduce too rapidly. These leukemic cells look different from normal cells under the microscope and are unable to do the job they were created to do. Other leukemia cells look just like normal cells, but they don't die when they should. Eventually, leukemic cells replace normal bone marrow, leaving insufficient room for "good" cells, which include red blood cells, nonmalignant white cells, and platelets, all of which are vital for the body to function properly.

This chapter first covers blood basics: normal blood components and how blood functions. Then we look at how leukemia begins and the resultant changes that occur in the blood. Next we discuss using blood samples to make the diagnostic determination. We focus on similarities and differences among the leukemias and, following that, we look at the different kinds of leukemias. We'll talk about some preleukemic conditions and other similar conditions that are not leukemia.

Information is based on Henderson and Lister's *Leukemia, Sixth Edition*; the National Cancer Institute's *Report on Leukemia*; the tenth edition of Wintrobe's *Clinical Hematology*; and resources listed in *Notes* at the end of the book.

Understanding how leukemia affects your blood cells and what the types of leukemia are will help you better visualize what is happening in your body, understand symptoms of the disease, and participate in treatment decisions.

If you've just been diagnosed, but you're not interested in medical details at this time, please skip ahead.

Understanding blood

Blood is made up of plasma and blood cells. Plasma is the straw-colored, clear fluid that carries the blood cells, also known as corpuscles. There are three different kinds of corpuscles in blood: the red cells (erythrocytes), the white cells (leukocytes), and the platelets (thrombocytes). White cells have nuclei, but red cells do not. Figure 1-1 shows the relative size and quantity of these three kinds of cells.

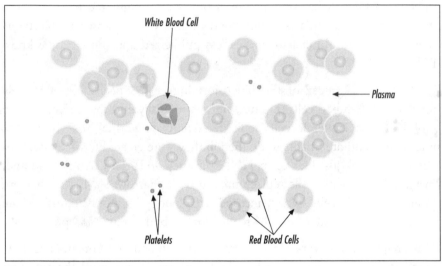

Figure 1-1. Blood cells in normal blood

Blood cells are formed in the bone marrow (the spongy tissue inside bones) from precursors called stem cells. Stem cells can become several types of blood cells: red blood cells, all varieties of white blood cells, and platelets. Each stem cell can reproduce (clone) itself and give birth to a number of immature cells (blasts) and cells that will mature into a particular type of blood cell (committed precursor cells). Stem cells can circulate and be collected as peripheral blood stem cells when they leave the bone marrow and enter the bloodstream.

Stem cells start out with the potential to become any type of cell. Specific hormone or hormone-like substances stimulate stem cells, committing them to either the lymphocyte cell line or the myeloid cell line. Figure 1-2 shows how stem cells progress to become particular types of blood cells. The particular types of cells are described in subsequent sections.

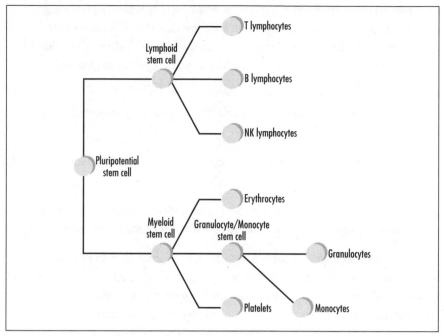

Figure 1-2. Progression of cell development from stem cell to definite cell line

If you'd like more information about how stem cells develop, see Appendix F, *Progression of Cell Development.*

Normal bone marrow is composed of many different cells all reproducing themselves and forming new cells that will, in turn, develop into red blood cells, white blood cells, and platelets. The normal marrow also balances the production of different cell types so they appear in the blood in proper amounts. In a leukemia patient, some blood cells develop in the spleen and lymph nodes as well. Blood circulates in the marrow and throughout the body.

Although the specifics of what cells make up blood, where blood cells are developed, and what kinds of white cells there are might sound abstract or complex at first, you'll become more familiar with what cells are affected by leukemia and how blood cell counts relate to treatment and your progress. As one survivor recalls:

When I was first diagnosed, I'd heard of white blood cells and red blood cells, but not much else. If I had thought, a year ago, that I'd be thrilled when my white blood cell count dropped or heartened when my red blood cell count was high enough for my next chemotherapy treatment, I wouldn't have believed it. I certainly wouldn't have believed that I would scan blood tests looking at how my lymphocytes or neutrophils were doing.

Since leukemia attacks my blood, I've become very interested in the health of my blood. I'm "rooting for" those little cells.

Another survivor recalls gradually becoming interested in her blood cells and counts:

At first, I wasn't at all interested in the different kinds of white cells and all the different terms. That was the doctor's business, wasn't it?

However, I quickly came to realize that the kinds and numbers of blood cells in my blood and bone marrow directly affected me. How many blasts (immature white cells) were developing in my bone marrow was an indicator that told me information about my health. My counts indicated if the treatment was working and whether I'd have chemotherapy as scheduled. Some counts tracked against how I was feeling; when my red cells were "up," I felt good.

I soon became a "blood watcher," too. The terms that sounded like Greek a few months ago are more familiar now.

Red blood cells

Red blood cells (erythrocytes or RBCs) contain hemoglobin, an iron-rich protein that picks up oxygen in the lungs and transports it throughout the body. Hemoglobin gives blood its red color. Red blood cells make up the largest proportion of blood cells in the body and approximately 45 percent of blood volume. When leukemia cells in the bone marrow slow down the production of red cells and not enough red cells are present, the patient develops anemia. Anemia can cause tiredness, weakness, irritability, pale skin, and headache. Some patients also report that they are short of breath when they are anemic.

White blood cells

White blood cells (leukocytes or WBCs) are fewer in number than red blood cells. White blood cells are part of the immune system; they scan for and destroy foreign substances in the body such as viruses, bacteria, and fungi. Different types of white cells have different roles, for instance, in fighting particular types of invaders. When there is an invasion of disease-causing cells, extra white cells are produced to combat the infection. Once the white blood cells have done their job, the white cell levels return to normal.

There are several types of white cells, including monocytes, lymphocytes, and granulocytes. Each has a specific function:

- **Monocytes (monos).** The largest white blood cells, these literally engulf and destroy invading bacteria and fungi. They clean up the debris left after other white cells have successfully overcome other invaders, and they clean up dying cells as well. When they enter tissues or organs, they are called macrophages. As they settle and mature in the tissue, they grow even larger and continue to destroy invading cells.

- **Lymphocytes (lymphs).** The smallest of the white cells, they are essential to the immune system. They fight viral infections and assist in the destruction of parasites, fungi, and bacteria. New lymphocytes grow continually in the bone marrow and the lymph nodes, and many clusters of lymphocytes grow in the spleen. There are several types of lymphocytes. Each cell has markers on its surface that tell if it is a natural killer cell (NK), a T cell, or a B cell and, if it is a B cell, what antibodies it expresses.

  Antibodies are proteins produced in response to the presence of foreign substances, known as antigens. B cells manufacture antibodies, or immunoglobulins, that coat invading microorganisms, making them easier to destroy. T cells are the body's main defense against viruses and produce substances that help regulate the immune response. These T cells also help B cells produce antibodies, and they control the activities of various other white blood cells.

- **Granulocytes.** These are the first defense against many types of infection. They take up bacteria and destroy them with potent chemicals. Granulocytes are divided into several categories:

  - **Neutrophils (polys or segs).** These are infection-fighter cells. They carry granules of bacteria-killing enzymes. Bacterial infections will likely develop when the neutrophil count is very low.

- Basophils (basos). These are the rarest and least understood of the white cells. They play an important role in allergic reactions, such as asthma, hives, and drug reactions.

- Eosinophils (eos). These attack infection and also play an important role in allergic reactions, particularly in conditions known as delayed hypersensitivity reactions.

The different types of leukemia are cancers of a specific white blood cell type. For instance, acute lymphoblastic leukemia affects only lymphocytes. The specific types of leukemia are explained later in the chapter.

Platelets

Platelets or thrombocytes are the smallest elements in the bloodstream. Platelets are essential to control bleeding. These cells allow your blood to clot and stop the bleeding when you are cut. When the level of platelets in the blood is low, small red dots called petechiae appear on various parts of your body, caused by the escape of small drops of blood. These minute red dots are a warning that platelet numbers may be abnormally and seriously low or may not be functioning normally.

Blasts

"Blast" is short for an immature white blood cell, such as a lymphoblast, myeloblast, or monoblast. Normally, less than 5 percent of the cells contained in healthy bone marrow at any one time are blasts. Normal blasts develop into mature, functioning white blood cells, and are not usually found in the bloodstream. Leukemic blasts remain immature, multiply continuously, provide no defense against infection, and may be present in large numbers in the blood stream.

Antibodies

Antibodies and immunoglobulins are proteins produced by B cells to act against a substance the body has identified as an invader. B cells make five different types of immunoglobulins (Ig) or antibodies (Ab). They are IgA, IgD, IgE, IgG, and IgM. More is known about some of these than others.

IgG is the best known of the immunoglobulin classes. It is highly reactive, increasing activity and specificity of the granulocytes and monocytes.

(Increased specificity means that pathogens are easier to target.) IgG is able to move into interstitial fluids (those that fill the spaces within a tissue) and other places with ease. It assists in making toxins more susceptible to destruction, which in turn further increases the action of granulocytes and monocytes. This activity can also cause disintegration of certain antigens all by itself.

When you are deficient in IgG, everything about your immune system works a little more slowly and less effectively. When you have enough IgG, simple everyday invaders, such as bacteria that routinely enter the bloodstream when you brush your teeth, are eliminated within minutes. When there is less—or less effective—IgG, there is more stress on the system and it takes a longer time for the same elimination to occur. Something that you might have shrugged off becomes noticeable.

How leukemia begins

Leukemia is a disease of the white blood cells. Each kind of leukemia involves a particular white blood cell and reflects the level of maturation of the cell. The blood cells involved mutate to become cancer cells.

When you are told that leukemia is a disease of white blood cells, it can be difficult to visualize what is happening. One patient remembers:

> *"You have leukemia," the doctor said. "It's a disease in which the white blood cells multiply until they take up all the space in your bone marrow, forcing out the healthy cells." At least I think I remember hearing that.*
>
> *All I could picture were white blood cells with evil faces running wild in my veins like a children's cartoon show on Saturday morning. Even in my shock, I knew that was far out. And once I could think again, I needed to know more about blood and more about this disease.*

In most leukemias, except chronic lymphocytic leukemia, white cells in the bone marrow and/or lymphoid tissues begin to reproduce uncontrollably. These rapidly multiplying cells start out in the bone marrow. They crowd out the useful cells. After a while they spill over into the blood stream and may be found in the vital organs. The most commonly affected organs include lymph nodes, the spleen, liver, or skin. Sometimes the kidneys, brain, or other parts of the nervous system are involved. Ultimately, all tissue and organs are susceptible to leukemic infiltration.

How leukemia is diagnosed

The initial diagnosis of leukemia usually will be made through evaluation of the blood work. The blood work may have been ordered because of symptoms you reported. Perhaps results that indicate leukemia might have appeared in a blood test panel taken for another purpose.

Early signs of the various types of leukemias are similar, so it requires laboratory analysis of blood samples to determine which particular leukemia is present.

Diagnosing leukemia can be difficult and confusing. Often the doctor will want to do sophisticated blood tests to discover which kind of chromosome or genetic pattern is present. Other tests, like biopsies (samples of tissue from an affected organ) may be needed. A bone marrow aspiration and biopsy may be used to verify blood test results.

Diagnosis will be based on blood test results, the patient's description of symptoms, pathology reports, and the doctor's findings after physical examinations. Family history and reports of occupational and environmental exposures may also be considered. Often additional information is obtained from x-ray examinations and body scans. Staging and risk levels will be determined at this time and serve as the basis for subsequent treatment decisions. Chapter 3, *Diagnosis*, details the process of diagnosis and some of the emotional responses to it.

Kinds of adult leukemia

Although there are different leukemia diagnoses, there are many similarities among the types. Leukemias all are characterized by excessive production of non-functioning white blood cells. They all come to medical attention with similar symptoms. They all can show genetic and chromosomal abnormalities. They all may share similar environmental exposure. These similarities are part of the reason why doctors sometimes encounter difficulties in making a diagnosis.

Differences among types of leukemia become clear when the blood work is evaluated. Genetic differences are seen in the cells. Chromosome patterns are not the same. Specific cancer cells are identified by their chemical composition or by unique arrangements of constituents on the cell surfaces and are found in certain patterns.

The two broad classifications of leukemia are:

- Acute leukemia (rapid progression)
- Chronic leukemia (slow progression)

The determination as to whether a type of leukemia is chronic or acute is based upon the level of maturation of the cells involved. The sections that follow describe the various types of leukemias.

A precise diagnosis lets your doctor select treatments that have been shown to be most effective for that type. Knowing the precise type of leukemia you have can also benefit you in a number of ways. It lets you exchange more meaningful information with other healthcare providers, lets you more accurately research existing treatment standards and clinical trials, and lets you know whether a journal article or line of research applies to your case. Knowing about the range of leukemia diagnoses gives you some idea of the differences among types and the complexity of diagnosis and helps you appreciate why your treatment or prognosis might differ significantly from that of another leukemia patient.

Acute leukemias

In acute leukemia the majority of cells are non-functioning blasts. The number of blasts increases rapidly, crowding out the working cells and worsening the disease. Treatment is needed at once or the disease is likely to be fatal.

Two major kinds of acute leukemia have been identified. They both come to medical attention with identical symptoms. The type of white cell involved determines a diagnosis of an acute leukemia. One is lymphocytic leukemia, affecting the lymphocytes, and the other is myelogenous leukemia, involving the granulocytes.

Acute lymphocytic leukemia (ALL)

Acute lymphocytic leukemia (ALL) is the most common form of childhood leukemia (75 to 80 percent of all childhood leukemias). Only 20 percent of all adult leukemias are classified as ALL. The number of individuals diagnosed increases significantly after age 50. ALL is characterized by extreme proliferation of lymphocyte cells in the bone marrow and in the lymphatic system. B cells or T cells may be involved.

Acute myelogenous leukemia (AML)

Acute myelogenous leukemia (AML) occurs in both adults and children, but is far less common in young people. It is also called acute nonlymphocytic leukemia because lymphocytes are not affected. The cells involved in AML are the myeloblasts that proliferate uncontrollably and prevent other needed cells from doing their jobs. AML affects only about 1.5 percent of people who have leukemia. The complex staging for this disease is covered in Chapter 5, *Subtype, Staging, and Prognosis*.

Chronic leukemias

In myelogenous chronic leukemias, some blasts are present, although blasts are usually not present in chronic lymphocytic leukemia patients. Often these cells have matured further and can carry out some of their duties for a longer period of time. The number of these cells increases gradually so this cell development pattern is called chronic. Treatment of chronic leukemias may be delayed until physical symptoms and blood work indicate that treatment is needed. The most common types of chronic leukemias are chronic myelogenous leukemia, chronic lymphocytic leukemia, and hairy cell leukemia.

Chronic myelogenous leukemia (CML)

Chronic myelogenous leukemia (CML) accounts for 15 percent of the adult leukemias. CML is also classified as one of the myeloproliferative disorders (see "The myeloproliferative disorders" section later in this chapter). CML is one of the chronic leukemias that eventually will move into an acute phase, becoming AML 70 percent of the time and ALL 30 percent of the time. A unique chromosome abnormality, known as the Philadelphia chromosome (Ph), is found in 90 percent of patients with CML.

CML can also be called chronic myeloid leukemia, chronic myelocytic leukemia, or chronic granulocytic leukemia (CGL). CML is a form of leukemia that affects the cells that make granulocytes and platelets. In its early stages it creates an increase in the numbers of granulocytes and platelets, yet these cells still function normally, and the patient may have no symptoms. This situation may continue for three or four years (known as chronic phase). Eventually the nature of the disease changes and CML starts to behave like other acute leukemias. The staging for this disease is covered in Chapter 5.

One patient remembers being confused by terms when first learning about CML:

> I already knew that I had chronic leukemia and that it affected the granulocytes. But when I tried to look it up, it was designated chronic myelogenous leukemia. Okay, so granulocytes and myelocytes were the same kind of cells, but the more I looked for information, the more confused I became about the many subtypes of the disease.
>
> But learning about it would help me cope, so I was going to master this information one way or another so I could understand what was happening and what the doctor was telling me.

Chronic lymphocytic leukemia (CLL)

Chronic lymphocytic leukemia (CLL) is the most common adult leukemia, comprising 25 to 30 percent of all adult leukemias. It affects 17 percent of people with leukemia. CLL has been considered a disease of elderly men, with a two-to-one ratio of men to women affected. Now, increasing numbers of younger people are also being diagnosed with CLL, possibly because routine blood exams are more common and may be facilitating earlier detection. In past years, treatment and research options were not undertaken, perhaps because it was believed that if you had CLL you would die of something else before you needed treatment. Today researchers are uncovering more promising treatment options.

CLL is a disease in which the affected lymphocytes mature partially, and divide slowly, in a poorly regulated manner. They live much longer than usual and over time are unable to perform their proper functions.

CLL is divided into subsets depending upon whether T lymphocytes or B lymphocytes are involved.

B-CLL involves B lymphocytes and is the most common subtype, making up more than 95 percent of all CLL cases. B-CLL has also been described as small lymphocytic lymphoma, and often a pathology report will say CLL/SLL when providing a diagnosis, because the same cell is affected in both diseases. In one instance, it behaves like a type of leukemia with a high white blood count, and in the other, it behaves like a lymphoma with lumps in the lymph nodes.

Less common subtypes of CLL include:

- **T-CLL.** Also known as large granular cell lymphocytosis. See the "Adult T-cell leukemia (ATL)" section.

- **CLL/PL.** A mixture of CLL cells and prolymphocytes (cells intermediate to lymphoblasts and lymphocytes) are present in the blood sample. Prolymphocytes account for 10 to 54 percent of the cells. See the "Prolymphocytic leukemia (PLL)" section.

- **CLL/mixed.** Variation in cell sizes is seen, with some cells larger than CLL lymphocytes. Some have irregular nuclei that appear to have clefts in them.

Other chronic lymphocytic leukemias

Many variants of lymphoid neoplasm (a new and unusual form of tissue or tumor) are known and recognized. They differ from true CLL in the picture they present under the microscope and in the surface markers of the specific cells that are proliferating. In hairy cell leukemia and splenic lymphoma with villous lymphocytes the cells have finger-like projections, like a veil, that look hairy under a microscope. Prolymphocytic leukemia, on the other hand, is believed to arise from larger cells called prolymphocytes.

A number of different diseases are now being recognized within the lymphoproliferative disorders of B and T lymphocytes. Through detailed analysis, it is possible to distinguish these disorders from chronic lymphocytic leukemia (CLL) and learn about their biology, natural history, and response to treatment. The main distinguishing feature between the B-lymphoproliferative disorders CLL and non-CLL shows up on chromosome studies using five criteria: immunoglobulin intensity and the presence or absence of CD5,

CD22, CD23, or FMC7 markings on the lymphocytes. (See Chapter 5 for information about cell markers.)[1]

Hairy cell leukemia (HCL)

Hairy cell leukemia accounts for only 2 percent of adult leukemias. The cells involved in HCL are lymphocytes with filamentous (hairy) projections from the cell surface. HCL is a chronic leukemia that rarely occurs. HCL may involve B cells or T cells, but the latter is extremely uncommon. In about one-half of HCL patients, marrow is scarred, so it is difficult to do a simple bone marrow aspiration, and it may require a core biopsy for diagnosis. Chapter 4, *Tests and Procedures*, describes these tests.

Splenic lymphoma with villous lymphocytes (SLVL)

This variant of CLL is associated with hairy cell leukemia, discussed in the previous section. Both hairy cell leukemia and SLVL always show spleen involvement. Villous lymphocytes have small protrusions, like veils or filaments extending from the cell membrane, that are wider and billowier than those seen in hairy cell leukemia. SLVL is also often confused with CLL, but the cell markers are more consistent with non-Hodgkin's lymphoma than with CLL. SLVL is a low-grade lymphoma that seems to correspond to splenic marginal zone lymphoma.

The main clinical and laboratory features of SLVL are enlarged spleen (splenomegaly) in 90 percent of cases, enlarged liver in 50 percent of cases, too many lymphocytes (lymphocytosis), too few healthy red blood cells (anemia), and too few healthy platelets (thrombocytopenia) in 25–30 percent of cases. When lymph nodes develop they may indicate transformation to a high-grade lymphoma, which may also occur in the spleen. The lack of cellular tissue in SLVL reflects the degree to which the spleen has grown, and the bone marrow may not be heavily compromised in the early stages of the disease.

The pattern of bone marrow infiltration is usually nodular, which means the leukemic cells congregate in nodes in the bone marrow. Bone marrow aspirate tests may sometimes yield less than 30 percent lymphocytes. A monoclonal band, immunoglobulin type M or type G, and/or free light chains in the urine is detected in 50 percent of cases.[2] (See Chapter 5 for a more detailed explanation of this information.)

This comment comes from Pat Gardiner, an SLVL patient:

> My oncologist has been watching very carefully and today has told me he has narrowed my diagnosis from the general type of CLL to a specific, rare strain of CLL called splenic lymphoma with villous lymphocytes, or SLVL. He said that, as with ordinary CLL, the wait-and-watch protocol was the best to follow at this stage. He says I will find almost no literature about it. However, I'm still curious to learn more.
>
> I am at stage zero, with a current white blood count of 23.9. It's been bouncing anywhere from 12 to 29. I have no other symptoms except an enlarged spleen, which is involved because it is a splenic lymphoma. Anyway, I am also so far one of the fortunate smolderers, with a slow growing disease, watching and waiting. I know other patients with more aggressive leukemias; I wish we could all be smoldering.

Another patient, Jim, explained his understanding of SLVL in this way:

> I talked with an expert from Royal Bournesmouth Hospital in Bournesmouth, England today. He called me and graciously spent a great deal of time with me telling me about my illness, splenic lymphoma with villous lymphocytes (SLVL). He stated that he was doing some sort of genetic research and that my offer to send blood was generous, but that blood does not travel well for the several days it would take to get to Great Britain.
>
> I learned that SLVL appears to be slow moving like CLL, that eventually the mutated cells can interfere with normal blood cell production by clogging the bone marrow. So it apparently acts very much like CLL.
>
> The doctor I talked to said that 78 percent of SLVL sufferers are alive at five years and that it rarely transmutes to another form of lymphoma. At age 50, it is rare to get it as, like CLL, SLVL normally strikes older individuals. Since I have had my spleen removed, he said that a major portion of the disease has been capped, that chlorambucil and fludarabine are the chemotherapy drugs available if and when my white blood

cells increase from their present 31,000 level and when I have other symptoms. For the present, I only continue to have monthly blood tests.

Prolymphocytic leukemia (PLL)

PLL comes to medical attention as a proliferation of larger cells called prolymphocytes. To sustain a diagnosis of PLL there must be more than 55 percent prolymphocytes in a blood sample. The spleen is involved, but the lymph nodes are not. PLL may affect either B cells (B-PLL) or T cells (T-PLL). The latter accounts for 20 percent of all cases of PLL. Sometimes both lymphocytes and prolymphocytes are involved. Then the disease is called CLL/PLL.

Although B-PLL is relatively rare, the disease is well recognized by the distinct presence of the circulating prolymphocytes. The clinical finding of an enlarged spleen without peripheral involvement of the lymph nodes, a high white blood count, and the strong expression of FMC7 and CD79b are indicative of PLL. Anemia (reduction in healthy red blood cells) and thrombocytopenia (reduction in healthy platelets) result from the combined effect of an enlarged spleen and heavy bone marrow infiltration in a diffuse pattern (the leukemic cells are spread widely throughout the marrow). The course of B-PLL is always progressive, with rising prolymphocyte counts and, not infrequently, systemic symptoms.[3]

A drug still in clinical trials, called 506U78 or ara-G, appears to affect B-CLL and T-PLL. The median survival for PLL was three years, but with new treatment options there is hope for increased survival rates.

Like many who encounter this rare disease, Dan Peiser has questions about his father's diagnosis of PLL:

> *My father, who has just turned 71, was diagnosed with prolymphocytic leukemia five weeks ago. As I am new to dealing with cancer, I'm not sure where this diagnosis, a relatively rare one, fits. Is prolymphocytic leukemia a subcategory of CLL?*

Ed Sakal was told that he had prolymphocytes but that his condition might never be diagnosed as PLL:

> *Four years after my CLL diagnosis, doctors discovered that I had a PLL population of 12 percent. I was told several things about that.*

First, it isn't really PLL until at least 50 percent of the cells are pro-lymphocytes (so mine is classified CLL/PLL).

Second, according to a study they did at M. D. Anderson, development of increased numbers of prolymphocytes may be a normal development in CLL as the disease wears on.

Third, if the prolymphocytes respond to treatment in the same way as the other CLL cells do, there is no concern. In my case they did respond and I had no evidence of PLL after several rounds of chemotherapy.

Adult T-cell leukemia (ATL)

Established as a distinct clinical entity in 1977 in Kyoto, Japan, this leukemia appears later in life, with frequent rashes, skin involvement, and lymph node and spleen enlargement. Sometimes the peripheral white cell count is elevated with abnormal lymphoid cells, but often there is only anemia, low platelets, and bone marrow infiltration. Patients show human T-cell lymphotropic virus type-1 (HTLV-1) as a causative agent. Exposure to the virus appears to occur in childhood. The disease then manifests itself after a long period of being dormant. The largest number of cases can be found in southwestern Japan.

Adult T-cell leukemia is associated with exposure to HTLV-1 (human T-cell lymphotropic virus) found primarily in oriental or Caribbean locations. This should not be confused with HTLV-3, the virus responsible for acquired immunodeficiency syndrome (AIDS).

The four subtypes are listed here: acute or prototypic ATL, lymphoma type ATL, chronic ATL, and smoldering ATL.

- **Acute or prototypic ATL.** This is characterized by high levels of lactic dehydrogenase (LDH), an enzyme that mobilizes the hydrogen of a substrate so that it can pass to a hydrogen acceptor; calcium and bilirubin are also usually present. Signs of ATL include increased numbers of ATL cells, skin lesions, systemic lymphadenopathy (swelling of the lymph nodes), and an enlarged liver and spleen. Chemotherapy is often ineffective in patients with acute ATL.

- **Lymphoma type ATL.** This comes to medical attention with prominent lymph node involvement but few ATL cells. No lymphocytosis (excessive numbers of lymphocytes) is present, with only 1 percent or less abnormal circulating lymphocytes.

- **Chronic ATL.** This used to be classified as T-cell CLL, but newer evaluations of the blood work have led to this separate classification. In this type, the white blood count (WBC) is elevated, skin lesions are present, and there is more than twice the maximum number of lymphocytes considered normal (lymphocytosis). Sometimes lymph nodes are affected, and the liver and spleen are enlarged, but the gastrointestinal tract, central nervous system (CNS), and bones are not involved.

- **Smoldering ATL.** This shows 5 percent or more abnormal T-cell lymphocytes in the peripheral blood for many years. Initial symptoms may include skin or pulmonary lesions. LDH and calcium levels are in the normal range. The central nervous system is not involved.

Diagnosis is based upon sophisticated blood tests with chromosome patterns proving a lymphocyte malignancy involving T cells. Antibodies to HTLV-1 are present along with abnormal circulating T lymphocytes (except in the lymphoma type) including flower cells and small and mature T lymphocytes with nuclei that have lobes and small incisions. The latter are characteristic of the chronic and smoldering types.

Preleukemic conditions

There are other diseases of the blood that are not cancer, but may become leukemia in the future. These diseases include primary myelodysplastic syndrome and secondary preleukemias.

If you have been diagnosed with a preleukemic condition, this does not mean that you will inevitably develop leukemia. It does mean that you should be aware of the condition so that you can tell future healthcare providers. Your doctor should track this condition through regular blood tests because a high proportion of patients with this condition eventually develop acute leukemia. Since you are at a higher risk for leukemia, you need to be followed closely. That way, if a preleukemic condition does become leukemia, you'll know about it quickly and can start treatment when the leukemia is most treatable.

Leukemia is serious, but try not to be overly concerned if you're now simply at greater risk for it. This is easier said than done, but learn what you can about the condition, make sure you get follow-up care, and take care of your general health.

Primary myelodysplastic syndrome or primary preleukemia (MDS)

About 2.5 percent of the population with a myelodysplastic condition (a developmental anomaly of the spinal cord) have primary myelodysplastic syndrome (MDS). Primary myelodysplastic syndrome may develop without a known cause.

In MDS there is a significant decrease in the numbers of all types of cells in the blood (pancytopenia) usually with increased blasts in the bone marrow. Most importantly, the bone marrow is hypercellular (has many more than the usual number of cells in any given place). MDS is a disorder in which a single stem cell has a malignant transformation, creating a clone of abnormal cells. It involves erythroblasts, myeloblasts, B cells, and platelets. Anemias, which are resistant to cure, generally fall within this grouping. These patients need to be closely followed by their doctors, since MDS has been known to develop into AML.

Secondary preleukemias or secondary myelodysplastic syndrome

Secondary preleukemias are conditions that develop from some other condition or treatment. The blood work of secondary preleukemias looks almost exactly like primary MDS, but shows chromosome breakage or cells that have been damaged by previous chemotherapy. Secondary preleukemias include several anemias, such as aplastic anemia, caused by previous chemotherapy. Anemia is a condition in which too few red cells circulate in the blood. Not enough of the red blood cell precursors mature to carry oxygen throughout the body. Secondary myelodysplastic syndrome usually is diagnosed following radiation therapy or chemotherapy for other diseases.

Genetic predisposing conditions

There is a group of diseases with specific chromosome alterations that have the ability to affect the blood. People who have such a condition are at greater risk than those in the general population for developing some form of leukemia. Down's syndrome is one such predisposing condition. Severe chronic neutropenia, known as Kostman's syndrome, in which there are not enough granulocytes (neutrophils) to fight off infection, is another. Congenital hypoplastic anemia, called Diamond-Blackfan syndrome, which is characterized by incomplete development of the platelets, is a third.

What leukemia is not

Some forms of leukemia have similarities, not only to other types of leukemia, but also to other types of cancers known as lymphomas. As noted earlier, it is possible for leukemia to be originally misdiagnosed as a lymphoma. Leukemia is different from lymphoma although the two diseases have many commonalities, which make diagnosis complex. Lymphomas include non-Hodgkin's lymphomas and Hodgkin's disease. Other disorders that affect the bone marrow may overlap with leukemia in their signs and symptoms.

Hodgkin's disease (HD)

Hodgkin's disease (HD) is a form of lymphoma, which usually manifests itself as a painless swelling of the lymph nodes in the neck, armpit, or groin. T lymphocytes in the immune system do not react appropriately. HD differs from non-Hodgkin's lymphoma in the types of cells seen by microscopic examination, in the patterns of spread of the disease in the body, and in the age groups of patients who are affected.

Non-Hodgkin's lymphoma (NHL)

In non-Hodgkin's lymphoma (NHL), lymph nodes are the most affected body part. Lymph nodes are small, encapsulated collections of lymphocytes ranging from the size of a pea to about the size of a lima bean. They are distributed throughout the body from the head to the feet. Tonsils and adenoids are also examples of lymphatic tissue. Lymphomas start in lymph nodes or other organs such as the stomach or intestines and spill over into the blood and marrow. For more information about this condition, see another Patient-Centered Guide, *Non-Hodgkin's Lymphomas: Making Sense of Diagnosis, Treatment, and Options* by Lorraine Johnston (O'Reilly & Associates, Inc.).

Multiple myeloma (MM)

Multiple myeloma is a disease in which cancerous plasma cells are produced. Plasma cells are a type of B cell that produces proteins called immunoglobulins, which circulate in the blood and function as antibodies. In multiple myeloma, plasma cells manufacture an excessive amount of abnormal immunoglobulins, which are ineffective in fighting infection. These plasma cells multiply abnormally, crowding out normal cells in the bone marrow. This can weaken the bones and lead to fractures. Anemia is common, and high blood calcium occurs as well. Kidney problems are seen because of damage caused by the abnormal immunoglobulin proteins.

The myeloproliferative disorders (MPD)

The myeloproliferative disorders (MPDs) are relatively rare hematological (blood) malignancies in which the stem cell that produces red cells, platelets, and some white cells loses the ability to produce blood cells in proper proportion. The key in MPDs is that the stem cell may proliferate rapidly or slowly. It may reproduce selectively (producing one type of cell) or totally (producing every type of cell).

MPDs are further classified by the kind of cell growth they induce:

- **Polycythemia vera (PV).** In the MPD variant polycythemia vera, the stem cells responsible for blood production make too many blood cells, most notably red cells, which literally causes the patient to have too much blood. The resulting increased blood volume and thickness lead to complications, such as thrombosis and periodic hemorrhage

- **Essential thrombocythemia (ET).** This occurs when an MPD variant characterized by platelet counts is greater than 400,000/µL (per microliter) of blood. ET patients may also have elevated white cell counts.

- **Agnogenic myeloid metaplasia (AMM).** This is a disease of the bone marrow in which the marrow becomes scarred (fibrotic). It is also referred to as myelofibrosis with myeloid metaplasia. In AMM, the spleen and lymph nodes take over their embryonic functions of making bone marrow cells. The fibrotic tissue inside the marrow cavity eventually takes over the spleen and the lymph nodes, leading to increasingly inefficient blood cell production and, ultimately, to bone marrow failure. In bone marrow failure, the good cells are pushed out and the marrow can't function to fight infection or create new cells. It is also possible to have myelofibrosis as a consequence of other myeloproliferative diseases such as PV, ET, or chronic myelogenous leukemia.

- **Subacute or chronic myelomonocytic leukemia (CMML).** This is a preleukemic form of the myeloproliferative syndromes. The affected cells are of the types that become granulocytes and monocytes, not lymphocytes. In this disease the spleen or lymph nodes may be involved in addition to red blood cells.

Joyce, first told she had polycythemia vera and then diagnosed with essential thrombocythemia, shares her experience:

> In 1988, at age 49, I was diagnosed with essential thrombocythemia after suffering a mild stroke that left me with difficulty speaking for about a year. My platelet count at time of diagnosis was 980,000 (WBC was also elevated at 27,000), and both spleen and liver were significantly enlarged.
>
> The period leading up to diagnosis was frustrating. For about a year, I had suffered from repeated bronchial infections. My white count kept climbing higher and higher despite repeated rounds of antibiotics. I was tired and had a host of little niggling complaints (tingling, transient numbness here and there but mostly in toes and fingertips, burning, etc.) I also was experiencing what my doctor referred to as "silent migraines" because I never experienced the severe headaches that go along with classic migraines. But I did have visual disturbances: light auras with temporary loss of vision for about twenty minutes as the auras filled up my sight, and these were usually accompanied by some nausea. I also was experiencing intense pain if I twisted the wrong way. Just simply putting on a seat belt brought me to tears. I later learned my spleen and liver were enlarged from my condition.
>
> Throughout this period, my internist kept brushing off my complaints saying, "It doesn't mean a thing, you're just heading into menopause." I can't believe now I was so stupid as to believe that. Rather, I think I was suffering from "I really don't want to know" syndrome.
>
> Once I snapped out of my "ostrich with head in the sand" period and got insistent about getting to the bottom of this, I was first sent to an

infectious disease specialist. He looked at my blood counts, poked around on my tummy, told me my spleen and liver were enlarged, called a hematologist and when he got off the phone pronounced, "You have polycythemia vera, you have around five years to live, try to enjoy them."

(If you have PV, relax, those statistics are now known to be untrue. You can live out a normal life span if you are properly monitored and treated.)

I was in shock! He then sent me off for a red cell mass test to confirm his diagnosis. This time my diagnosis was essential thrombocythemia. By the time all the testing was done the diagnosis was ET with secondary myelofibrosis and myeloid metaplasia.

Waldenstrom's macroglobulinemia (WM)

Waldenstrom's, like CLL, is a disease of older individuals and frequently involves the lymph nodes and spleen. The malignant lymphocytes have some plasma cell features. Some symptoms of the disease occur due to the presence of abnormally high amounts of a large immunoglobulin, an antibody-like molecule, in the blood.

CHAPTER 2

Signs and Symptoms

If you're reading this book, you probably already have a diagnosis of leukemia. However, once most people are diagnosed, they look back on what led up to the diagnosis and understand signs and symptoms in a new light. They also probably wonder if they experience the same symptoms as others with the same condition.

The signs and symptoms of leukemia are confusing and vague. Understanding that many other, more common conditions share some symptoms with leukemia might help reassure you if you are second-guessing yourself or your doctor, wondering why the leukemia took so long to diagnose. Being familiar with the signs of leukemia also gives you more surety in monitoring yourself for any signs of recurrence and reporting to your doctor.

This chapter talks about bringing symptoms to your doctor, honoring your instincts when the body isn't behaving as it normally does, and ensuring that your doctor understands your concerns. It also looks at physical symptoms that may be causing you concern, as well as the unexpected results of a routine physical and how they relate to the various types of leukemia.

Bringing concerns to your doctor

Although there are different kinds of leukemia, many share similar symptoms: fatigue, painful swelling of lymph nodes or spleen, pressure pain, nausea, back and joint pain, night sweats, and weight loss. Any one of these symptoms may also result from stress, nagging respiratory condition, virus, the flu, or menopause. They may mean nothing special or they could indicate problems. The important thing to discover is from what condition the symptoms arise.

Leukemia can present with one symptom or several at the same time. For example, one person who goes to the doctor might be feeling tired and run down, find it hard to get up in the morning and make it through a whole day of work. Another might catch every virus that seems to be going around and have the illness hang on for a long time. Lymph nodes, which are usually indistinct, might suddenly become visibly enlarged or palpable in the neck, groin, and/or under arms. Pressure pain may be caused when an enlarged node or organ pushes against a body part; drenching night sweats may also occur.

On the other hand, leukemia might be present with no symptoms at all. For example, a person might go to the doctor for a routine physical examination, including blood tests. This patient might feel fine and have no reason to suspect that anything is wrong. When the blood tests results come in, however, the doctor has startling news: "There's something unusual showing in these tests, perhaps we should run them again." Perhaps the doctor notes that white blood cell counts are high or red blood cell counts and platelet counts are dropping. There may even be some odd-looking cells showing up in the slides.

Making sure symptoms are given credence

One problem that leukemia patients report is that some doctors do not take their concerns about unusual health phenomena seriously. In their defense, doctors are rushed, overbooked, and haven't the luxury of time to simply listen to patient complaints. Some doctors haven't been taught how to listen "between the words" to understand what they are actually being told. On the other hand, some patients don't know how to explain their symptoms efficiently or they sense a doctor's haste and don't mention those nagging concerns that might help to make the picture more complete. When the doctor is aware of only part of the problem and vital information is not shared and therefore not considered, the patient's legitimate concerns are not totally addressed.

At times doctors wave aside or even negate patient concerns by saying, "I wouldn't worry about that." Some will simply ignore those concerns. Such behavior is likely to infuriate some patients. It will make other patients feel insecure, implying that they are wasting the doctor's time with trivia. Even worse, such dismissal of the patient's concerns can cause the patient not to share what may be important diagnostic information.

Before diagnosis, during treatment, and after treatment, it is important that you make your doctor aware of your nagging concerns and unusual health experiences. You need to document them by giving very careful descriptions of what has happened, and then bring to the doctor's attention just how anxious those situations make you. If you mention a concern in passing, with an "Oh, by the way," it is less likely to be taken seriously than if you state clearly, "I am really worried about this. Please give me your opinion about it. It is very important to me." Even if you are not sure how important the information may be, it is wise to share it with your doctor.

On the other hand, sometimes doctors seem uncaring, but if every doctor fully investigated every vague symptom as if it were leukemia, it would create havoc. So give your doctor the benefit of the doubt. Most of the time your doctor will tune in to the symptoms that are indicative of problems.

Honoring your instincts

If something is happening to your body, you are the first one who will be aware of it. Others can't necessarily see it or know it is occurring, but that doesn't make it any less real. When several things are happening that cause you concern, you may have a feeling of dread. Many people try to ignore the feeling, hoping the symptoms will go away. Some deny that symptoms are happening. A few watch and document symptoms before speaking about them to their physicians.

Although these responses are normal, it is important not to hide what is happening with your body. Trust your feelings. Trust also that when you report these symptoms, your doctor will recognize you as a reliable informant and take what you say seriously. Then work to make sure that happens.

The stories in this chapter speak of the often lengthy periods between first noticing symptoms and diagnosis. Patients describe symptoms that may be ambiguous, and both patients and doctors may attribute the symptoms to other conditions.

Acute leukemias

Acute leukemias usually begin abruptly with intense symptoms. The early signs of acute lymphocytic leukemia (ALL) and acute myeloid leukemia (AML) are identical and can be easily confused with common infectious illnesses. Most symptoms of acute leukemias are caused by the decrease in healthy blood cells as the immature, malignant blood cells (blasts) multiply, crowding out the healthy cells.

Symptoms of acute leukemia include:

- Fever and feeling as if you have the flu, which are usually the first signs

- Fatigue, pale color, weakness and dizziness, which are all related to lack of red cells

- Easy bruising and slow clotting, from platelet depletion

- Frequent infections, which occur when production of healthy white cells decreases, impeding the body's ability to fight off bacteria, fungi, and viruses

- Bone and joint pain

Leukemia blasts themselves cause some symptoms as they invade the spleen, lymph nodes, and liver. These lymph nodes enlarge and press against other organs, adding to your discomfort.

The spleen and/or liver may become enlarged and painful as they press against other organs, resulting in shortness of breath and a feeling of fullness. Leukemia cells may also invade the central nervous system (brain and spinal cord). If leukemia has entered the central nervous system (CNS), your symptoms might also include headache, blurred vision, confusion, altered thinking patterns, and unexplained fevers. Sometimes, family members of elderly patients might ascribe these changes simply to "aging" or have concerns about Alzheimer's disease or other neurological disorders.

Symptoms of acute leukemia are similar to those of a variety of non-malignant diseases; therefore, those possibilities must be investigated first. Mononucleosis, lupus, aplastic anemia, and AIDS all must be ruled out, and so must lymphoma and chronic leukemia.

Sharon Foster tells about the range of symptoms shown by her husband over a period of several months, before he was diagnosed with ALL:

> *My husband was diagnosed on July 21st. During the first part of the year Tony had some joint problems. His foot hurt for a while and the doctor sent him for some diagnostic and then orthopedic assistance, but Tony's foot got better. Then his knee started playing up. He was limping for a short while, then that cleared up. Next he had a vein on the inside of his leg going from mid-thigh to mid-calf come up all red. The doc looked*

at it and told him it was just a surface vein and prescribed some anti-inflammatory tablets. He told us it was nothing to worry about despite the fact that Tony had high blood pressure. No tests were done on his blood. This would have been around April.

Tony started getting hot sweats at night around the end of May. As it was quite humid here in Toronto and he was a big lad (245 pounds and 5'11" tall), we just thought it was pretty normal for him. The sweats didn't really improve and Tony found himself lacking in energy in a big way. In fact he had lacked energy from about the beginning of March that year.

The symptoms got more severe in the week before the diagnosis:

Finally around mid-July Tony started feeling very sweaty all the time, and tired. He fell asleep at work a couple of times but didn't tell me about it at the time. He had no other symptoms but severe tiredness and sweats until around July 19th when he started being sick. The family had had stomach upsets recently so no one really thought anything was strange. Tony had history of being severely sick with stomach upsets when everyone else would be sick for a few hours. Tony's sickness could go on for several days.

Finally, Tony was taken to the emergency room, when symptoms became even more acute. There, a diagnosis was made:

It wasn't until the morning of July 21st when Tony fell asleep at the breakfast table and was holding his stomach (spleen area) that I finally insisted he go to the emergency department at the local hospital. They said they wanted to do some tests. The sickness turned out to be ALL (acute lymphoblastic leukemia, T cell) and by then his white count was at 170,000.

Arthur Flatau, PhD, a computer engineer, described what he experienced on his way to a diagnosis of acute myelogenous leukemia. The period between the onset of symptoms and when they became more pronounced was shorter than Tony's. However, there were still several weeks of confusing symptoms before diagnosis:

I felt tired for several weeks before my diagnosis, but I had put that off to too much work, two little kids, and trying to play rugby again (training two evenings a week, and games on Saturdays, many out of town).

The two weeks before my diagnosis, I often felt cold at work and really started to feel tired. I also had a lot of bruises from rugby games, although I did not think much about that.

The week before diagnosis, I started running low-grade fevers (99–100) and I was really run down. On Saturday we had a rugby game in which I played a few minutes (perhaps fifteen). Fortunately I was too weak to really get into the action. I did get a very minor bump near my eye during the game. This bump later developed into a really major black eye.

On Sunday, I again was very tired—too tired to do much of anything. I also started to run a higher fever (101+). I took ibuprofen for the fever. I also had taken some during the week (not the best choice of anti-fever medicine in my condition, but what did I know). That night I also had some bleeding in my gums that really scared my wife. She wanted me to go to the emergency room that morning, but my calmer (and stupider) mind prevailed and we just went to see our family physician later that morning.

At the time, I had not put the bruising and the fevers and fatigue together. I thought something I had not had before was causing the fatigue and fevers. I thought the bruises were something else. Diagnosis was acute myelogenous leukemia.

Chronic leukemias

In chronic leukemia, at first white blood cells continue to function as they should, but as the disease progresses they become less functional and more abnormal. Chronic leukemias have a range of symptoms similar to those of acute leukemias; the symptoms, however, can take longer to show up or come on more gradually.

Chronic lymphocytic leukemia (CLL)

About 25 percent of individuals with CLL are diagnosed as the result of a routine blood test and show no symptoms at all. However, some patients do report feeling symptoms, and even several of those who didn't think anything was wrong often report, with hindsight, that they should have realized that they were having some degree of symptoms. Symptoms of CLL may include:

- Fatigue
- A feeling of ill health
- Lack of energy
- Night sweats
- Loss of appetite and weight loss
- Series of infections
- Constant bruising that is slow to heal
- Shortness of breath or a feeling of fullness when eating, sometimes caused by an enlarged spleen pressing against other organs
- Enlarged lymph nodes

Tom McCune, who was diagnosed with CLL while still in his 30s, describes his symptoms this way:

> As to the symptoms that lead to my seeing a doctor for my B-cell CLL diagnosis, I had just two large lymph nodes, on both sides of the jaw. Subsequent symptoms included my "heart attack," which turned out to be my massive spleen. Many enlarged lymph nodes developed later. Otherwise, I always appeared to be fine.

David Covell, a member of the Association of Cancer Online Resources (ACOR) CLL Internet support list shared his symptoms with the group:

> My diagnosis should have happened years earlier. Seven years ago, while my wife was still in the US Air Force, I saw a military doctor about constantly swollen lymph nodes on both sides of my neck. I was told it was "probably nothing" and despite my request, a biopsy was not performed.
>
> Medical records from that visit show that my white blood count was 12,000 and I also had swollen nodes in the groin. I had also mentioned to the doctor that I was having periodic shingle-like irritations to the skin along nerves on my chest and back, always on just one side, but never erupting into lesions. The doctor didn't put two and two together, though.

*Two years ago I began experiencing tightness in my chest and fatigue
and became concerned about possible heart problems, which run in the
family. I saw my primary care physician, who did a complete blood count
and other routine checks. I got a call the next day saying something had
gone wrong with the test and I needed to come back for another sample.
No concern yet.*

*The doctor called me that afternoon and said that both tests showed
white blood counts of 100,000 and that I should see a hematologist for a
"leukemia-like condition." I made an appointment for the following week,
at which point I had my first bone marrow biopsy and flow cytometry
test. Results indicated CLL, and I began the usual watch and wait.*

When you look back at a long period of time during which symptoms were
discounted—particularly if doctors were the ones discounting them—you
may feel regret or bitterness. You might regret not having been listened to or
regret not having gotten treatment sooner. David, who had symptoms for
years before diagnosis, says:

*In retrospect I realize I had many of the classic symptoms but didn't
know what to make of them: fatigue, frequent colds, night sweats, shingle-
like episodes, and numerous swollen nodes. I mentioned these symptoms
to various doctors during the years that my CLL was developing, but not
one of them ever pursued it. I guess I'm a little bitter that nobody ever listened; recurring shingle-like episodes combined with permanently swollen nodes should have made someone curious enough to investigate.*

Chronic myelogenous leukemia (CML)

In CML, abnormal granulocytes multiply, but they usually retain their ability
to function properly. In later stages of the disease the cells lose their ability
to mature and blast cells begin to build up in the blood and bone marrow.

Most CML patients are diagnosed during the chronic (first) stage of the disease, which may last from a few months to several years. After that, the disease moves into the accelerated phase during which more blasts and fewer
normal cells appear in the marrow. Finally, it moves into the blast or crisis
stage when more than 30 percent of the cells in the marrow and the blood
are blast cells. In this stage, collections of blasts may form tumors in the
nodes, bones, or, more rarely, other sites. Blast crisis occurs three to five
years after diagnosis and resembles ALL. At this point, 90 percent of CML

patients have an enlarged spleen. Median survival has risen to five or six years. (This means that half of the people with CML live longer than five or six years.)

Some common early symptoms of CML are:

- Tiring easily
- Fatigue
- Loss of appetite and weight loss
- Headaches
- Sweating
- Fever
- Bone pain or tenderness
- Bleeding

One patient describes her symptoms this way:

> Like many chronic leukemia patients, my symptoms were initially very vague and varied. Over a period of approximately one year, I noticed a general feeling of fatigue, which I attributed to work and home pressures. I had stopped hill walking (10–15 mile hikes) because of this tiredness and a pain in my hip, which came during the walks. I thought the pain could have been the onset of osteoporosis. I had also noticed three tiny "spots" of raised reddish skin that did not heal. This was odd because I have always had very good skin.
>
> Three months prior to diagnosis, while in Germany at a conference, I slipped in the bath and had a number of very large bruises on the inside of both my thighs. Although this was very unusual, I merely felt very cross with myself. On reflection, the bruises were different. In the past I rarely bruised myself. When I had, the bruises were usually small and the color was usually yellow/blue, not the deep purple/black and blue bruises I had this time.
>
> I eventually began to find it difficult to eat, with constant indigestion. I described this feeling to my doctor as similar to when I was pregnant. I later learned this was due to an enlarged spleen. It was measured on diagnosis as 13 1/2" long—and I am a small lady (5' 2"). I went to the doctor a number of times over approximately eight weeks. I was given a

variety of medications for the heartburn and indigestion. I had an x-ray for the hip pain and finally a blood test was taken by the nurse, resulting in the diagnosis of chronic myelogenous leukemia.

I also had nosebleeds. Only minor nosebleeds when I blew my nose, but I had never had a nosebleed before. I still have a slight problem.

Hairy cell leukemia (HCL)

Hairy cell leukemia starts slowly. Symptoms of HCL include:

* Weakness

* Frequent infections

* Discomfort from enlarged spleen

Some symptoms of hairy cell leukemia are documented in the following patient's story:

I am currently 64 years old. I guess you could say my symptoms started when I was about 45 years old. I went in for a fairly thorough physical about that time, since I had not had one for many years. The doctor noted that my white blood count was lower than normal, but just a little below the lower limit for a normal count. He did not see any reason for alarm.

Over a period of years, I had some minor heart problems, which were treated with three different drugs over a period of time. My heart doctor noted low WBC, although he never took a blood panel.

I eventually consulted with my internist about my low blood counts and he recommended a hematologist.

The hematologist/oncologist monitored my blood for several years, and we watched as my count kept going down. There was no apparent reason for this and I felt healthy. My doctor was perplexed. Bone marrow tests did not show anything (although I think they might have missed hairy cell leukemia on the first test). My hematologist once used the term "myelodysplastic syndrome" early on in my visits to him.

For years during this course of events, I also saw a dermatologist for skin problems, and one symptom was acne rosacea on the face. This was pretty painful at times, and they used tetracycline, which did not really help. I could never get either my dermatologist or oncologist to consider the low white counts as being tied to the acne and HCL. It turned out that it was. A second bone marrow biopsy showed the presence of HCL. I have not had the acne problems since the treatment for HCL.

CHAPTER 3

Diagnosis

Making an accurate diagnosis is a process. With a disease whose symptoms are often vague at first and which could indicate a wide range of more common conditions, leukemia is rarely the first condition considered. The process of getting to a diagnosis of leukemia is usually emotionally harrowing. Getting a precise diagnosis is necessary, both for your own certainty and for your healthcare team to recommend an optimal treatment plan for your individual situation.

In this chapter we first describe the general process of diagnosis: which medical specialist to see, where to go for testing, and what comprehensive blood testing is and how to make sense of the resulting information. We then look at the deep emotional responses that diagnosis usually brings up.

This chapter can help you understand the process that you've been through, including the length of time it took you to realize that there was something seriously wrong and/or for the doctor to pinpoint what was wrong. Knowing more about the process and the specific diagnostic criteria for various leukemias can help you find questions that you might now want to ask your doctor.

Diagnosis by blood work

There is one major consistency in a leukemia diagnosis: the blood work will tell much of the story. Leukemia is diagnosed by examination of a blood sample under the microscope. Sometimes that sample comes from a finger stick or from blood drawn from an arm vein. For many years the determining factor was the bone marrow aspiration and biopsy. Cells would be removed from the patient's bone marrow (aspiration), and a core sample of the bone marrow would be taken as well (biopsy). This material would be sent for evaluation. The cells from the bone marrow aspirate and from the core sample would be examined under the microscope and, if possible, the diagnosis would be made. Hairy cell, acute myelogenous, and adult acute lymphocytic leukemia may not have leukemia cells circulating in the blood at diagnosis. For such diagnoses a bone marrow biopsy is still required.

Today, although analysis of the bone marrow remains the "gold standard" for the diagnosis of leukemia there are more sophisticated techniques, which simply require a sample of blood from the arm. The benefits of these methods are that they are easier on the patient, they give the doctor a wealth of information that he or she never had before, and they help provide a more confident diagnosis. However, these methods of analysis require sophisticated and expensive flow cytometry equipment run by trained clinical laboratory scientists, so they cost more.

The options you have for diagnostic testing depend on where you live and the kind of healthcare services available to you. Some people have access to comprehensive cancer centers and are fortunate enough to have medical plans that accept these centers as an integral part of their treatment system. Other people use a nearby general hospital with no special cancer expertise; a number of the tests will be done right in the local hospital laboratory, in the doctor's office, or in a reference laboratory that may be across the country. Still others struggle to get adequate care and information.

The experience with individual doctors also varies. Some people are lucky enough to find a caring doctor who has experience with the disease and who can communicate with patients, as the patient and family require. Many go through several doctors before finding the one with whom the patient and family can relate and give their trust.

A diagnosis doesn't always follow the initial test results. Daryl Rutherford tells about his frustrations in getting to diagnosis:

> I had low white blood cell counts that kept decreasing for a period of several years. The oncologist I was visiting was perplexed by this, because I seemed to be feeling well otherwise. The only other clue was that I had a considerable amount of acne rosacea on my face and forehead. This was quite painful at times, and it was considered quite separate from the blood count problem.
>
> I had also contacted a dermatologist during this period and discussed the problem of my blood counts. It seemed that I could not get either doctor to consider the possibility of some relationship between my skin problems and my strange blood counts.

I had a bone marrow biopsy that showed "nothing." A couple of years later a second bone marrow biopsy showed hairy cell leukemia to be the cause for my low white blood count. Now that really enlightened me about the acne. I had discussed the possible relationship between the blood count and acne, but neither doctor gave it any credence. Subsequent treatment with 2CDA for the leukemia cured my blood problem and the acne problem.

My recommendation is that if you feel there is a possible link between other physical problems and your white count, don't give up searching for the answer.

Another patient, Danielle Simons, gives the following account of what she went through while trying to get to diagnosis. You will see that there were a number of tests done that were repeated several times, and there still were questions as to what was really happening with her:

I am a 37-year-old female who sought medical help after a menstrual period continued for three weeks. All gynecological tests were normal. After a few more weeks, I began spotting rectally and had a minor nosebleed. The vaginal bleeding did not cease.

After a complete blood count test (CBC) showed some abnormal results, I was sent to a hematologist who ordered an electrocardiogram and chest x-ray (both normal) and a bone marrow biopsy. It took three months for the health maintenance organization to approve the biopsy. By that time, the vaginal bleeding had continued without interruption for eleven weeks. It stopped right before the biopsy. During this time my weight dropped from 110 to 92 lbs. When the biopsy was performed, all counts except the mean corpuscular value and neutrophils were in the normal range. My red blood count had dropped to 39, down from 50 in my previous blood work.

Some abnormalities were found, including two nuclei in some cells, variability in cell appearance, abnormal granulation in the cells, and too many segmented neutrophils. There were too many leukocytes, macrocytes, and a few others. Development was progressive in all cell lines with variable numbers of cells.

My hematologist felt the drop in the red blood counts had been reactive to the bleeding, and unfortunately the biopsy results were inconclusive for the same reason. We adopted a "watchful waiting" policy with a follow-up CBC to be done in 30 days.

Even with a hematologist performing regular tests and with access to good screening technologies, blood abnormalities may be difficult to diagnose precisely:

> *In the four months following, I have had three CBCs and no bleed-ing, except normal menstrual periods. After the first 45 days, all the CBCs have shown increases in counts and the hematocrit has been rising about 1.5 points a week. The last was hematocrit 47, hemoglobin 15.5, white blood count 12,000, MCV 120.2, neutrophils 10 (82 percent), but the lymphocytes were dropping quickly, from 27 to 14 in a month (nor-mal for my lab is 20–50). Other tests (for B-12, folate levels, thyroid, liver and kidney function) were normal.*
>
> *My hematologist and I are trying to decide where to go from here. He is very open to suggestion. He wonders if this could be a myelodysplastic disease or a myeloproliferative one. It doesn't appear to be a leukemia.*

This patient is presently undiagnosed and only by following her medical experience over time will the diagnosis perhaps become clearer.

Who to see for testing

Once your doctor suspects leukemia, you will be referred to another doctor who deals in blood cancers with whom you have probably never spoken before. This medical specialist is called a hematologist/oncologist.

Many people hear the word hematologist and have no clue what it means. If you don't know about the specialty, you may visit this doctor expecting to be given some pills, and be told to rest and that all will be well. Other people hear the word hematologist and immediately get a sinking feeling, because they fear the news won't be good.

When you are referred, you need to make a key decision and make sure that the specialist you will see is right for you. Important factors to consider are:

- **Access.** Find a doctor who is part of your managed care plan or who will be fully or partially reimbursed by your insurance company. You'll want to find a doctor whose practice is conveniently located and is affiliated with a hospital recognized for its state-of-the-art facilities and skilled personnel; a comprehensive cancer center connection would be wonderful.

- **Expertise.** Find someone who has the necessary credentials and has worked with other leukemia patients. It is even better if the doctor has dealt with many cases of your particular type of leukemia.

- **Communication.** You should feel free to speak honestly and openly with the doctor, and the doctor is able and willing to answer your questions. Poor communication, unfortunately, can occur for a number of reasons, such as a lack of chemistry between doctor and patient, conflicting cultural backgrounds, or the doctor's limited availability.

It is very important that a good relationship evolve between the doctor, patient, and his or her family members because a hematologist is likely to be your long-term doctor. Your relationship doesn't have to be exclusive, however, because older patients have more health problems in general and often need follow-up treatment in other areas: for example, in osteoporosis or prostate or gynecological concerns. Your oncologist may not be able to deal with those problems in a busy hematological practice, so you will also need a good internist.

One patient expressed her concerns about a doctor to whom she had been referred, saying:

> There I was, a middle-aged woman. I was at one of the top cancer research centers in the country so I knew the equipment was cutting-edge and the doctors were well trained and knowledgeable. I was well informed for a patient and I was asking lots of questions about the procedure I was about to experience. The doctor came from an Arab country where women are not looked upon as equals, and he couldn't maintain eye contact with me. All of his comments were made to my husband who had accompanied me to the clinic.
>
> Unfortunately, my husband, while supportive, had no idea what questions to ask, what follow-up information was needed, or what research I had done that needed addressing. I had always taken care of that part of my disease. My requests for information were met with silence and a shifting of the doctor's feet. It was clear that he was very uncomfortable whenever I attempted to enter the conversation.

When we left the clinic, I felt upset because I was no better informed than when we had come. My husband felt no better, because he knew I was frustrated. I knew then that we were in trouble unless we found another doctor with whom I could communicate directly. It was a very difficult situation, because this man was a leader in his field and had come very highly recommended by someone in whom I had infinite trust.

This patient had several problems to handle. First, there was the male-female cultural problem, and then there was the inability to get answers to questions that were important to her and her family members. She rightfully concluded that she would not be comfortable if she continued to attempt to work with this doctor. Moreover, she knew that she would have to go back to the referring doctor to explain why she couldn't continue seeing this person and request another referral.

Questions for a first visit

When you are referred to a hematologist/oncologist, your doctor will send your medical records ahead of time or perhaps you will hand-carry them to the appointment. Medical records include blood work, slides, pathology reports, x-ray films or radiographs, and all relevant scans.

At your first appointment, you will probably be nervous about what will occur and might have a litany of questions running through your head. A large group of patients was asked what questions they wished they had asked their specialists. The following questions were suggested:

- Do conditions other than leukemia have similar symptoms and blood-test results? Which ones are they?

- How do you differentiate among these conditions to determine that I have leukemia?

- What do the blood test results mean?
  - What are the normal ranges for blood tests?
  - How do my results compare to the normal ranges?
  - Why might the tests be showing these differences from the normal ranges and what does that mean?
  - What sort of changes should I be looking for in the future?
  - How often should I expect to have blood tests?

- What other tests are needed for you to reach a diagnosis?

- What kind of leukemia do you think I have?

- In what stage do you think I fit at this time?

- Can other annoying health problems that I have experienced recently be related to my leukemia? (These might include sinus infections, bone and joint pain, and other symptoms that you haven't previously reported or that you think you should have mentioned, but didn't think were important before.)

- How many cases of leukemia are in your practice? How many have you treated who have this kind of leukemia?

- What changes can I make in my daily living to improve my situation? Are there herbal treatments or other treatments that will help me at this time? Are there specific fitness activities that I should be doing?

- What symptoms should I watch out for in the future?

- What information can you give me about this disease?

- Where may I find additional information?

- How often do you want to see me and when do you want to see me again?

- What treatments are you recommending for me?

- What clinical trials are available to me and where are they located?

You will notice that questions about prognosis are absent. It is usually the main question on everyone's mind at first, but it is difficult to answer with a high degree of accuracy. If you won't be comfortable leaving the appointment without asking for life prognosis statistics, go ahead and ask. But remember that the data changes with each new advance in treatment and the information you receive is likely to be already out of date because of rapidly changing scientific advances. No two individuals react in exactly the same manner to any treatment protocol so nothing is guaranteed.

Comprehensive blood testing

The doctor you first go to with symptoms or for a general physical usually does initial testing. The tests led to concerns about blood counts and possible leukemia. You were probably asked to come back to repeat the initial tests to ensure that the results were accurate.

It usually takes a while to get from referral to actual appointment with the hematologist/oncologist. So, when you finally visit the oncologist, the original blood tests will probably be repeated. This is done to allow the oncologist to see if there are any significant changes from the original blood tests during the interval between initial testing and this second round. Moreover, this is the point at which sophisticated blood sample evaluation may well be done to look for markers on the cells and for chromosome patterns that differ from normal. Generally, a larger blood sample than you are used to providing is needed for this additional testing.

If you described or if your doctor found lymph node enlargement, the doctor will likely order further tests to check for lymph node involvement. Specific tests are described in Chapter 4, *Tests and Procedures*.

Blood tests may be used to answer many questions, so many such tests exist to meet those needs. Two major types of testing—cytogenetic and immunophenotyping—look at the chromosome patterns and the cell markers and are of great importance in making diagnostic decisions.

After blood tests and evaluations, the pathologist sends a comprehensive pathology report to the oncologist. The report shows which antigens the blood sample has been tested for and which specific antigens the cells in the sample express. From this information the pathologist determines which type of leukemia is shown. Then your hematologist/oncologist makes the diagnosis.

With the information from the pathology report, your input as to symptoms, and the results of your physical examination, a precise diagnosis can be reached. It helps a great deal that the doctor has experience in dealing with the suspected disease. Patients are unique and all diagnoses are not based on exactly the same presenting information. It takes good skills and lots of knowledge to come up with the correct diagnosis.

In some cases a patient is diagnosed with one form of leukemia and later his doctor discovers that the patient has another form entirely. Acute lymphocytic leukemia may be confused with acute myelogenous leukemia, hairy cell leukemia, or non-Hodgkin's lymphoma. The symptoms of lymphomas and leukemias often overlap in their initial presentations. Hairy cell leukemia and mantle cell lymphomas are also often misdiagnosed as chronic lymphocytic leukemia.

For precise treatment recommendations, the oncologist considers the sub-type of leukemia and the staging of the disease so that both doctor and patient have some idea of where the patient stands in terms of the severity of the disease and the prognostic indicators. These determinations play a large role in treatment decisions. Chapter 5, *Subtype, Staging, and Prognosis*, describes in more detail some of the evaluations done on blood samples to determine subtypes and staging.

Hearing the diagnosis

All of the information from the tests has now been received. Tests providing confusing results have been repeated until the results are convincingly the same. Basic blood work has been redone, so everyone is convinced that a virus, common infection, or allergy is not causing the abnormal counts. Sophisticated blood analysis evaluations are in. The doctor has ruled out maladies that are not leukemia. Now the patient meets with the doctor to hear the diagnosis.

This is a difficult meeting for the doctor. No matter how professionally the doctor handles it, no matter how carefully the doctor chooses words to blunt the impact, you receive frightening news that you don't want to hear. If your doctor is a warm and caring individual, he or she has probably carefully thought about how to deliver the diagnosis. Even if the doctor is starchy and aloof, with an emphasis on keeping a professional distance, the information is not easy to present. Oncologists say that giving a cancer diagnosis is one of the most difficult tasks they face in their medical practice.

Both patient and family are having a very difficult time as well. By now they suspect that the news is definitely not what they want to hear. They have been under stress throughout the time it has taken to reach diagnosis, with horrible scenarios playing out in their minds as they waited. "Will this be a death sentence?" is the main question in the patient's and family members' minds.

"You have leukemia," the doctor says, and the patient's mind shuts down and shock takes over. Generally, only about half of the rest of the conversation is heard and probably almost none will be remembered. A family member who is with you may be able to recall what was said a little better. But even that isn't always good enough. This is why a tape recording of the visit is a bless-ing. With the doctor's approval, taping the visit will give patients and caregivers a resource for later, so they can listen to the doctor's words after the shock of the initial diagnosis has been absorbed; they will better assimilate discussion of staging and treatment options.

The following story is a classic example of what can happen when the stress level is high and people aren't really thinking straight:

> When my husband and I walked out of the meeting with the hematologist we were really shook up! We had expected the diagnosis of leukemia, but there was so much new information to be absorbed. The doctor said I should start treatment at once, and I asked, how I could do that and get ready for Jan's wedding next month?
>
> "That's not what I heard," my husband said. "She said that you could wait until after our daughter's wedding next month to start treatment. That's why your next appointment isn't for three weeks."
>
> It was a good thing we had a tape recording of the meeting, because clearly, although we had been in the same room, we hadn't been to the same meeting.

Chronic leukemia patients and families may be somewhat comforted to hear, "This is a chronic disease and the best medical practice indicates that we should just keep track of your progress and wait to see how things develop." Unfortunately, patients with acute leukemia seldom hear such comforting words.

Diagnosis of acute leukemia

Acute leukemia patients need treatment almost immediately, so it is wise to schedule another appointment with the oncologist very soon after the first one. At this meeting, ask the doctor to go over the information that was covered in the first meeting. Then get further information about the disease and discuss staging and treatment options. Again, it is very wise to tape the meeting and to have another person with you, so that you can compare notes afterwards and make sure that you heard what the doctor really said.

Diagnosis of chronic leukemia

What chronic leukemia and hairy cell leukemia patients do not want to hear and are told all too often is, "If you have to have cancer this is the best one to have." Patients would rather be told that this is a slow progressing leukemia and that there is time to enjoy life. They come to accept and learn to live with it before anything needs to be done. No one wants to hear that they have the best cancer, when no cancer is good!

Elizabeth Hawes describes the cavalier manner in which she was told that she had chronic leukemia:

> I was diagnosed by accident in May of this year. I had complained to my primary care physician (PCP) because she didn't believe in performing routine complete blood counts. She figured if something was wrong, the patient would know and she could react accordingly.
>
> This time I did not leave without vowing to change physicians after I got the results of the blood work she had ordered to see if perhaps I was anemic. The day after I saw her for my annual physical, she left a message on my machine telling me I needed to get in touch with her about the results. When we finally caught up with each other, she said, "Well, I'm leaving for a few days tomorrow, but I just wanted you to know that you have chronic lymphocytic leukemia and you're anemic."
>
> There was a long pause on this end of the phone. "Uh, what— exactly—does that mean?"
>
> Chuckle from her: "Well, you don't have to draw up your will tomorrow."
>
> Yuck, yuck! Now you know why she's my former primary care physician.

A long-term testicular cancer survivor who was in remission tells about finding out that he must live with a chronic leukemia:

> I went for my annual check-up about nine days ago. The chest x-ray showed two small "somethings," and blood work showed a high white cell count of 15,100. The red blood count and platelets were down.
>
> My doctor ordered a CT scan that showed two BB-sized things in my left lung and something else in the center of my chest. I had testicular cancer six years ago and have been clear, so he sent me to my oncologist. The oncologist ordered a lower CT scan and a pelvic as well. I went back last week for results. I was prepared to be told about the next step in diagnosing the spots. Instead he told me I have CLL. The CT scan showed a swollen spleen and lymph nodes, and second blood tests showed my

white count slightly higher than before. I have been having night sweats and bleeding under the skin.

The oncologist took the first bone marrow aspiration and biopsy. It was very painful and I cannot forget that experience. That's where I am. I go back next week to talk about chemotherapy. He said chemotherapy would be three days a month for four months, but I can't remember what drugs he said it would be.

Emotional responses to diagnosis

Patients usually react to leukemia diagnosis with shock. No matter how prepared one is to hear those words, the shock is still there. Cancer? Me? No, it can't be! Make it not have happened! A purely emotional reaction takes over. The doctor may as well not have gone on to provide the subsequent information. The patient is too traumatized and focused on the emotional blow just received.

There is a range of normal emotional responses to a leukemia diagnosis.

Fear

Any leukemia diagnosis brings with it a secondary reaction of fear. Fear of dying, fear of what the future will hold as the disease progresses, fear of what treatment will be like, and fear for the family all come in a rush. Parents of young children become frantic about what will happen to the little ones. You can't deal with all of those fears at once. Nevertheless, the fears will surface during a momentary loss of focus. In addition, patients face fear of the unknown and fear of physical limitations caused by the disease and its treatment. You also may be facing insurance problems; you may be fearful of high financial costs. Additionally, you may have a fear of being a burden upon loved ones.

Distress arises with the first suspicion of leukemia and is most prevalent while patients and family are waiting for diagnosis, fearful of what will be discovered. This is probably the period during which patients cry the most and respond most emotionally.

If you are a family member or caregiver, think of the shock of associating leukemia with yourself and you may begin to understand the overwhelming emotional response of the patient. Patients and family members need to be kind to one another as they learn to accept that leukemia is part of their lives.

Some people have described the emotional pain and anguish by saying they felt isolated, set apart, totally alone even when surrounded by friends, family and well-wishers. They describe feeling stigmatized just by the concept of leukemia being related to them.

Physical pain is a continuing fear for patients. Patients may still remember old stereotypes. You may have heard of physical pain that comes with leukemia or have read books or seen films where the patient dies in great pain. That old stereotype makes it even more difficult for the leukemia patient. Pain control is available and used more freely today to keep patients comfortable and pain-free.

The side effects of treatment are also very frightening to contemplate, especially if you or a family member has had a bad experience with the medical industry or with medical procedures in the past. Everyone has heard horror stories of noxious side effects of chemotherapy, radiation, and other cancer treatments. Even contemplating the inevitable blood draws, with the accompanying vein sticks, can be downright nerve-wracking to someone who hates needles and fears being stuck.

You may also fear how you will fare in the workplace. Will you be able to continue to work? Will the diagnosis change the way you are perceived on the job, keeping you from well-earned promotions? Will you be stigmatized by colleagues and treated differently because the diagnosis makes others aware of their own mortality, of their inability to find the right words to say what they feel, of their fear that if this happened to you, could it happen to them as well?

Adding to the fears concerning the workplace are fears about insurance and payment for medical treatments. Costs can be very high, and if there is no insurance or limited insurance or a poor managed care program, the problems can become real very rapidly.

Anger

Anger comes right along with fear. "Why me? I've always been a good person and tried to be kind to others, so why me?" Of course there is no rhyme or reason for this, but there are loads of books and publications out there that try to put the blame for getting cancer right back on the patient. You didn't eat the right diet. You didn't exercise enough. You are too heavy. You are too thin. You color your hair. You don't take care of yourself. It goes on non-stop and is infuriating.

The National Cancer Institute trumpeted that too much fat in the diet aided in developing breast cancer. A whole campaign was launched to teach women to eat right. A few years later, studies showed that the amount of fat in the diet has nothing to do with breast cancer. Look at the vegetarians who work out religiously, who get plenty of rest, and still get cancer. Yes, patients get angry!

Every day scientists learn more about genetic involvement in cancer and viral effects on genetic structure. Even though patients are learning about that, some still feel they have been given a heavy burden to carry, one made all the heavier by the "you are responsible for your own cancer" mongers.

Guilt

Guilt is a response to diagnosis in some patients. Many people assume that if they had just eaten right, exercised more, slept less or more, moved away from power lines, chosen a different job, and on and on, they wouldn't have leukemia now. This is dangerous thinking. Many patients want someone to come along and tell them there is a magic pill that will cure their disease. Perhaps it will go away if the patient just sends money, eats exotic foods, or... Both the patient and family need to realize that just as diet didn't give the patient leukemia, a change in diet will not necessarily cure it.

Patients have enough to deal with. They definitely don't need a sense of guilt to add to their burden. More complex is the guilt associated with finding a familial predisposition to leukemia and the concern about having passed it unknowingly to children.

There is guilt because of what the diagnosis and ultimate outcome will do to the family. Relationships are strained to the limits. Often the family caregiver becomes the patient and relationships are turned around. This change in roles doesn't always work so there is added stress on everyone involved. Children become frightened and worried and may begin to act out. Parents have to deal with children's fears, which makes for additional guilt.

Denial

Denial is a protective reaction meant to slow the absorption of painful information.

Some people simply won't accept that they have leukemia. That's easier for those who have a chronic leukemia and go through a long period of watch and wait with only periodic check-ups. For years, some people are able to get away with practically forgetting about the disease and living a normal life, almost as if they had never been diagnosed. They are often surprised by the onset of new symptoms and repeated infections as the disease progresses.

Denial as a method of coping is more problematic with acute leukemias, which require treatment almost immediately. In fact, for those who use denial as a defense mechanism, the speed with which treatment proceeds becomes an emotional trauma in itself. One day, things are fine and life is normal. A week later, the patient may be fighting for his or her life in the hospital, having to rely on everyone.

Sadness and emotional pain

Many people who are actively dealing with leukemia become very sad and have difficulty dealing with the emotional pain they experience. Psychological distress, negative attitudes, constant concern that each little twinge or sniffle signifies disease involvement, and anxiety about separation and death, all become part of their lives. Concerns about health, work, family, and friends affect quality of life. Fatigue often makes it even harder for patients to deal with the emotions they encounter.

Different individuals have different coping skills, which make a huge difference in the way families and patients are able to cope with the disease. It often takes a while for life to return to some semblance of what it was before diagnosis. This is one instance when the expression "my world turned upside-down" is not a cliché.

Acceptance

It may seem ludicrous to talk of acceptance, as if you may or may not accept a diagnosis of a malignant disease. But in truth, most patients do come to acceptance. They accept that they must live with this disease and with the problems that it brings to them and their loved ones. Most patients don't reach this point easily or quickly, and some never do. But if the patient can accept the diagnosis and the idea of living with leukemia, steps can be taken to learn about it, to cope with it, and to plan for the future.

Gary Moon, an AML patient and engineer, described his eventual acceptance of having leukemia, a year after receiving the diagnosis:

> This past year has been a roller coaster ride for my family and me. The most traumatic part of my year was when I was told I had AML. My wife and children were devastated.
>
> I made up my mind that I was going to beat the odds. I was given only a 20 percent likelihood that I'd be alive two years from diagnosis. As a systems engineer I determined that I had to learn about a new system: a biological, electrical, mechanical system, with which I was intimately connected. This is not something I would recommend for the general population, but if you are dealt the entry cards for this experience, you must play the cards to the best of your ability with the restrictions given.
>
> I developed some thoughts during the first traumatic 48 hours that helped me focus on what had to be done to attempt a sane survival of the disease and treatment.
>
> Knowledge is power. Learn everything you can about your disease and its treatment. Don't be afraid to ask questions.
>
> This is a team effort to get you well, and you are the most important member of the team. It's your body! You have a vested interest in its well being.
>
> Get and try to keep a positive attitude. Be willing to adapt to changing situations.
>
> I believe that these concepts helped me survive the treatment with my sanity intact. They also made it easier for care team members to see me as a real person, and it was less stressful for my family.

CHAPTER 4

Tests and Procedures

When your doctor suspects that you have an illness that may be leukemia, he or she will order tests in an effort to arrive at a definitive diagnosis. After diagnosis, several of these tests may be repeated throughout your treatment in order to gauge how well you are responding to treatment, and several will be given again after your treatment to confirm continued remission or a recurrence.

This chapter begins with a description of general preparations for all procedures. Then, we list tests and procedures alphabetically. For each test, we state whether it is done on an inpatient or outpatient basis. We describe what the test or procedure accomplishes, tell how to prepare for the test, and detail how it is administered. Further, we share how most people feel about how painful or uncomfortable the test may be, discuss recovery issues, and outline any possible risks.

General information

It's most important that you receive a correct diagnosis of leukemia type (and subtype where appropriate) before treatment starts. Some of the tests are performed to determine exactly the kind of leukemia you have and to identify the best possible treatment options open to you.

A biopsy procedure requires communication between your oncologist and the pathologist at the hospital in order for the necessary diagnostic tests to be performed correctly. This includes the doctors agreeing in advance as to how the tissue samples should be prepared—for example, by freezing or by fixation within a paraffin block.

There are required retention times for pathology specimens that hospitals must meet according to the Clinical Laboratory Improvement Amendments of 1988. Although many institutions attempt to keep some tissue samples in perpetuity, this cannot be guaranteed, because space limitations and maintaining the proper environment for specimen storage may be a problem. Specimens used in national clinical studies are usually kept for many years in a central repository. If your pathology specimens and blood slides are not in a central repository, it would be well to send a written request asking that, at such time as your slides are likely to be disposed of, they be sent to you. This may be very helpful if your leukemia converts to another form of the disease, or transforms into a different disease, and your oncologist needs to compare a newer sample to the original. You may be glad that the sample is still available should some question arise later regarding the original diagnosis. Perhaps, too, you may be considering one of the newer emerging treatments that could require an analysis of the previous cell sample.

You have a right to request copies of test results. It is wise to ask for, and make sure you receive, your own copies of all records. That way, if you go for a consultation you have the information you need at your fingertips. Some patients keep track of blood test results on spreadsheets that they update each time they have blood work done. This ensures that they have a complete record and can keep track of how the counts are moving. There is no need to keep tabs on this information. Your doctor will do it for you, but having records of test results does come in handy when you want to see how you're progressing or track a remission or relapse.

One patient who tracks and charts her blood work explains how it helped during a consultation:

> I walked in with all my previous records—in a stack about four inches high. I saw the look on the consulting doctor's face, and quickly I said, "If you don't have time to get through all these records just now, I have been tracking my blood work and any major problems I've had and medicines I've been on since I was diagnosed. It's here in a two-page spreadsheet. Will this help you?"
>
> The doctor reached for the spreadsheet and I saw the relief in her face. "Yes, this is most helpful and gives me a feel for where you started and what you have been through. Thank you. I'll go through your records later, but at least this gives us a starting point."
>
> My relationship with this doctor has been cordial and she has been most helpful to me in making treatment decisions as a result of that consultation. These days she automatically reaches for my spreadsheet because she knows she can rely on the information it contains.

It is not unusual to feel nervous about upcoming tests. You have the right to know if a test may be painful, and to ask in advance about options for controlling pain. You have the right to ask for and receive pain medication before a painful test or procedure is performed. The various pain-controlling medications can be requested in advance, such as the injected relaxant Demerol; the brief amnesiac Versed, which is also injected; the topical cream EMLA, which contains the drug Xylocaine familiar in dental care; or the short-acting anti-anxiety tablet Ativan.

Lobby for pain-relievers, and become informed about less invasive procedures. Be aware of alternatives. For tests about which you feel unsure or uneasy, ask the following:

- Why is this procedure or test necessary? Will it determine or change my treatment plan?

- Is there a safer or more comfortable alternative?

- What are the risks and side effects?

- How will pain be controlled?

- Will you please explain this procedure to me, or provide me with literature that describes it thoroughly?

- How experienced is the technician or doctor performing this procedure?

To spare yourself agonized waiting, you should discuss in advance with your oncologist how test results will be communicated. Some patients mistakenly assume that their doctor will take the initiative and contact them, when in fact the doctor's policy may be that the patient should take the initiative and call for results. If you know that your best method of coping includes acquiring as much information as possible as quickly as possible, tell your oncologist that you appreciate timely communication, and offer to expedite communication by making yourself available. Be aware that some oncologists are reluctant to leave test results on an answering machine without assurance from you that this is not a violation of your privacy. In addition, many ancillary doctors involved in your testing may choose for ethical reasons to communicate only with your primary oncologist, unless instructed otherwise. Discussing these issues in advance with your oncologist is wise and helpful.

Never assume that the hospital staff members administering the test are fully aware of your circumstances. Always tell the technicians doing the test that you are a leukemia survivor. Always tell them of any other health problems or allergies you have—such as previous allergic reactions to the iodine in shrimp—and of any prescribed or over-the-counter medications you are taking. If you have had a bone marrow transplant, be sure to tell them that as well.

Make comfort a priority. Many of the tests done today require that you lay on a hard table for extended periods while cameras and x-ray machines do their imaging. Take advantage of this opportunity to nap by asking for extra blankets for comfort and then finding a position in which you can remain pain-free for long periods. Ask for pillows to support your back and knees if you suffer from back pain.

If you are going to a hospital or testing center other than the one you usually use, take copies of previous test reports, slides, and x–ray films with you when you go. That will help the consultant understand clearly what your original doctor has noted and the current problems you have. It is very likely that the second hospital, cancer research center, or testing center will want to repeat the tests using their own equipment, so be prepared if that should occur.

The tests that are described here are those most commonly used for leukemia. However, your doctor may order additional tests not described in this chapter. An excellent resource for finding information about other tests is *Everything You Need to Know About Medical Tests*, published by Springhouse, written by more than 70 medical experts, and describing more than 400 tests. See Appendix A, *Resources*, for other recommendations.

Keep in mind that even if you are familiar with test procedures, your own reaction to the tests can vary. Here is how one leukemia survivor's reaction to a simple blood test changed over the years:

> When I was diagnosed with myelodysplastic syndrome about 30 months ago, I went through a lot of needle sticks in order to draw blood for tests. The phlebotomists at that time remarked on what great veins I had and always got their blood easily. These same remarks persisted throughout two years of blood tests and transfusions.
>
> However, after my bout with acute leukemia, the remarks have changed, and during my last two blood draws the phlebotomists have had to stick me several times to get blood. Maybe this is just a result of the chemotherapy and my low counts, or maybe it is due to the progress of my disease. In any case, it's discouraging.

Specific tests

The following section lists tests and procedures alphabetically, and state whether they are done on an inpatient or outpatient basis. Each test is accompanied by a description of what it accomplishes, how to prepare for it, and how it is administered. Also included are explanations of how most people feel about the pain and discomfort of the tests, recovery issues, and risks.

Blood product transfusion

This outpatient procedure is a means of replenishing your red blood cells and platelets if chemotherapy and/or radiation therapy have caused red blood cells and platelets to die or if they have inhibited the bone marrow's ability to produce new blood cells.

Preparation: Check the blood product brought to you for infusion to be sure it matches your blood type. Platelet matching may also become necessary after many platelet transfusions, as the body gradually becomes sensitized to and attacks donated platelets. Be sure to tell the nursing staff if you have ever before had an allergic reaction to donor platelets. Also, if you have had a bone marrow transplant, make sure the staff knows that you must have irradiated, filtered blood cells. This will ensure that there are no white cells in the blood that might raise a likelihood of graft-versus-host disease.

Method: An intravenous (IV) line is inserted into a vein in your forearm, or into your central venous catheter if you have one. The blood product to be transfused is hung from an IV pole and is dripped over a period of about four hours.

If you have no catheter and an IV line is inserted into your vein, you may feel mild pain during its insertion.

Recovery: If you have had a catheter inserted, be sure that sufficient pressure is applied for a minute or two upon removal, since that will prevent the development of large black and blue marks at the site. There are no recovery issues following transfusion. On the contrary, you can expect to feel much less tired almost immediately after red blood cells are infused.

Risks: There is a risk of serious allergic reaction if donated blood products are not properly matched to yours. If you have chills, fever, or difficulty breathing during a transfusion, notify the nursing staff immediately. This may be the beginning of an allergic reaction. Should the connection between the catheter and the vein loosen, you will see swelling and a buildup of blood at the site. This is usually accompanied by mild pain, and must be called to the nurse's attention at once so the catheter may be removed. In this case the pain is a warning that you should appreciate. If you have had a bone marrow transplant, look carefully to make sure the cells that you are to receive have been irradiated and filtered. There is a slight risk of infection at the site of IV insertion.

Most patients have no problems during blood transfusions and the experience is usually uneventful. Occasionally one encounters a problem. This leukemia survivors tells a story about such an occasion—having an allergic reaction during a blood transfusion:

> "You need a transfusion right now," the doctor said. "I'm sorry, but you're not going to work. You're going to the treatment center for blood."
>
> Within an hour the blood typing was done and the nurse had set up the intravenous drip. I was hooked up to an IV pole. The first pint of blood went in, as it should have. The second pint of blood came in a small pouch and a second nurse came in to check numbers and blood types with my nurse, just as they had done with the first pouch.
>
> About an hour and a half into the infusion I had a wildly allergic reaction to the blood products. It started with a mildly upset stomach— lunch didn't look at all appealing. Then it quickly changed so I was feeling incredibly cold. I had uncontrollable shivering despite three or four blankets that were provided, and violently chattering teeth that I couldn't stop no matter how hard I tried.
>
> My body was out of my control and when the nurse took vital signs I was running a fever. I was immediately given a Benadryl shot and they tried to give me acetaminophen, but I couldn't stop chattering long enough to sip some water. They finally gave me a shot of Demerol and that seemed to work. After about a half-hour I was more or less back to normal, but I was still shaky, tense, and emotionally drained. The nurses made sure that I was in good shape before they let me leave a few hours later.

Blood tests

Various blood tests detect different conditions. The purpose of each blood test is discussed following the name of the test. All are outpatient procedures.

Preparation: Most blood tests require no preparation. Some, however, may require overnight fasting or cessation of certain medications for a few days. Always tell your doctor and the staff administering the test about any drugs, prescription or over-the-counter, that you are taking. Ranitidine, for example, can suppress platelet production and could cause an inaccurate result in a complete blood count.

Method: Most blood tests are performed by drawing blood from the vein just inside the elbow. If your veins have been damaged by chemotherapy, if they are hard to find, or if they roll, the technician (phlebotomist) may use a vein on the back of the hand or on the back of the lower forearm. Some implanted catheters can be used for blood draws (see "Catheter insertion").

You can make your veins easier to access if you:

- Ask the phlebotomist to lay a wet, warm cloth on the vein just before blood is drawn, or ask to use a restroom to soak the forearm in warm water.

- Gently pump the muscles in that arm just before the draw. Too vigorous pumping will cause incorrect results in blood counts and some chemistry tests, and may cause coagulation problems as well.

- Hang the arm lower than the rest of the body for a few minutes just before the draw.

Once a vein is accessed successfully, a blood draw takes under three minutes.

Pain: Most people report minor pain or no pain during a blood draw. If, however, you are afraid of needles, of needle pain, or of the sight of blood, you are not alone.

Here are a few tips for reducing fear and pain during a blood draw:

- Slap or rub the injection site just before the draw so that you will be less likely to feel the insertion. Be aware, however, that this may actually cause incorrect results, since it changes the environment of the vein.

- Ask the phlebotomist to use a butterfly needle if possible. It's the smallest needle available for drawing blood.

- Ask for EMLA cream to use two hours before your appointment. Keep the site covered with an airtight bandage until your draw.

- Ask the phlebotomist, most of whom are quite skilled at reducing pain, to stretch the skin at the injection site.

- Look away while the blood is drawn.

- Think of someone who delights you and makes you smile.

- Practice taking long, slow breaths and concentrate on counting to ten before exhaling slowly through the mouth. Not only will this relaxation method divert your attention, it actually does a better job of stabilizing the blood.

- Make small talk with the phlebotomist to ease your tension. "So, how's business?" is a good opener.

- A good phlebotomist is worth his or her weight in gold. Make a friend and you know that the friend will make things as painless as possible. Phlebotomists know that the job they perform is unpleasant. Do not insult them by likening their profession to "vampires," even in jest.

- For some, blood draws can be an especially difficult ordeal. It might be possible for the technician to do a finger-prick or draw from the earlobe after the area has been numbed with EMLA cream if only a small amount of blood is needed.

Recovery: Most blood draws entail no recovery, but you may have slight, painless bruising at the injection site the following day. Stretching the skin to make the blood draw less painful may increase this chance of bruising. Steady pressure on the injection site for 60 seconds or more, directly after the needle is withdrawn, facilitates clotting, and can reduce the chance of bruising.

Probably the most common cause of bruising or pain after phlebotomy is carrying a pocketbook or briefcase. While the blood has clotted at the site, it has not yet formed a strong seal, so reaching for, or toting a heavy load with that arm may cause the clot to weaken and possibly leak.

Risks: Unless you have blood that won't clot normally, there are only minor risks associated with a blood draw, such as the possibility of painless bruising.

Specific blood tests: Blood tests are listed alphabetically (find normal values for these blood tests in Appendix B, *Normal Blood and Marrow Test Values*):

Alkaline phosphatase

This product's value may be abnormal if liver function is affected, or if bone is being lost, for example, when calcium levels are out of balance.

Antibody screening

See "Coombs direct or indirect," later in this list.

Bcl-1, bcl-2, or bcl-6 gene rearrangements

Gene rearrangements are detected using sophisticated tools that analyze the DNA in our chromosomes. Patented procedures such as polymerase chain reaction (PCR) may be performed first to provide a sample large enough for analysis. Bcl-2 gene rearrangements might be detected in either blood or bone marrow.

Beta-2 microglobulin (B2M)

B2M, a product of white cells, is thought to be a measure of how successfully leukemias will respond to the treatments in use today. Beta-2 microglobulin is a nonspecific tumor marker. Its levels are elevated in solid tumors and lymphoproliferative disease such as B-CLL, non-Hodgkin's lymphoma, and multiple myeloma. It is not useful in monitoring response to treatment. Its levels in spinal fluid are useful for detection of diseases involving the central nervous system. It has recently been considered that low B2M scores (below 2.5) are good prognosticators for B-CLL. B2M is said to be an indicator of the degree of aggressiveness of CLL.

Bilirubin

As with other liver products, the level of this substance is a reflection of the liver or bile duct function.

Complete blood count (CBC)

This test measures the three blood cell types and reports on their proportions, age, and the iron content of red cells. During chemotherapy and radiation therapy, white counts in particular can drop and make the patient susceptible to infections.

See Appendix B for a sample of normal values. Be aware that norms differ from one lab to another so it is wise to create a chart of your own normal highs and lows.

Coombs direct or indirect

These tests are used to look at antigen-antibody complexes on the surface of the red blood cell membrane. This test helps detect antibodies in the bloodstream to ensure that donor and recipient are compatible when blood is being transfused. It also alerts the doctor when rho (D) immune globulin needs to be given and help confirm diagnoses of hemolytic anemia. One of these tests is likely to be ordered when the Hct and Hgb drop, despite the support of red blood cell transfusions.

Creatinine (serum creatinine)

This substance helps indicate how well the kidneys are working. Nodes can press on the ureter—the tube leading from kidney to bladder—and impair kidney function. Creatinine can be elevated when there is muscle-wasting since it is a product of skeletal muscle breakdown. It is normally excreted by the kidneys, so an elevated creatinine level in the blood indicates impairment of kidney function.

Differential (Diff)

The differential measures the percentage of different kinds of white cells in the blood sample. This enables the doctor to determine the absolute cell count. Multiply the percentage of cell type by the total white blood count to get the absolute cell type count. Appendix B, Table B-2, "White Count Differential of the CBC," shows you the cell types, normal percentages, and normal numbers of cells in a sample.

Doctors watch the absolute neutrophil count (ANC) to see when patients' counts are so low that they are likely to develop infections. Patients with lymphocytic leukemias follow the differential so they can determine their absolute lymphocyte counts.

DiSC assay

DiSC assay (differential staining cytotoxicity) is a test in which the patient's cells are collected and exposed to the proposed treatment drug. Briefly, mononuclear cells are isolated from blood, lymph node, bone marrow, or fluids and cultured with the drug to be used in therapy for four days. Then cells are cytocentrifuged onto slides, stained and apoptotic cell death is assessed morphologically. This tells if the cells are responsive to the drug to be used. At present this test is not in general use, but some patients will request that it be done.

Electrolytes

Levels of various minerals in the blood are sometimes a reflection of problems related to tumor metabolism, or to chemotherapy, and most often to levels of hydration. Even a mild bout of diarrhea can change these values. It's always a good idea to make sure that you are properly hydrated, regardless of whether or not there are blood tests planned on a given day. Levels of sodium, calcium, potassium, magnesium, iron, and other electrolytes can be modified by disease or by its treatment.

Erythrocyte Sedimentation Rate (sed rate)

This test measures how quickly red blood cells settle when a sample is placed in a glass tube. Red blood cells that settle quickly indicate an inflammation within the body, usually because levels of fibrinogen and globulins in the blood cause the red cells to settle faster. This test is not reliable, however, if you have anemia, since fewer red cells will fall faster.

FISH (Fluorescence in situ hybridization)

See "ISH," later in this list.

Flow cytometry

This method of examining tissue exploits two principles: first, cancer cells can be tagged with chemicals and so be made to look different than normal cells. Second, these cells can be forced to flow single file through a narrow tube so that they can be counted one at a time, much like children returning from recess. The tagged cancer cells are counted as they flow through a light beam or other tool for detecting whatever tagging agent was used. In this manner, bone marrow and blood can be examined for very specific features that indicate cancer, such as a single damaged gene. Hematologic tumors can be studied using a battery of monoclonal antibodies that identify the cell from which the immunoglobulin leukemic cells are being cloned.

Immunoglobulin studies (IgM, IgA, IgD, IgG, IgE)

Immunoglobulins are one of the weapons in the body's immune system arsenal. They are classes of proteins produced by a special category of B cells (plasma cells), which ordinarily function as antibodies to protect against infectious diseases or other foreign substances. Tests for immunoglobulins commonly detect the quantity of the specific immunoglobulins in the blood. These tests also attempt to determine if increases in immunoglobulins are produced by many different cells (polyclonal) or by a single clone of cells (monoclonal). Elevations of monoclonal immunoglobulins are commonly seen in certain malignancies such as multiple myeloma, Waldenstrom's macroglobulinemia, or non-Hodgkin's lymphoma. Inherited immune system disorders may also have characteristic patterns of immunoglobulins in the blood.

ISH (in situ hybridization)

This test of the DNA contained in blood or other tissue uses chemicals to mark specific gene sequences. The chemicals consist of molecules (probes) constructed to match exactly the gene being sought. The probe untwists the two strands of DNA and, when a match exists between the chemical probe and a gene, attaches itself to one piece of DNA—thus the term hybridization. By using probes that have been tagged and processed further, the pathologist or geneticist can look into the microscope or on x-ray films to see the gene, its breakpoint, any crossing over with other genes on the same or on other chromosomes, and so on. This is an exquisitely sensitive technique for differentiating certain lymphomas and leukemias.

Lactate dehydrogenase (LDH)

Testing for high levels of LDH in leukemia survivors is useful because LDH is released when certain body tissues break down for any reason. Although by itself it is not reliable for diagnosing leukemia, it is a surrogate for tracking tumor burden in patients who have been diagnosed by other means. It is usually done for those who are said to have bulky disease. Elevated LDH can be seen in non-malignant hematological disorders as well as in leukemia, lymphoma, and liver failure.

Liver enzymes

The liver enzymes are SGOT (AST) and SGPT (AST). Unusual amounts of liver enzymes correlate loosely with both the presence and extent of disease, or alterations in liver function from other causes. Some drugs have liver toxicity as a side effect.

Northern blot assay

See "Southern blot assay," later in this list.

Polymerase chain reaction (PCR)

PCR can use many different source tissues as long as they contain genes and chromosomes Deoxyribonucleic acid (DNA,) Ribonucleic acid (RNA) or specific proteins. Blood and bone marrow are two such likely sources, particularly for lymphomas and leukemias. PCR is a method, not a test or substance. It involves taking a very small amount of genetic material and replicating it over and over, so that enough is produced to run tests that will require larger amounts of genetic material.

Reverse transcriptase –Polymerase chain reaction (RT-PCR)

This method is similar to PCR with the substitution of a viral enzyme, reverse transcriptase, which permits amplification of RNA rather than DNA as the initial substrate. Sometimes it is the specific gene-product, RNA, which is easier to detect than the gene itself, composed of DNA, in the cell chromosomes.

Southern blot assay

This hybridization technique is used when searching for a specific DNA fragment. Named after its inventor, E. M. Southern, and like the PCR test, it is designed to detect DNA. It can identify specific genes or onco-genes in specific tumor cells. It is used when doctors are attempting to ensure that specific B cells are no longer present in the blood sample and is considered extremely reliable. A similar technique done with samples of RNA instead of DNA is called *Northern blotting.* Continuing with the geographical metaphor, if protein is the substance to be detected (by specific antibodies, not hybridization,) the test is called a *Western blot* procedure.

T-lymphocyte and B-lymphocyte assays

These methods help determine primary or secondary immune deficiency diseases. They also help differentiate between benign and malignant lymphocytic proliferative disease and monitor response to treatment for immune deficiency diseases.

Uric acid

Uric acid is the substance formed from the breakdown of the contents of the cell nucleus. The kidneys ordinarily excrete uric acid, so levels may increase when the kidneys are impaired or when production of uric acid in the body exceeds the capacity for excretion by the normal kidney. Rapid destruction of cells caused by chemotherapy produces large quantities of uric acid in the blood. If it is allowed to persist, it can damage the kidneys and other tissues in which it may be deposited by the blood, resulting in a condition called pseudogout, which is so named in order to distinguish it from the inherited disease gout.

Bone marrow aspiration/biopsy (BMB)

By examining the aspirated cells or the solid core of bone marrow under a microscope, a pathologist can assess the production of normal cells in the blood. When the bone marrow contains abnormal cells, the effects of chemotherapy or radiation can be evaluated and the extent to which the bone marrow is involved can be determined in leukemias, lymphomas, and other cancers. In addition, it can be determined if other non-malignant conditions, such as myelofibrosis (scarring) or an infectious disease, such as tuberculosis, may be present.

Bone marrow aspiration involves drawing a small amount of bone marrow or small number of cells into a narrow needle. Bone marrow biopsy involves drawing a piece of bone and its attached, intact marrow into a larger needle called a trephine. Although in most people all bones are capable of producing marrow, for these tests the large bone of the hip is usually used. As one gets older, blood cell production in the bone marrow tends to concentrate more in the bones of the skull, ribs, spine, and pelvis, rather than in the long bones of the extremities. Bone marrow aspiration and biopsy is usually, but not always, an outpatient procedure.

Preparation: A sedative and/or an amnesic drug may be given to you in advance. Bring a heating pad with you, and ask the staff if you can place it over the hip area for ten minutes or so beforehand, as some patients report that this reduces pain afterward. If you have had biopsies in the past and prefer the technique of a particular staff member, try to obtain an appointment that matches his or her schedule. Be sure your sedative or local anesthetic has become fully effective before allowing the staff to proceed.

Method: A local anesthetic is injected over the back of the hipbone and a very small incision is made. Into this incision, the needle or trephine (or each in turn, if both aspiration and biopsy are being done) is inserted to penetrate the bone. For a marrow aspiration, the blood and marrow is drawn into the needle by the quick suction of a syringe and the needle is removed. For a biopsy, the trephine is pushed through the bone and rotated to collect a core of bone and its attached marrow and is then removed. If not enough marrow can be obtained, a second insertion through the same incision, but into a different area of bone, will be attempted. Pressure is applied over the insertion point for a few minutes to stop bleeding. A small dressing is applied.

Pain: Many patients report moderate to severe pain during this procedure. Be sure to ask for a sedative, or an amnesic such as Versed if you know from past experience that you prefer being very much unaware of any pain. In all cases, make sure the doctor/technician uses enough local anesthetic and waits long enough for it to deaden feeling in the area before he begins the procedure. You may feel a unique pressure as the needle is pushed through the bone, especially if your bones are very dense. You may also feel the pressure as the marrow is drawn into the needle. You may feel pain if the needle slips across the bone surface as it is being inserted.

Bone marrow biopsies are usually one of the least liked tests that leukemia patients face. One patient used information she gathered from the technicians who do this test at M. D. Anderson Cancer Center to create a humorous recipe for a painless bone marrow biopsy and she swears that it works:

> *Let me introduce you to my recipe for a reasonably livable BMA/ BMB (bone marrow aspiration/bone marrow biopsy):*
>
> 1. *Remind the doctor to be sure to use enough local anesthesia to numb the area completely.*
>
> 2. *Ensure that the doctor uses enough local anesthesia to numb the area completely and thoroughly.*
>
> 3. *Insist that the doctor waits long enough so that the local anesthesia numbs the area completely.*
>
> *Step to supersede Steps 1 through 3: engage the doctor in conversation after you've been given the local so that you both need to concentrate on what you're discussing and the doctor can't work while you wait for the area to numb.*
>
> *The technicians at MDACC who do the painless bone marrow biopsies told me exactly what they do:*
>
> 1. *They use lots of lidocaine—lots and lots.*
>
> 2. *They wait until it numbs the area fully.*
>
> 3. *They talk us through the procedure so we know what to expect as they do it.*
>
> 4. *They are careful to stay within the numbed area when they work.*

> *I have never had a painful bone marrow aspiration and biopsy using this combination.*

Many patients who have "been there, done that" try to give other patients the benefit of their experience with bone marrow biopsies. Some find it helpful to take medication to ease the anxiety caused by the procedure. Mark Freymiller has ALL and is the veteran of a number of bone marrow biopsies. He responds to a question from a new patient with CLL, facing her first bone marrow biopsy and wondering about how much pain is involved. He also echoes the advice to make sure to take advantage of adequate medication and avoid unneeded pain:

> *I was diagnosed with ALL in May 1998 and have had at least six bone marrow biopsies. Doctors have good medicines to make the experience not so bad, but my bone marrow biopsies have definitely been more painful than "having a tooth worked on."*

> *You will very likely need to have more bone marrow biopsies in the future to verify how effective your treatment is against the CLL. Since psychologically it is easier to go in for a second biopsy if the first one went well, I'd recommend getting some good drugs prior to the procedure. If the procedure goes great and next time you feel like you need fewer drugs, then you can reduce the drugs for next time.*

> *I now take 2 mg of Ativan (lorazepam) one hour prior to any bone marrow biopsy. It is a prescription antiemetic drug that also functions as an anti-anxiety drug for me. It also helped me a lot with the nausea related to receiving IV teniposide and Ara-C. Two mg is a high dose for me and someone else drives me home from the procedure and then I sleep off the drug for the next four hours. Patients don't need to just accept the pain as a necessary part of the treatment. The bone marrow biopsy is one of those times that I am quite pleased to avoid some of it.*

Recovery: Unlike a bone marrow harvest, during an aspiration or biopsy very little marrow is removed, so subsequent lightheadedness and fatigue are rare. Afterward, your hip may feel sore for a few days. This can usually be relieved with Tylenol-type medications. The patient is asked not to get the dressing wet or to remove it for at least 24 hours.

Risks: There is a slight risk of infection at the incision site.

Bone marrow harvest

A bone marrow harvest is usually an inpatient procedure with its own preparation and a longer period of recovery than that for bone marrow biopsy. It is discussed thoroughly in Chapter 9, *Transplantation*.

Catheter insertion (central catheter, central line)

This procedure can be done on an inpatient or outpatient basis. A central catheter or line is a flexible tube that is threaded into a very large vein near your heart. Its presence in a large vein dilutes chemotherapy drugs amidst a large volume of blood. That makes chemotherapy safer and more easily tolerated. Moreover, depositing chemotherapy drugs near your heart will distribute them more quickly and more evenly to all parts of your body than is possible when chemotherapy is infused directly into an arm vein. Using a central catheter can eliminate damage to arm veins during chemotherapy and can eliminate somewhat painful penetration of arm veins for blood testing and for administering other drugs.

Preparation: You need to decide whether a catheter is the right choice for you and which kind of catheter you prefer. You will also need to decide whether to get an external catheter (with tubing emerging from the skin) or a subcutaneous catheter (under the skin). Your oncologist may already have very strong opinions on this topic.

Some advantages of catheter use are:

- Chemotherapy is safer when diluted by lots of blood.
- Chemotherapy is spread throughout the body more quickly and evenly with a central catheter.
- Vein damage is minimal or nonexistent.
- Some models can be used for blood transfusions.
- Some models can be used for hemapheresis, the collecting of stem cells for a stem cell transplant.

Note that with an external catheter there are no needle sticks that hurt, but with an internal catheter, no periodic cleaning is necessary.

Some drawbacks of catheter use are:

- Surgery is required to install a central catheter.

- External catheters must be cleaned and flushed daily or tri-weekly, and kept dry.

- Infections can lodge in a catheter. Their treatment may entail use of very strong antibiotics, with risky side effects, such as permanent vertigo, or may require surgical removal with a third surgery for reinsertion at a later date.

- The external types that emerge from the skin of the neck or chest can appear unsightly and make the patient feel uncomfortable.

- It is necessary to wrap them carefully when showering and bathing so they do not get wet.

- If your catheter is not perfectly placed, it may be necessary to shift positions often and to sit up or lie down to enable them to function more effectively.

- The types that do not emerge from the skin still require somewhat painful skin penetration to access the port.

- Central catheters can break and travel through the vein to your heart.

Central catheters can kink and make drug infusion difficult. Nevertheless, despite the drawbacks, once you have lived with a catheter that functions well, you will appreciate the fact that you don't have to go through treatment with peripheral vein catheters and the problems that may ensue. Just think, no needle sticks each time blood must be drawn, no needle in the arm while you go through a four- to eight-hour treatment session, and best of all, no multiple needle sticks while the nurse tries to capture your rolling, hiding veins.

When you have a catheter inserted, you may be given the choice of a local or a general anesthetic. If you choose a general anesthetic, preparation for and recovery from this procedure may be more complex. On the other hand, some individuals who chose a local anesthetic report that they could still feel deep pain during the procedure.

You will be told to fast for twelve to eighteen hours before surgery. The risks associated with this surgery will be explained to you, and you will be asked to sign a consent form. If in the past anesthesia has made you nauseous during recovery, tell the anesthesiologist. You will be given antinausea medication in that event.

Method: After donning a hospital gown, you are taken to a surgical suite. A local anesthetic is injected in the skin near the vein that will be used for the general anesthetic, and an intravenous line (IV) is inserted once the area is numbed. An oxygen mask may be fitted over your face while you are still awake. A general anesthetic is injected into the IV line to make you fall asleep. Afterward, you may be kept asleep with gas anesthesia.

After the anesthetic has taken effect, two areas, both on the chest, or one on the chest and one on the neck, are cleansed and two incisions are made. The surgeon accesses the large vein near the heart through one of these incisions. The central line is threaded through the large vein until it rests near your heart. The other end is threaded beneath your skin and, for an internal port, secured there. For an external port, it is threaded through the surface of the skin with an anchor just below the surface. The incision is then closed layer by layer. Surgical staples or stitches are used to close both internal and external layers of tissue. Dissolving synthetic fabric layers may be used internally to prevent a form of internal scarring called adhesion.

Pain: Directly after surgery you are given intravenous pain medication. Sometimes the hospital staff looks for signs that you have awakened from general anesthesia before administering pain medication, which once again makes you sleepy. This precaution is taken to ensure that you are not overdosed. Be sure to make clear your need for pain medication as soon as you are awake if you are experiencing pain, as excessive pain can interfere with healing. Most patients report pain at the incision site, a sore throat from the breathing tube that was previously inserted for anesthesia, and a few report sore throat upon awakening.

When you are discharged, you are given a prescription for oral pain medicine. Many patients report a lingering dull ache in the area beneath the incision for weeks afterward.

Some who have had a central line implanted report pain when moving their arms or when lying in a certain position for several weeks following implantation. Some who elect local anesthesia report feeling deep pain during the procedure.

Recovery: When you wake, you will have the catheter attached to an IV line, which is now supplying you with saline, nutrients, and painkiller. In general, the sooner you rise from bed and walk, the sooner you regain full function of all body organs, as movement aids the healing process.

See "Node biopsy" for recovery issues after local anesthesia.

If you have chosen an external catheter, you will be taught how to clean, flush, and care for it. Redness, swelling or bleeding that persists at the incision site should be reported to your doctor, since this could signal an infection.

The length of hospital stay varies based on the patient's condition and the type of insurance in effect. If you feel you need to stay longer in the hospital, but your insurance policy limits your stay, be sure to make this need known to your doctor and to the nursing staff.

Sometimes having a catheter installed can be a mixed blessing. The following leukemia patient had a catheter inserted but only slowly came to the opinion that it was, on balance, worthwhile:

> I was really unhappy about having the central venous catheter
> installed in my body. Just the idea of installing anything foreign was dis-
> concerting. Then, when I awoke from the procedure, I was really upset.
> The lumens were protruding from the upper part of my breast, my breast
> was black and blue, and it appeared that there were scars all over my
> upper chest. I felt like an alien and I hated what they had done to me.
>
> Even worse, I could not lie down in bed for the first few days and had
> to sleep with my arm raised to shoulder level on the back of the couch.
> That eventually went away, but I sure was unhappy while it was going on.
> The leukemia wasn't bad enough? Now I had to deal with pain and dis-
> comfort as well. Tylenol was their idea of a painkiller. I think that per-
> haps some of the doctors who do this procedure need to have some experi-
> ence in going through it!
>
> Adding insult to injury, I couldn't shower casually. It took careful
> preparation and lots of tape to keep the area around the insertion point of
> the catheter clean and dry, and the lumens as well. I packaged myself as
> well as I could, but it was definitely not something I appreciated having to
> live with.

On the other hand, once the catheter was installed, there were no more sticks with needles for blood draws, and chemotherapy was certainly easier. I suppose if I had to balance having a catheter or not having one, the catheter would win by a very narrow margin.

Risks: There are a number of risks associated with surgery done under general anesthesia, including excessive bleeding from the incision site, such as accidental penetration of a major vein, and a very small risk from the anesthesia itself. Your doctor and the hospital staff will explain fully the risks that apply most closely to your surgery.

See "Node biopsy" for a description of preparation for local anesthesia. Having a catheter placed into your body can be very disconcerting. People who have exterior catheters may find the presence of the lumens (the exterior tubes through which chemotherapy and blood products will pass) hanging from their chest very difficult to handle.

CT scan (computed tomography, "CAT" scan)

An outpatient procedure, computed tomography is a series of many very narrow x-rays taken at varying depths of tissue from different angles around your body. These x-ray images are then analyzed and reassembled by a computer into an image of your internal organs. CT scans differ from traditional x-ray imaging in that x-ray imaging can't readily distinguish organs that are lying behind other organs. Imagine looking at several veils, hanging one behind the other, each painted with a different design. You can imagine how difficult it might be to discern the design on the farthest veil. CT scans, on the other hand, are able to delineate even those organs that are obscured by other tissue.

Preparation: You may be asked to fast overnight, to use a laxative, or to come early to drink a contrast agent if a CT scan of your abdomen and/or pelvis is planned.

Your scan may require an iodine-based contrast agent. Be sure to tell your doctor and the staff doing the test if you have thyroid disease or are allergic to iodine in seafood or other sources. A non-iodine contrast agent can be substituted. Because the iodine contrast agent used may cause a sensation of heat, skin flushing, or rapid heartbeat, be sure to tell the technician if you have heart disease, high blood pressure, or any additional health concerns.

If you have internal staples from a previous surgery or pieces of metal embedded in your body from a previous injury, tell the technician. They represent no danger to you during the scan, but may appear on the film as unexplained phenomena.

CT scanners are open, doughnut-shaped machines that generally do not cause patients to feel claustrophobic.

Method: CT scans are performed while you are lying in a carefully chosen position that has been aligned with the machine. It is important to maintain the position that was chosen until the technician says you can relax. Most CT scan sessions include a fast, initial pass with no contrast agent, followed by a second, slower scan with a contrast agent. The first scan images the entire body to use as a frame of reference for the rest of the scanning. During the first scan, you'll feel the table you're laying on move smoothly through the doughnut hole of the machine, without stopping and starting.

While the second, slower scan is underway, you may be asked to hold your breath briefly over and over. Some scanning machines take ten to twenty minutes to scan, depending upon how much of the body is being scanned. During this time, the contrast agent is slowly dripped into your vein. The part of you being scanned is positioned inside the doughnut hole, which is about twelve inches thick. You'll feel the table you're laying on move slowly through the machine a few centimeters at a time, stopping and starting. Some people try taking a nap at this point.

Newer scanners can do the entire scan very quickly, in about twenty seconds. For these machines, you may have to hold your breath for the entire twenty seconds, and if a contrast agent is injected, it will be pushed rapidly into your vein instead of slowly dripped. This quick administration of the contrast agent may cause stronger feelings of heat and faster heartbeat, sensations that are not considered an allergic reaction. You will feel the table you're laying on move smoothly through the doughnut hole of the machine without stopping and starting.

For some scans of the stomach or bowels, you may be required to drink a contrast agent just before the scan is taken.

Pain: CT scans are painless; however, when a contrast agent is used, it is injected into a vein, perhaps causing minor discomfort. See "Blood tests."

Recovery: If you have had a scan that required drinking a contrast agent, you may experience gas, diarrhea, or constipation for one to three days afterward. Drinking large amounts of water will hasten the removal of the contrast agent from the digestive tract. If you have had a contrast agent injected, you may have a harmless and temporary discoloration of the urine or skin for several days afterward. If you are sensitive to iodine or have a thyroid condition, you may feel fatigue for several days after receiving an iodine-based contrast agent.

Risks: A CT scan, if repeated over and over for many years, may deliver enough radiation to body tissue to cause health problems later in life, such as lung, thyroid, or breast cancers. However, as CT scanning technology has improved, the amount of radiation delivered has been lowered.

FISH (fluorescence in situ hybridization)

See ISH under "Blood tests."

Flow cytometry

See "Blood tests."

Gallium scan (scintigraphy, gallium scintigram)

This outpatient test exploits the fact that some affected lymphatic tissue will absorb more of a substance than will surrounding tissue or healthy lymphatic tissue. Your doctor will choose a scintigraphic agent that works best for the type of node involvement you have, and its location. Different scintigraphic agents may be used because:

- Low-grade tumors sometimes absorb thallium more readily than gallium.

- T-cell tumors may absorb gallium more readily than B-cell tumors do.

- Abdominal tumors of several types may be hard to distinguish from normal tissue with either gallium or thallium.

When a node or other lymphoid tissue absorbs gallium well, it is called gallium-avid. If a tumor is suspected not to absorb gallium well, any one of a variety of other radioisotopic agents, such as technetium-99m or Indium-111, may be used instead. Tumors that are not gallium-avid may be so because the lymphatic ducts are blocked, because internal tumor pressure is too great to allow the substance to enter, or because surrounding tissue is inflamed and takes up just as much gallium, thus reducing contrast.

Sometimes this procedure is repeated using a camera that is sensitive to the emission of a single positron. A positron is a particle given off (emitted) by the radioactive tracer that is used. This is called a SPECT or SPET scan, and works on a similar principle. The gallium makes your tissue more visible to the camera. The gamma camera, if it is used, is not a doughnut-shaped solid thing like a CT scanner. It's more like a shield that moves back and forth in half circles starting at the top of the body and working down. It moves close to the body, but does not touch it.

Preparation: An enema or laxative will be necessary the day before the test. After lying down on the camera table, get comfortable because you must hold this position for about one hour.

Method: Gallium-67 is injected into a vein in the forearm and the needle is then withdrawn. Depending on the agent used, the patient may be scanned repeatedly in 2, 4, 24, 48 or 72 hours, or a combination of these times. For the repeated tests, the patient must return to the hospital. No second injection is required before the second scan. Scanning is done fully clothed, lying on a camera table that is sensitive to the energy emitted by the injected agent. It is important to hold still for the duration of the film exposure. Some patients are embarrassed to note that, although they are fully clothed, the computer-assembled image on the screen is of the naked body.

One patient described his experience with the gallium scan this way:

> *I've had a couple of gallium scans. Other than having to have an injection of radioactive (they said it was low-dose) gallium a couple days earlier, it is very much like a CT scan. You just lie there and let the machine move a small distance (an inch?) at a time for each part of the scan.*
>
> *My understanding is that the gallium is absorbed by rapidly dividing cells, so that the bright spots on the scan shows where, and how active, the cancer is. They said my first one lit up like a Christmas tree, but today I'm cancer free.*

Pain: You may feel a slight sting when the scintigraphic agent is injected. You won't have to stay away from others later to avoid exposing them to radioactivity, as is necessary after receiving injections of some other isotopes. Allergic reactions are extremely rare.

Recovery: There are no recovery issues associated with this test.

Risks: As with other imaging techniques, there are risks of false-positive and false-negative readings with gallium. The amount of radioactive exposure with these procedures is almost negligible and the scintigraphic compounds decay quickly.

MRI (magnetic resonance imaging)

This outpatient test uses large magnets and radio waves to cause the different atoms that make up our cells to vibrate at different speeds. The different speeds are then mapped by a computer into an image of the body part being examined. MRI is better than a CT scan for imaging soft tissue, such as cartilage or the brain. There is no exposure to radiation when having a MRI.

Preparation: You will be asked to lie on a table that moves in and out of the tunnel-shaped MRI machine. The body part being scanned will be positioned within a basket-like brace to help maintain the position chosen by the technician.

MRI machines make hammering noises because the magnets are being repositioned constantly while the images are being generated. The technician supplies you with disposable earplugs.

A contrast agent may be injected for imaging certain organs. Ask the technician about the risk associated with the agent being used, and tell him or her if you have any allergies or problems with blood clotting. Also, it is imperative that you inform your doctor, as well as the technician, if you have any metal implants in your body. For example, you may have a metal plate in your head, hip, leg, or a ball and socket joint. Staples also should be mentioned.

Some people find the enclosed models of MRI machines claustrophobic. Certain MRI machines have an open gazebo-like design to reduce claustrophobia, with the magnets overhead supported on pillars. Others are made of clear plastic.

If you're claustrophobic, there are several things that can help alleviate panic, such as knowing that there is a speaker inside the machine so that the technician can hear you if you ask for help, and that you, in turn, can hear her. There is also a hand-held beeping summons that you can press if you feel overly tense. Most facilities have a sound system and will let you choose the music. You may also notice that relaxing photographs have been taped to the inside of the machine. Fans circulate fresh air into the tunnel at all times. It's also possible that, unless your head is being imaged, only part of your body will be within the machine and your head may not. If you still feel that claustrophobia will be a serious problem, ask your doctor whether a sedative taken beforehand would interfere with the imaging process.

Some people, on the other hand, report that the MRI experience is comforting, like a return to the womb. In fact, a friend reports that he likes to have an MRI because it's the only place where nobody can interrupt him.

Method: An initial scan to set benchmarks is done rapidly using no contrast agent. A second scan for finer detail is then repeated at slower speed. If a contrast agent is to be used, it is injected into a vein in the arm before the second scan. Although earplugs help mute sounds, you will hear hammering noises that vary in speed and pitch. While being scanned, one must remain as still as possible, but breathing is not restricted as it sometimes is during a CT scan.

A scan, in general, takes about 40 minutes. After scanning is complete, there is a five- to ten-minute wait while the computer analyzes and maps the signals generated by the magnets. The technician will check the resulting images to be sure they are readable.

The imaging process is painless, although you may feel a slight sting or warmth during injection if a contrast agent is used.

Recovery: If a contrast agent is used, temporary changes in the color of skin, urine, or feces is possible.

Risks: There may be risks of an allergic reaction associated with specific contrast agents; ask your doctor or the technician. As always, there is a very slight risk of infection at the injection site, and a risk of minor, painless bruising at the injection site.

MUGA scan (multiple gated acquisition scan, gated blood pool scan, radionuclide ventriculography [RNV])

This outpatient test is used following certain chemotherapies to determine if the heart has been damaged so that an assessment can be made regarding how much additional chemotherapy can be administered safely.

Preparation: You may be asked to restrict food or caffeine intake for about three hours prior to the test. Wear comfortable clothing because you may be walking on a treadmill or riding a stationary bicycle for about fifteen minutes.

Method: A safe, mildly radioactive contrast agent such as technetium-99 or thallium is injected into your forearm and subsequently collects in the heart, arteries and veins. Sometimes a binding agent for the contrast agent is injected first. Alternately, a small amount of blood may be drawn and the contrast and binding agents mixed with this blood and reinjected. You may be resting, or exercising for fifteen minutes, or both while this test is performed. The scanning camera will be placed above your chest if you are lying down, or in front of your chest if you are exercising. For the resting scan you must hold quite still.

An electrocardiograph machine may be used at the same time. If used, its electrodes will be attached to about six areas of your rib cage using sticky bandages.

Pain: Minimal pain is possible at the injection site. If you experience chest pain during this test, tell the technician immediately.

Risks: There is a very slight risk of developing cancer associated with the very small amount of radioactive material used; more so if you have had many previous X-rays, CT scans, radiation therapy and other procedures that use radioactive agents, as radiation dose is cumulative.

There is a slight risk of infection at the injection site.

Needle biopsy (fine-needle aspiration, CT-guided needle biopsy, percutaneous biopsy)

This outpatient test is a means for retrieving a tissue sample from a lymph node or any body organ without requiring an incision or more extensive surgical exploration. Needle biopsies are commonly used to examine the thyroid, kidney, liver, lung, breast, prostate, pancreas, salivary gland, spinal fluid, and bone marrow. Bone marrow biopsies and spinal taps will be discussed separately.

Needle biopsies produce a small core of tissue about 1 to 3 centimeters in length and 1 to 2 millimeters in diameter. Needle aspirations produce a sampling of cells but without the supporting framework of tissue. In that instance, only the cells can be evaluated, but not their architectural or structural relationship to each other.

This is not considered a good choice for identifying leukemia or lymphoma within a node. The architecture of the entire lymph node contributes important information for the diagnosis, helping the physician determine if he is looking at leukemia or lymphoma.

Preparation: You may be asked to fast for twelve hours before the procedure if a sedative or general anesthetic will be used, or if the tissue being biopsied is part of the digestive system. Blood or urine samples may be collected prior to the biopsy. Bring comfortable clothing to wear afterward, and plan on not being able to walk or drive alone after a sedative or general anesthetic is used.

Method: You will be lying flat on a table for most such biopsies, although lung biopsies may be done while you're seated. The skin will be cleaned. A local anesthetic will be injected, or a sedative or general anesthetic may be given by injection or inhalation, or, if a fine-needle biopsy is planned, no anesthetic may be used. Directly before the biopsy, the area of interest may be imaged by CT scan or x-ray, and the skin above it may be targeted with ink or dye. Depending on the organ being examined, you may be asked to regulate your breathing or to hold quite still during the biopsy. A tiny incision is made and the biopsy needle is inserted through the incision. For kidney biopsies, a guide needle may be used first. A small amount of tissue is drawn (aspirated) into the syringe. The needle is withdrawn, pressure is applied to halt bleeding, a bandage is applied—no stitches are required—and the tissue is sent to the pathology lab for analysis.

For breast biopsies, stereotactic needle biopsies, which are computer-guided and very rapid, are sometimes performed. While you are lying facedown on a table equipped with an area to accommodate the breast, the tissue of interest is mapped from several angles. The automated biopsy needle enters and exits the breast within seconds.

Pain: A slight sting from the injected anesthetic or fine-needle biopsy is common. Depending on which organ is being biopsied, you may feel pressure, a brief, sharp pain, a dull, deep ache, or cramping. For liver or other digestive tract biopsies, you may feel pain in the shoulder. Tenderness or bruising may occur at the site of the biopsy and within any intervening muscle tissue for three to seven days. Some physicians prescribe Tylenol or Tylenol/codeine combinations for relieving the aftereffects.

Recovery: Following kidney biopsies, you may be asked to lie on your back for twelve to twenty-four hours, and you may note the presence of red blood in your urine for 24 hours.

Risks: Possible risks involved include organ failure while under general anesthesia, infection, internal or external bleeding at the site of the puncture, or injury to adjacent organs. For lung biopsies, risk of a collapsed lung exists, thus any difficulty breathing should be reported immediately to your doctor. For kidney biopsies, blood in the urine may persist beyond 24 hours and this should be reported to your doctor.

Node biopsy (excisional biopsy)

This test is the best means for the diagnosis of lymphoma or other cancerous involvement in the lymph nodes. It is another way of helping the doctor determine if the patient has lymphoma or leukemia.

It is generally, but not always, an outpatient procedure. An inpatient stay usually is necessary if the node being biopsied is in the abdomen or chest.

Preparation: No physical preparations are necessary.

Method: While lying flat on a table, the area above the node will be cleaned and a local anesthetic will be injected. Rarely, a general anesthetic is given by injection or by inhalation. An incision is made, the entire node is removed, and the incision is stitched. The node is sent to the pathology lab for analysis.

The surgeon and the pathologist must coordinate the preparation of the node for pathology after its removal.

Pain: A slight sting from the local anesthetic is common. The site may feel tender for three to seven days.

Recovery: You may be instructed to keep the incision dry until the stitches are removed. Stitches usually are removed in seven to ten days.

Risks: A slight risk of organ failure while under general anesthesia exists. A slight risk of infection or bleeding at the site of the incision exists.

PCR (polymerase chain reaction)

See "Blood tests."

Sonogram (ultrasound, sonography)

An outpatient procedure, sonography creates a map of how your body structures appear when sound waves echo from them. The sonography equipment includes a wand that generates sound waves and a microphone for sensing the echoes the sound waves generate. The wave signal is passed to a computer that reformats the signals into a picture of body organs on a screen.

Bone interferes with sonography, so scanning the brain is not successful using the equipment readily available today.

Color Doppler ultrasound is specialized sonography that can detect the speed and direction of blood flow within the body. The differences appear as different colors. This is useful because some tumors commandeer a large blood supply, and this excessive blood supply may be visible and meaningful using color Doppler ultrasound. A common use today is for the visualization of the ovaries to be able to distinguish cysts from tumors.

Preparation: For a pelvic sonogram, you may be asked to drink large quantities of water, because the urinary bladder acts as a window for sound waves when the bladder is very full. If you sometimes experience urinary incontinence, you should make the technician aware of that fact before the test is performed.

Method: You will be lying on a table while the technician gently presses the wand over your body. Depending on what body part is being imaged, you may be asked to remove certain items of clothing and to wear a sheet in their place. The technician will first apply warmed gel to your skin to make the wand move smoothly. She may ask you to tilt your body and to maintain the tilt with your muscles, or she may brace the tilt with pillows under you.

For a transvaginal ultrasound, she will apply warm gel to a special wand and ask you to insert it comfortably into your vagina. Once in place, she will guide it from side to side to visualize the uterus and ovaries. This specialized wand is quite long, which means that the technician's hands are not very close to your private body parts, and, with your body covered by a sheet, you probably won't feel overly exposed to a stranger.

If you are having pelvic sonography along with a second sonographic scan, ask the technician to do the pelvic scan first so that you can empty your bladder.

Many sonography facilities have an overhead screen so that you can see the same image the technician is seeing.

Pain: Sonography is not painful. Having to maintain a very full bladder for a pelvic sonogram is uncomfortable.

Recovery: There are no recovery issues following sonography.

Risks: There are no known risks associated with sonography. No one has ever ruptured a bladder even though it is markedly distended.

Ultrasound (ultrasonography, sonogram)

See "Sonography."

X-rays (radiographic studies)

X-ray imaging may be used early in the diagnostic process to detect unusual masses and determine the extent of disease. During treatment, x-ray images can be used to locate intestinal blockages caused by certain chemotherapies, and to detect enlarged nodes. x-ray imaging is diagnostic, and is different from x-radiation therapy in that it delivers much lower doses of radiation to tissue. X-ray studies are an outpatient procedure.

Preparation: You may be asked to fast overnight, to use a laxative, to purchase and drink a contrast agent, or to drink copious amounts of water if x-ray imaging of your colon or kidneys is planned.

If your x-rays will require an iodine-based contrast agent, as is used for certain x-ray studies of the kidneys, be sure to tell your doctor and the staff doing the test if you have thyroid disease or are allergic to iodine in seafood or other sources. A non-iodine contrast agent can be substituted.

If you have internal staples from a previous surgery, or pieces of metal embedded in your body from a previous injury, tell the technician. They represent no danger to you during the x-ray session, but may appear on the film as unexplained phenomena.

Method: X-ray films are taken while you are sitting, standing or lying in a carefully chosen position that has been aligned with the x-ray machine. It is important to maintain the position that was chosen, and to remain very still, until the technician says you can relax.

For some studies of the stomach or bowels, you may be required to drink a contrast agent while the x-ray films are being taken.

For some bowel studies, an enema may be administered to fill the lower bowel with a contrast agent. Hospitals with the latest equipment will help you retain the fluid with an inflatable bulb that is part of the enema package and is inserted just inside the rectum and painlessly inflated when correctly positioned. If this newer equipment is not available, you will be expected to retain the contrast agent using rectal muscles alone for up to ten or fifteen minutes. While not painful, this may be uncomfortable, because in these circumstances the urge to empty the bowel is quite strong.

Pain: X-ray studies are painless; however, if a contrast agent such as dye is needed, it may be injected into a vein causing minor discomfort. See "Blood tests." Some studies require positioning of the body that may be temporarily uncomfortable, if, for example, you suffer from back pain. If you are having a barium enema, ask the technician to let you remove the nozzle of the enema yourself when the test is complete to reduce the chance of rectal discomfort.

Recovery: If you have had a study that required a contrast agent in the stomach, small intestine or large intestine, you may experience gas, diarrhea or constipation for one to three days afterward. Drinking large amounts of water will hasten the removal of the contrast agent from the digestive tract. If you have had a contrast agent injected, you may have a harmless and temporary discoloration of the urine or skin for several days afterward. If you are sensitive to iodine or have a thyroid condition, you may feel fatigue for several days after receiving an iodine-based contrast agent.

Risks: X-ray studies, if repeated over and over, may deliver enough radiation to body tissue to cause health problems later in life, such as lung, thyroid, or breast cancers.

CHAPTER 5

Subtype, Staging, and Prognosis

The type of leukemia—chronic lymphatic leukemia, hairy cell leukemia, etc. —is not the only information that needs to be ascertained about your disease. After the type has been determined, the doctor also has to consider subtypes of that leukemia and staging of the disease.

Differentiating among subtypes and stages is necessary so that both doctor and patient understand the severity of the disease and the prognostic indicators. This knowledge plays a large role in making treatment decisions. For example, the doctor might be able to recommend a therapy more likely to be helpful or to avoid a therapy not likely to be helpful. Or a doctor might recommend more aggressive or less aggressive treatment based on certain prognostic factors.

This chapter focuses on more specific information that doctors can glean about each person's disease and gives some background on how that information can impact treatment decisions. It is not easy material. In fact, you may decide to skip this chapter because you don't want to go into such depth about the disease at this time. However, if you are a "tell me everything" kind of person—if you want to understand some of the language in your pathology report, you want to communicate more effectively about treatment options, or if you want to know some questions to ask—this chapter contains informational support.

The chapter first looks at what can be learned from blood work and what techniques are used for doing so. It then describes subtypes and staging for each type of leukemia. Acute leukemias are listed first, followed by chronic leukemias, and then hairy cell.

Blood tests yield subtype and staging information

When the blood work is completed, the oncologist will receive a comprehensive pathology report. It tells the number and percentages of cells in the sample, as well as which antigens the blood sample has been tested for and which specific antigens the cells in the sample express. The oncologist reviews the cellular morphology (cell form and structure) and the information about histology (the identification of the minute structure, composition, and function of tissues). Appendix D, *FAB Staging of Acute Leukemia*, gives the French-American-British (FAB) classification scheme for acute leukemia. This method of classification is used universally. The reports the doctor receives serve as a key to the markers expressed by the cells.

Scientists are continuing to be able to glean more information from blood testing. With the knowledge that we are gaining from the human genome project, we are able to be more precise in identifying the kind of cell that has become leukemia and the origin of the leukemic cells. Our knowledge of blood cells and their functions is increasing rapidly and we learn more daily about how cells grow, react, and do their prescribed tasks. This new knowledge also allows us to be more specific in diagnosis and will ultimately lead to treatment options that are based upon the likely response of the specific leukemic cell to the treatment substance.

Susan Leclair, Professor of Clinical Laboratory Science at University of Massachusetts, Dartmouth, describes it this way:

> *In the future, blood analysis will be done with increasing precision as we are able to go deeper into the structure of the cell. First we'll do a microscopic evaluation, as we do now, and we'll identify the cells that are abnormal and describe their differences, just as if we were taking someone's family name (i.e., Lambet) and describing that person as part of the family of Lambets.*
>
> *Then using flow cytometry, we'll further identify you by your first name but still as a member of the Lambet family. So we'll be able to describe you by the antibodies that appear on your lymphocytes and whether the cells all come from the same original cell or from different ones.*

Then as more sophisticated, additional testing is done, we'll be able to distinguish where the change originated and figure out when and why it happened, just as a genealogist can trace back many generations to find specific incidents in the family history.

Cytogenetics and karyotyping

Cytogenetic testing is one of several types of evaluations done on patients' blood samples. Genetics is the study of heredity. Cytogenetics is the branch of genetics concerned with those parts of the cell involved in heredity—the chromosomes. Each chromosome contains tightly packed strands of deoxyribonucleic acid (DNA), one set from the mother and one from the father. There are 46 rod-shaped chromosomes in normal cells, 22 pairs numbered from 1 to 22, and two sex-determining chromosomes—two X's for females, an X and one Y for males.

The cytogeneticist looks for chromosome abnormalities. Since 1977, attempts have been made to discover consistent chromosome anomalies in leukemias. It is now well established that specific chromosome abnormalities show such a close association with particular subtypes of leukemia that they clearly have diagnostic and prognostic significance. Cytogenetic information also helps in determining treatment protocols for leukemia patients.

The individual chromosomes are separated, identified, and laid out in a specific arrangement on paper. This is called a karyotype. Then the chromosomes are photographed. The karyotype is a reference tool for understanding chromosome abnormalities and transpositions.

Cytochemistry

In order to see cells from blood or bone marrow under the microscope, thin films or smears of the cells must be placed on glass slides. Then the cells must be stained with dyes that impart color to the structures of the cells.

The routine stains permit the distinction of the nucleus and its components from the rest of the cell (cytoplasm). The cytoplasm contains granules, which themselves contain chemicals, enzymes that can be specifically identified using special techniques.

The methods that are used, that employ specific staining reactions to identify these particular cellular constituents, comprise the field of cytochemistry.

Cytochemical reactions are particularly useful in distinguishing among the varying forms of acute leukemia.

Molecular analysis

Molecular genetic analysis is a sophisticated tool for analyzing cellular function, gene expression, and human disease. It looks at the precise relationship between observed disease traits and specific changes in the cell's DNA. A specific gene and an alteration in that gene can be related to a particular disease with certainty, not just by inference.

The technique of molecular analysis is usually geared toward finding specific changes in the genes that make up chromosomes called clonal rearrangements of the immunoglobulin gene in B-cell malignancies or of the T-cell receptor gene in T-cell malignancies. These rearrangements are too subtle to be detected by conventional cytogenetics.

Immunophenotyping

Immunophenotyping is the process of classifying cells based on structural and functional differences (the ways different types of cells are put together and what those types of cells do).

In the case of leukemia, immunophenotyping is complex testing done on white blood cells from a blood sample. Molecules on the surface of the white blood cells are examined for antigens—any protein that stimulates the body to produce antibodies. Molecules are identified by patterns in these antigens. The patterns are called clusters of differentiation (CD).

A little history will explain how these clusters of differentiation were discovered. In many laboratories scattered throughout the world, researchers identified antigens on the surface of white blood cells and antibodies. (Antibodies are proteins produced by the body to fight foreign substances, otherwise known as antigens.) Every so often, at international meetings, it became clear that antibodies identified and named in different labs were actually the same molecule. At that point, the antibodies would be assigned a CD number. Thus, the antibody (and by loose association, the molecule to which it binds) might be referred to by one of several laboratory names or by its CD number. For example, antibodies that recognize the identified characteristic B-cell molecule might be called alternatively L26, B1, Leu16, or CD20. The CD number (in this case, CD20) provides scientists in different labs a "common language" to describe antibodies.

The profile of the cell—the arrangements of groups or clusters of specific molecules on the cell surfaces—determines how the cell is classified. Diagnosis by immunophenotyping depends upon the number of cells expressing the specific markers that are normally present in small numbers. See Appendix E, *Genetic Classification of the Lymphocytic Leukemias*, for genetic descriptions of each of the leukemias.

Immunophenotyping is complex, and there are few black-and-white rules. According to the Department of Pathology, State University of New York at Stony Brook[1] here are the basic types of cells that immunophenotyping identifies:

- **Lymphoid cells.** Most are reactive for CD45 (leukocyte common antigen, or LCA).

- **B cells.** Almost all of these are reactive for CD19, CD20, and CD22. Certain low-grade B-cell lymphomas are reactive for two markers otherwise found only on T cells: CD5 and CD43. Acute lymphocytic leukemias are frequently CD10 (+) (CD10 markers are present), but is normally not true of CLL.

- **T cells.** Pan T-cell markers (present on almost all T cells) include CD2, CD3, CD5, and CD7 (the early childhood leukemia markers). Most mature T cells mark with CD4 (helper cells that help T cells fight infection), CD8 (suppressor cells that stop infection-fighting activity), or cytotoxic cells (cells that kill invading cells).

- **Natural-killer cells.** Natural-killer cells are specialized white blood cells that can kill tumor cells without having been previously exposed to the cell and without the tumor cell having antigens most other white cells require to attack. Natural-killer cells are frequently associated with CD16, CD56, or CD57. Leukemic cell-marker analysis lets researchers or pathologists establish where the leukemia cell originated and thus help identify the cell. B cells develop in the bone marrow. T cells develop in the thymus.

Immunophenotyping is especially useful for determining subtypes of B-cell leukemias that express surface immunoglobulins (and most of them do).

Acute leukemias

Diagnosis of acute leukemia has traditionally been done through identification of the predominant cell type in the bone marrow. Prior to the latter half of the twentieth century, there were only two acute leukemias known: myeloblastic and lymphoblastic. With the advent of newer techniques for cell study, differentiation among leukemias has become clearer. Immunophenotyping has led to the identification of biphenotypic (two or double involvement) leukemias. Biphenotypic leukemias are composed of malignant blasts of lymphocyte and myelocyte types. It is believed that many types of adult acute leukemia express markers from more than one type of leukemia. Presently, acute leukemias are described as myeloid, T-lymphoid, B-lymphoid, or biphenotypic. At this time, there is no staging system for biphenotypic leukemia.

Acute lymphocytic leukemia (ALL)

Acute lymphocytic leukemia is classified according to the number and type of lymphoblasts (immature lymphocytes) present in the blood sample. Size, shape of cell nucleus, and maturity are the criteria. About 25 to 33 percent of adults with ALL have the Philadelphia chromosome. This is explained further in the discussion of CML, later in this chapter.

Scientists from several countries of the world have agreed on the categories of ALL so that there is consistency in diagnosis. The French-American-British (FAB) classification of ALL recognizes three categories: L1, L2, and L3. The determinations are made based upon the size of the blast cells and certain features of the nucleus of the blast as it is viewed with the microscope. The pragmatic significance of the FAB classification of ALL in adults is not yet clear, but remissions appear to be more complete in patients of L1 type.

B-cell ALL accounts for 25 to 35 percent of adult ALL.

T-cell ALL accounts for 15 to 20 percent of adult ALL. This is a form of leukemia that is most often seen in Japan, Jamaica, Trinidad, and Tobago, but it appears in Europe and North America as well. T-cell ALL shows changes in the T-cell receptor gene (TCR) markers. T-cell ALL also expresses nuclear TdT (terminal deoxynucleotidyl transferase) in over 90 percent of cases.

The following list names the types of ALL and the CD markers that are most commonly associated with each. The presence or absence of these markers will appear on your pathology reports and help the doctor arrive at the most accurate diagnosis.

So, if your pathology report shows that your blood work has lots of CD1, CD3, CD5, and CD8 markers, you are more likely to have T-cell ALL. Each of these CD markers may be either present (+) or absent (−) and may be bright or dull in expression. The concern is not with individual test results, it is the pattern of positivity/negativity that is important.

B-cell markers include:

| CD10 | CD19 | CD20 | CD21 | CD22 | CD24 | Surface Ig |

T-cell markers include:

| CD1 | CD2 | CD3 | CD5 | CD7 | CD4/CD8 |

The bright or dim expressions reflect how much of the CD marker is present on the cell surface. Whether a patient responds to a given monoclonal antibody depends on how intensely the positivity is expressed rather than the percentage of cells that are positive. For example, a person whose blood work shows 70 percent of cells expressing CD20 with bright expression might respond much better to a monoclonal antibody than a person whose blood work shows 90 percent of cells expressing CD20 but very dimly. Unfortunately, most labs presently only measure the percentage of CD positive cells and not the number or intensity of CD molecules on the cell surface.

Anyone who desires a more complete explanation of the cell differentiation process should read a good medical hematology text. Suggestions may be found in Appendix A, *Resources*.

Acute myelogenous leukemia (AML)

Acute myelogenous leukemia is the most common of the acute adult leukemias. The blasts of AML are most often larger than lymphoblasts and have greater differences in size and shape. Chromosome abnormalities can be detected in most cases of AML. Each normal chromosome pair shows long and short arms. Abnormalities in both the long and short arms are seen, as well as translocations (a piece of one chromosome moves to another chromosome), inversions, and insertions of genetic material. A diagnosis of AML is called for when more than 30 percent of cells with visible nuclei in the bone marrow are blasts. Cell markers play a lesser role in AML and often diagnosis is associated with the absence of the lymphocytic markers.

The classification structure of this disease is complex, but has been agreed upon by an international group of scientists. The FAB classification of AML has eight categories:

- M0. AML with minimal differentiations on the cell surface. CD13, CD14, or CD33 and CD34 antigens are expressed on the cell surface of at least 20 percent of the cells.

- M1. Acute myeloblastic leukemia without maturation. Large, poorly differentiated myeloblasts represent 90 percent or more of the blood cells, which aren't red blood cells. Predominantly granulocytic differentiation is seen.

- M2. Acute myeloblastic leukemia with maturation. This type is seen most often in young adults. Rod-shaped granules called Auer rods may be present in the myeloblasts. Predominantly granulocytic differentiation is seen.

- M3. Acute promyelocytic leukemia (APL). This disease affects young adults and the elderly. Bundles of Auer rods may be present in the myeloblasts. Predominantly granulocytic differentiation is seen. MC3v is a variant of this category in which very small granules (potent chemicals that kill other cells) are found.

- M4. Acute myelomonocytic leukemia (AMML). Less than 80 percent of the nonerythroid cells are of monocytic lineage (coming from the same monocyte). M4E or M4Eo are variants that involve the eosinophils.

- M5. Acute monocytic leukemia showing more than 80 percent of nonerythroid cells to be of monocytic lineage. This category has two variants, M5A and M5B.

- M6. Erythroleukemia where more than 50 percent of nucleated cells are erythroblasts and 30 percent or more of the nonerythroid cells are monoblasts.

- M7. Acute megakaryocytic leukemia. The blasts are identifiable as megakaryoblasts (platelet precursors).

Malignant cells in almost all AML cases express CD13, and/or CD33. CD34 is usually expressed in cases with less-differentiated morphology.

A patient with AML learned more particulars of his diagnosis over time as the results of more sophisticated blood work became available. The particulars included a chromosome pattern that showed a better prognosis for his disease.

AML has a number of different subtypes. Sometime during that first week, my doctor told us that the bone marrow biopsy had shown myelomonocytic (M4) leukemia, and that I had an inversion in chromosome 16. I would later learn from him and other sources that the prognosis for AML with an inversion in chromosome 16 is better than most cases of AML.

Chronic leukemias

Chronic leukemias include a broad spectrum of disorders, which makes it hard to define them and determine a diagnosis. These leukemias are diseases in which too many mature white cells are produced and build up in the body. At first these cells function as they should, but over time they stop performing their necessary tasks and simply reproduce without dying as they should.

There are no staging systems for prolymphocytic leukemia, splenic lymphoma with villous lymphocytes, or any of the preleukemias.

A reminder about cell counts: all cell counts are done based on a specific volume of whole blood. The smallest volume—the microliter—gives a count in the thousands (for example 4,000). In the scientific notation used in the United States, that is written $4.0 \times 10^3/L$ although verbally one still uses the "thousands" term. Many laboratories report counts using the internationally accepted scientific notation based on the liter. As a consequence, the report might read $4.0 \times 10^9/L$. Notice that the important number, the "4," remains the same and only the description at the end changes. This chapter refers to the numbers in thousands since that is the way most American physicians use them.

Chronic myelogenous leukemia (CML)

Chronic myelogenous leukemia is known also as chronic granulocytic leukemia. Characteristics include high platelet counts, usually over 400,000, and a high granulocyte count, of more than 30,000 cells, maturing in an orderly fashion. In fact, the marrow is usually packed with mature and maturing large granulocytes. Chromosome analysis of these cells shows the presence of the abnormal Philadelphia (Ph) chromosome, which is considered a diagnostic indicator of CML. The Philadelphia chromosome is an abnormal chromosome that results from an exchange of DNA material between the normal chromosomes 22 and 9. It is present in over 90 percent of CML cases. There is a small percentage of patients in whom the Ph chromosome is not present. This is described as Ph-negative CML.

Closer examination of the Philadelphia chromosome shows that it results from a translocation of the bottom part of chromosome 22 onto the bottom of chromosome 9 to create a hybrid gene called bcr/abl. The technical nomenclature is t(9;22)(q34;q11). More precisely, in chromosome 9, there is a gene called c-abl (named for its discoverer, Abelson). A break occurs beside this gene and it is translocated to a site on chromosome 22, called breakpoint cluster region (bcr). Next these two pieces of DNA fuse, creating fusion gene bcr/abl. This fusion gene is involved in the pathogenesis of CML. It also serves as a molecular marker of Ph-positive cells.

Sometimes the product of the translocation can be found. It is a protein called P210. This protein is also known as a tyrosine kinase, and some drug treatments are focusing on destroying this protein. Ph-negative CML patients almost always display the bcr/abl fusion gene. In fact, the bcr/abl fusion gene is present in 95 percent of CML patients.

Chronic lymphocytic leukemia (CLL)

Blood test results show high white counts in CLL patients. In asymptomatic patients, counts are usually below 50,000, but in symptomatic patients counts can be from 100,000 to 1,000,000. The circulating cells are small, mature lymphocytes.

A diagnosis of chronic lymphocytic leukemia requires an absolute lymphocyte count of greater than 5,000. More important is evidence that all the malignant B cells in the clone must have arisen from a single precursor cell. This is called monoclonality. It is critical to the diagnosis that there be monoclonality of lymphocytes with the characteristic CD markers and expression of only a single immunoglobulin light chain on the cell surface—either a kappa or lambda chain. Small monoclonal bands are noted in 5 to 10 percent of patients with B-CLL and the bands are usually immunoglobulin M. Chromosome abnormalities may be present. Deletions in 13q14, 11q23 and 6q21 are characteristic of CLL. Deletion 13q14-23 is the most common. In addition, trisomy 12 is found in about 30 to 50 percent of CLL patients. Trisomy is the term for three chromosomes present where there should be only two. Deletions or mutation of the P53 tumor suppressor gene can be seen. There is also a novel suppressor gene called DBM (disrupted in B-cell malignancy).

Overexpression of the bcl-2 gene is present in more than 70 percent of cases of CLL. A protein called bcl-2 usually is beneficial to cells. Manufactured by the gene bcl-2, it protects cells from a lifetime of insults, including infection and toxins. But some cancer cells have too much of the protein. They resist dying, so CLL cells are said to have a defect in apoptosis (normal, genetically programmed cell death.) The CLL defect in apoptosis allows the uncontrolled proliferation of more mature cells in this disease. In some cases, the cells resist chemotherapy drugs when too much bcl-2 is present.

Platelet counts, hemoglobin, and hematocrit are usually in the normal ranges until white counts become so high that the leukemic cells drive out the red cells and take over the marrow and the lymph nodes. Hemolytic anemia (red blood cell destruction) and decreased normal immunoglobulin production may also be present.

The absolute lymphocyte count (ALC) is a figure defined as the percent of lymphocytes in the blood sample multiplied by the total white blood count times 100. See Appendix B, Table B-3. The ALC is used in calculating lymphocyte doubling time—the rate of increase of the absolute lymphocyte count. Lymphocyte-doubling times of more than one year are considered an excellent prognostic indicator. Doubling times of less than twelve months are cause for concern.

The following list names the types of CLL and the CD markers that are most commonly associated with each. It is important to remember that each of these CD markers may be either present (+) or absent (−) and may be bright or dull in expression. The concern is not with individual test results, it is the pattern of positivity/negativity that is important. The presence or absence of these markers will appear on the pathology reports and help the doctor find the most accurate diagnosis.

B-CLL markers include:

CD5+	CD103−	CD19+	CD20+	FMC7+/−

CD10 (typically negative, but occasionally positive)   CD52+

CD22+	CD23+	CD25+	CD11c+/−

CLL is CD5+, as is mantle cell lymphoma, but all other B-cell neoplasms, such as hairy cell leukemia and follicular lymphoma, are CD5−. CD5 must be recognized as a T-cell marker that is appearing in a B-cell neoplasm. That is a real help in making a diagnosis. In addition, B-SLL (small lymphocytic lymphoma) is often practically identical to B-CLL and quite often the diagnosis comes back as B-CLL/SLL.

T-CLL markers include:

CD2	CD3	CD5	CD7

Criteria for diagnosis of CLL

Doctors come to a CLL diagnosis in different ways. Several different staging systems have been in use throughout the years. As we learn more about the cytogenetics of CLL, we can expect to see the staging systems evolve to include new genetic information. However, the following staging systems are in use at this time.

Staging systems

The stage of a disease is a statement of measurement of the extent to which the disease has spread in the body.

There are two staging systems for CLL in widespread use by practicing physicians at the time of this writing: the Rai Staging System and the Binet system. There is also a combined staging system, which uses both the Rai and Binet systems. The combined staging system is listed in parentheses next to the equivalent stages in the Binet system.

The first system, developed by Dr. Kanti Rai and his collaborators, is known as the *Rai Staging System*. Patients are staged according to the findings in the peripheral blood, marrow, and physical examination of body organs as follows:

- **Stage 0.** Absolute lymphocytosis (more than 15,000 lymphocytes per cubic millimeter of blood) is the only finding

- **Stage I.** Absolute lymphocytosis and enlarged lymph nodes (lymphadenopathy)

- **Stage II.** Absolute lymphocytosis and lymphadenopathy with either enlarged liver or spleen

- **Stage III.** Absolute lymphocytosis and anemia (hemoglobin less than 11. 0 g/dL,) with or without lymphadenopathy, enlarged liver, or spleen

- **Stage IV.** Absolute lymphocytosis and thrombocytopenia (platelets lower than 100,000 per cubic millimeter of blood), with or without symptoms of anemia, lymphadenopathy, enlarged liver or spleen

Another staging system used with CLL is the *Binet system*. This system is based on the number of involved areas and the level of hemoglobin and platelet count. The five areas of lymphoid involvement are head and neck, axillae (underarms), groin, palpable spleen, and palpable liver. The stages are as follows:

- **Stage A.** Hemoglobin greater than 10g/dL and platelets greater than 100×109 /L and fewer than three areas of lymphoid involvement (Rai stages 0, I, II)

- **Stage B.** Hemoglobin greater than 10g/dL and platelets greater than 100×109/L with involvement of more than three areas of lymphoid or nodal involvement. (Rai stages I and II)

- **Stage C.** Hemoglobin less than 10g/dL and/or platelets less than 100 ×109/L regardless of the number of areas of lymphoid enlargement (Rai stages III and IV)

It should be noted that both the Rai and Binet staging systems set the hemoglobin required for advanced stage disease much lower than the lower limit of the normal range. One reason why they chose that number is that most patients do not experience any signs or symptoms of anemia until the hemoglobin values get that low. The belief is that any fall in hemoglobin is an adverse prognostic factor.

Prognostic factors for CLL

Prognostic factors may be used in determining how aggressive a therapy might be tried or in choosing therapies to avoid because they are unlikely to be helpful. Positive prognostic factors include beta 2 microglobulin (B2M) scores of less than 2.5 percent of normal, absolute lymphocyte doubling time of one year or more, non-diffuse patterns of bone marrow involvement, the absence of translocations in chromosome 11 and 7, and low presence of soluble CD23.

CLL cells are known for their failure to achieve normal, orderly programmed cell death, or apoptosis. That is one reason there are so many CLL cells in a blood sample. Bax is a protein that appears to promote apoptosis. Bcl-2 is thought to be an apoptosis inhibitor. The balance of the combination of these two proteins may be most important in stimulating or inhibiting apoptosis. While no clear pattern has emerged, abnormal levels of bcl-2 are common in CLL and bcl-2 to bax ratios are also commonly disturbed. Bcl-1 levels are commonly increased in B-CLL as well. The presence of elevated bcl-2/bax on chromosomes appears to be a consistent feature of apoptosis resistance in B-cell CLL and may be correlated with chemoresistance. See the section on antisense therapy in Chapter 10, *Clinical Trials and Beyond* for more information.

The prognostic value of the presence of immunoglobulin type VH (IgVH) gene mutations and of CD38+ cells in CLL patients is being studied. Those with unmutated VH genes appear to display higher percentages of CD38(+) B-CLL cells than those with mutated VH genes, who appear to have lower percentages of CD38(+) cells. Patients in both the unmutated and the greater than 30 percent CD38(+) groups respond poorly to continuous multiregimen chemotherapy (including fludarabine) and have shorter survival. In contrast, the mutated and the less than 30 percent CD38(+) groups require minimal or no chemotherapy and have prolonged survival.[2]

CLL/mixed

Another type of CLL shows the same variety in cells, but the cells are intermediate in size. They are not prolymphocytes, but they do show increased notching or clefting in the cell's nucleus. This type is known as CLL/mixed.

CLL transformations

Several CLL transformations exist. In contrast to chronic myelogenous leukemia (CML) where transformation into the acute blastic phase is the rule, transformation of CLL into acute leukemia is rare. It is much more common for CLL to develop into a diffuse, large cell lymphoma, or into a more prolymphocytic cell population. In rare cases, patients develop multiple myeloma. Secondary myelodysplasia and AML in CLL patients is extremely uncommon.

Richter's transformation or Richter's syndrome

Richter's syndrome is the transformation of CLL to diffuse large cell lymphoma, which is one of the non-Hodgkin's lymphomas. It is a form of lymphoma that evolves from CLL through major changes in the same population of cells as CLL. In this case, it is considered a transformation. If the lymphoma arises from different cells, it can be regarded as a secondary cancer arising by chance.

Richter described the transformation of CLL cells into large granulocytic lymphoma in 1928. At that time the disease was known as reticulum cell sarcoma. About 3 to 10 percent of CLL cases may develop Richter's transformation.

Clinical features include systemic fever, weight loss, night sweats in more than half the cases, below normal lymphocyte counts, progressive development of enlarged lymph nodes, extranodal involvement of the cells, and the abnormal proliferation of lymphoid cells producing immunoglobulins (monoclonal gammopathy). (The gammopathies include multiple myeloma, macroglobulinemia, and Hodgkin's disease.) The strongest evidence that Richter's syndrome is derived from the CLL population is the immunoglobulin gene rearrangement pattern.

Patients at all stages of CLL are at risk for this transformation, and so are those in complete remission. There are no obvious causes for the transformation of CLL to Richter's syndrome. Some patients develop Richter's shortly after a CLL diagnosis. It makes no difference which, if any, treatments were given—alkylating agents or purine analogues. The median survival time for these patients is five months despite vigorous treatment for large granulocytic lymphoma. Patients who respond to lymphoma treatments have a prolonged survival.

Prolymphocytic leukemia (PLL)

CD markers for B-CLL are similar to B-cell prolymphocytic leukemia and for small lymphocytic lymphoma. B-PLL shows more cells called prolymphocytes and is CD5 negative, so it is easier to tell it from B-CLL. The FMC7 marker is also helpful in identifying prolymphocytes. When a patient with a history of CLL begins to show prolymphocytes his doctor will follow that closely. When the reports come back indicating that between 10 and 55 percent of the cells look like prolymphocytes, the diagnosis can be CLL/PL (CLL with prolymphocytes). When there are greater than 55 percent prolymphocytes in the sample this is known as the CLL/PLL transformation, because the CLL is transforming into prolymphocytic leukemia. If the patient is newly diagnosed with prolymphocytes of more than 55 percent, the diagnosis is simply prolymphocytic leukemia. Prolymphocytic leukemia has no staging system at this time

Hairy cell leukemia

Hairy cell leukemia is named for the filament-like (hairy) surface projections on the edges of the cells visible under the microscope. This is almost always a B-cell disorder, but rarely it will appear as a T-cell disorder. The cells are moderate in size with erratic oval nuclei and variable prominent nucleoli. Nucleoli are specialized structures within the nucleus of the cell. Most of the nucleus is composed of DNA while the nucleoli are composed of RNA so they stain differently. As a rule, nucleoli are not seen in mature cells so their presence and prominence is a characteristic of immature cells.

Common CD markers associated with hairy cell leukemia are:

CD5–	FMC7+	CD11c+	CD19+	
CD25+	CD23–	HC2+	B-ly-7+	CD103+

HCL is also classified by the high frequency of abnormalities in chromosome 5. HCL cells also show positive cytochemical staining for tartrate-resistant acid phosphatase (TRAP). Acid phosphatase is an active enzyme in the the cell and is not affected by tartrates (cream of tartar is one), so it can be detected with the microscope as a specific color in the cell cytoplasm when a special stain is used.

The peripheral blood shows anemia, a reduced number of leukocytes, and fewer than normal platelets. A depression of all the cellular components of the blood is present in 70 percent of HCL patients. Granulocyte and monocyte precursors are profoundly reduced. Bone marrow is difficult to aspirate successfully and in 5 percent of cases yields insufficient cellular material for evaluation. Immunoglobulins are usually normal but are elevated in 40 percent of the cases. Liver tests are usually normal. There is no staging system for hairy cell leukemia. It is described as untreated or progressive.

CHAPTER 6

Risks and Causes

It's only human to wonder what causes disease. After a diagnosis, you may ask, "How in the world could this have happened? What caused me to get leukemia?" Nobody knows. There are many theories and ideas about what causes leukemia, but no hard and fast answers.

In this chapter we look at what is known now. First we will look at 1973–1996 SEER Cancer Statistics Review statistics about who gets leukemia and briefly discuss the limitations of applying general statistics to your particular case. Although the principal causes of leukemia are still unknown, we look at a possible link with viral infections as well as a range of more speculative causes. Some people wonder if they have done anything to cause leukemia or if other family members are at risk, so we describe what is and isn't known about prevention.

Who is at risk for leukemia

In 1993 about 10 per 100,000 Americans were newly diagnosed with leukemia. It is heartening that incidence rates of all leukemias dropped by 5.3 percent from 1973 to 1993. This drop was seen across genders and ethnic groups. Similarly, mortality rates dropped 6.2 percent during the same period. More efficacious methods for diagnosis and a much wider variety of treatment options have made this possible. More understanding of possible causes and areas of concern also impacted the statistics.

Although percentages have dropped, as the population has grown, the number of people affected has risen slightly in the past few years. In 1999, an estimated 27,900 adults were diagnosed with leukemia. That's up from 23,100 in 1995. More common use of blood tests has made early detection of these diseases possible. To put the numbers in some perspective, in 1999 in the United States of America alone, about 1,221,800 new cases of all kinds of cancer were diagnosed. Yet graphs of new leukemia diagnoses have remained pretty flat for the last five to eight years.

Leukemia rates vary by ethnic background, gender, and age. Caucasians are diagnosed with leukemia more often than African Americans, Hispanics, and Asians. Men are diagnosed more frequently than women.

Leukemia diagnosis rates climb as people age. In America, 10.3 of 100,000 people, of all ages, were diagnosed with leukemia in the years 1992 through 1996. However, where about 5.8 per 100,000 people below the age of 65 were diagnosed, the rate jumped to 51.4 people per 100,000 aged 65 and older, as Figure 6-1 illustrates.

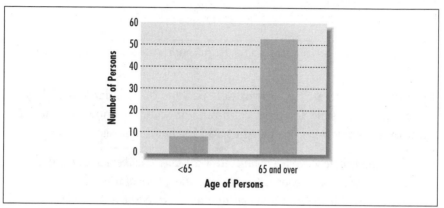

Figure 6-1. Incidence of Leukemia per 100,000 persons, as a function of age

Survival rates are rising. The one-year survival rate for patients with leukemia was 63 percent as of 1997. Survival drops to 43 percent at five years after diagnosis, primarily due to the poor survival of patients with some types of leukemia, such as the acute myelocytic form. Nevertheless, there has been a dramatic improvement in survival statistics for patients with acute adult lymphocytic leukemia—from a five-year survival rate of 4 percent for people diagnosed in the early 1960's, to 38 percent in the mid-1970s, to 55 percent in the late 1980s. Figure 6-2 shows the increase.

Causal information

Leukemia was first described only about 150 years ago. Since then there have been substantial advances in diagnosis, tracking of cases, classification, and treatment. Developmental, physical, environmental, and other factors that may cause leukemia are not yet known. It is most likely that the principal causes for leukemia have yet to be discovered. This is what the present literature is saying.

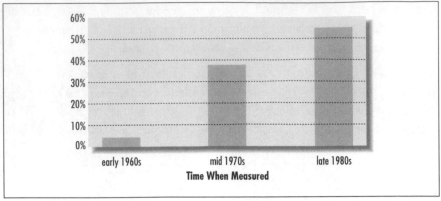

Figure 6-2. Five-year survival statistics for patients with acute adult lymphocytic leukemia (ALL)

Even though there are no clear causes, patients do wonder. Often they feel somehow responsible for their condition or want to know how to make sense of it. Here is what one patient said after her diagnosis:

> I immediately wanted to find out what caused leukemia. Could it have resulted from mononucleosis or radiation, both of which I had in college in 1949? It seemed very important to find a reason at the time....

Viral links to leukemia

Two viral diseases have been implicated in the development of leukemia. One is the Epstein-Barr virus (EBV); the other is the human T-cell lymphotropic virus (HTLV-1). While most people who get either of these viruses do not subsequently get leukemia, enough people do to indicate a link. There is also some evidence to implicate the human immunodeficiency virus (HIV) in causing leukemia.

The Epstein-Barr virus is a herpesvirus with a host range of B lymphocytes and nasopharyngeal cells. HTLV-1 is the virus that is closely associated with the T-cell lymphocytic leukemia found in Japan, Africa, and the Caribbean, as discussed in Chapter 5, *Subtype, Staging, and Prognosis*. Only a small fraction of those infected—no more than 4 percent—with this virus develop leukemia.

Both viruses leave residual traces in the cell markers. People who catch Epstein-Barr early in life are thought to be at increased risk for B-cell lymphoid tumors. EBV-infected B lymphocytes have an increased proliferation rate, increasing the likelihood of genetic error during DNA replication. Altered lymphoid cells with specific chromosomal transformations give rise to leukemic clones. These translocations rearrange elements of immunoglobulin genes, resulting in B-cell ALL in children and adults. Epstein-Barr is also implicated in CLL, but not directly involved. The illness most commonly associated with EBV is infectious mononucleosis.

Patients generally seek causative information when they are initially diagnosed. Since the cause isn't yet clear, patients might come across new bits of causative information during treatment and as research evolves.

The following patient reconstructs a conversation she had with her doctor, during which she gleaned causative information without ever asking for it:

> When I was diagnosed with CLL ten years or so ago, my doctor said to me, "Well you know, you test positive for having had the Epstein-Barr virus."
>
> "That's interesting," I replied. "What is Epstein-Barr and what does that have to do with lymphocytic leukemia?"
>
> He answered, "It's a B-lymphocyte herpesvirus that starts out like a respiratory infection. But once you've had it, the traces stick around for life. You probably got it when you were a very young child."
>
> Then he went on to tell me that it is associated with leukemia, lymphoma, and chronic fatigue syndrome, and that most of his leukemia and lymphoma patients showed traces of it in their blood work
>
> I'm a 50-year-old mother of three, and here we are discussing a childhood disease that I probably had before I was ten. I was supposed to believe this was a cause of my leukemia at this time?
>
> The doctor was very careful to explain that the Epstein-Barr virus is an indicator that is found in many patients. He made no claim that it was a cause of the disease. By the time he was finished talking, however, I was anxious to research other possible causes of the disease.

Speculative causes of leukemia

Certain genetic disorders predispose individuals to leukemia. Certain viruses are closely linked to leukemia. However, most of the other risk factors for leukemia are poorly understood. There is much discussion of ionizing radiation and occupational and environmental chemical exposures, some known and some just thought to be responsible for development of leukemia. The following sections list some risk factors speculated to increase one's chances of having leukemia. Most possible causes are currently under study.

Ionizing radiation

Radiation is the best known and most studied risk for leukemia. Studies have been done of people exposed to radiation in war, on the job, or as part of medical treatment. CLL is one leukemia that has not been linked with radiation exposure. The other three major leukemias were found during studies of ionizing radiation in survivors of the atomic bombing in Japan. Survivors developed leukemia at a minimum of two years after exposure, and at an average period of ten years after exposure. People receiving high doses of radiotherapy for solid tumors are at relative risk for leukemias as well. Further, the risk of subsequent leukemia is also increased for patients receiving radioactive iodine for thyroid cancer or radioactive phosphorus for polycythemia vera.

Nonionizing radiation

Nonionizing radiation, in the form of extremely low frequency electromagnetic field exposure induced by electricity has been suggested as a possible risk factor for leukemia. This suggested cause has been linked to adult ALL for those working in occupations where they have steady exposure. Power linemen, utilities workers, electronics workers, and other such workers are most often mentioned as possibly at risk. There have been studies showing an increased risk for these occupations, although results are not clear-cut. However, for electromagnetic exposure in the home, all but one study of the hazards to adults has been negative.

Occupational exposure to benzene

Exposures to certain known chemicals and certain occupations have been linked to increased risk for leukemia.

Various implications have been made about leukemias resulting from occupational or environmental exposure to benzene. Relative risks have been reported to be as low as 1.9 or as high as 10.0 among workers exposed to benzene. This means that, depending on the study, people exposed to benzene were from two to ten times as likely to be diagnosed with leukemia as were people who were not exposed to benzene. Categories of occupations at risk include petroleum manufacturing, chemical manufacturing, rubber manufacturing, shoe manufacturing, printing, and painting. AML is most strongly linked to benzene exposure, but CML may also be linked to benzene exposure. There also is a link with CLL. It must be noted that the industrial use of benzene has been outlawed in the US since the end of World War II. However, it is still used in some developing countries.

Other chemicals have also been linked to leukemia. Fewer studies have been done, but exposure to styrene and butadiene correlates to higher rates of lymphoma and CLL. Hairdressers, garage and transport workers, rubber workers, sawmill and wood products workers have all been exposed to some form of chemical that may be perceived as a leukemia risk factor.

Studies looking for an increased risk of leukemia in farmers have been suggestive but inconclusive. Some studies of farmers and farm workers have revealed elevated leukemia risks from 10 to 40 percent. Still, others have shown no increase in risk for agricultural workers at all. Among farmers in those studies where the results were positive for raised rates of leukemia, almost all types of leukemia increased. Exposure to pesticides, herbicides, fertilizers, diesel fuel and exhaust, and infectious agents associated with livestock have all been listed as possible risk factors.

The bovine leukemia virus produces transformed B lymphocytes in cows, so farm workers and veterinarians may be at some risk for this virus. Feline leukemia virus disease, when present in cats, has no relationship with human disease.

Antineoplastic agents

Antineoplastic agents are substances that prevent the development, growth, or proliferation of malignant cells. Many chemotherapy agents are antineoplastic agents.

Some people have been exposed to chemotherapeutic agents destructive to bone marrow cells, primarily alkylating agents such as Leukeran (chlorambucil) and Cytoxan (cyclophosphamide). Some people are given these agents to combat other malignant and nonmalignant disorders, such as rheumatoid arthritis and other autoimmune diseases. These agents increase the relative risk of subsequent leukemia. Increased AML has been consistently reported among patients treated with alkylating agents for many solid tumors and blood and lymphoproliferative malignancies. The terms used here are more fully described in Chapter 7, *Treatment Options*.

Lifestyle risk factors

Lifestyle risk factors, shown to be important for many patients with solid tumors, have received little attention or appear to play a very small part in the development of leukemia. Several studies of the possible effects of diet or alcohol consumption on leukemia risk have shown nothing definitive.

Cigarette smoking is linked to leukemia. Cigarette smoking has been recognized as a potential cause of leukemia only since 1986. Since then, more than twenty studies have been analyzed or re-examined to look into this assumption. A few studies have shown increased risk for lymphoid leukemia among cigarette smokers, but most show a relationship to myeloid types. Indeed, recent evaluations of these studies indicate the risk is greater for myeloid leukemias, perhaps raising risk by as much as 15 to 22 percent. Nevertheless, total leukemia incidence has not risen over time, while the use of cigarettes and exposure to cigarette smoke has climbed steadily. Lung and other smoking-related cancers have rising incidence rates that can be directly attributed to smoking. Therefore, leukemia risk attributed to cigarettes might have been overestimated.

Immune suppression

Immune suppression can lead to leukemia or lymphoma transformations. Bone marrow transplant, chemotherapy, and radiation attempts may control leukemia but may also cause immune suppression, which can also lead to transformations. This will be discussed more thoroughly in Chapter 7. Renal transplantation and heart transplantation are associated with immunosuppressive drugs implicated in secondary leukemias.

Familial predisposition

Inevitably, patients will ask if there is a familial predisposition to leukemia, both because they want to understand the cause of their own disease and because they are concerned about risk to other family members. Many times the answer from medical researchers and professionals is, "We still don't really know." As more molecular analysis is performed and researchers have more of a database of results, relationships between heredity and leukemia will become clearer.

The types of leukemia constitute a highly heterogeneous group of disorders in which inherited characteristics may occur in a low percentage in the general population. However, the inherited characteristics can be quite high in individual families. It is likely that as we learn to do more molecular analysis, we will learn more about heredity and leukemia. This is different from genetics, since in this instance, genetics looks at the genetic make-up of the malignant cells.

Of all the major hematological malignancies, CLL shows the highest family influence, suggesting a genetic component to the cause of the disease. By definition, familial CLL occurs when the disease is present in parents or siblings. There have been reports of CLL striking two siblings in one generation as well as reports of CLL in the same family in two generations. Reports of CLL in three succeeding generations are rare. The clinical path that the disease takes in such familial situations is extremely variable. There is also the likelihood that CML, hairy cell leukemia, ALL, or NHL may be found in families with CLL. Active research into the question of inheritability is ongoing in the US and Great Britain.

It is increasingly evident that familial leukemia can be associated with inherited chromosome instability. People with CLL or hairy cell leukemia, and some people with AML M6 seem to have a greater predilection for familial leukemias.

Age

Some researchers believe that the greatly increased incidence rates for leukemia in people over age 65 may be related to a general weakening of the immune system that comes with age. Research to come to some definitive conclusions about this needs to be done. Other researchers feel that the increased incidence rates in older individuals may be the result of the society in which we live and that genetic damage from substances in an industrialized society accumulate over time, becoming more powerful as we get older and are less able to deal with them.

Prevention and reducing risk

The question, "What should I have done to prevent this?" has no answer. Many people also ask what they can do immediately following diagnosis to help make a difference in the outcome of treatment and to prevent recurrence after remission.

There are some general recommendations for taking care of yourself to which you can pay attention. For example, if you smoke, it's logical to stop. If exposure to toxic chemicals is part of your daily life, see what kinds of changes can be made. If you are operating under considerable job-related or family-related stress, make efforts to reduce daily strains. Eating right and getting exercise are strongly recommended for everyone's good health. It's especially important for those who have been diagnosed with cancer. Patients often report a lack of appetite and weight loss associated with leukemia symptoms.

However, you have no control over some factors that might have placed you at risk. You can't change your genetic make-up. You can't change your ancestors and the chromosomal patterns that you have. You can't change the social structure into which you were born. Also, it isn't practical to avoid exposure to everything that is considered a possible risk for leukemia. Life isn't fair, and developing a malignant disease is one of the most unfair things that can happen to anyone.

Diet

Many people receive a leukemia diagnosis and immediately want to make dietary changes in an attempt to slow the progress of the disease. Some blame themselves for eating incorrectly in the past. Current nutritional theory strongly recommends a diet high in fruits and vegetables, whole grains and cereals. It suggests you eat meats and dairy products only moderately and that you cut way back on sugars, fats, alcohol, and salt. However, healthy eating neither causes nor changes the progression of leukemia.

Some individuals change their whole eating pattern upon finding out they have cancer. For example, they change to a macrobiotic diet, eating only vegetables and eschewing meat. Since a cancer patient in treatment often needs supplemental protein and iron, that may not be the best choice. Some patients feel that a few cups of green tea daily may prove beneficial.

Some believe a low-fat diet and/or cutting down on sugar may be effective. It is wise to talk with a trained dietician when treatment time approaches.

Nutritional recommendations for leukemia patients may be different than general nutritional theory because the recommendations are designed to build your strength and help you withstand the effects of treatment. Some patients are anemic and really benefit from increased red meat or high protein intake in their diets. Some have diarrhea or mouth sores and should avoid foods containing high fiber, which aggravate those symptoms.

If you have leukemia and are undergoing treatment or are simply not feeling well, it is often difficult to get enough nutrients to remain well nourished. A healthy eating pattern is important so that your body works as well as it can. If you go into treatment eating a healthy diet, you'll have reserves to help keep up your strength, prevent body tissue from breaking down, to rebuild tissue, and maintain defense against infection. Eating well helps you cope with side effects of treatment, and in some cases treatment is actually more effective if the patient is well nourished and eating sufficient calories and protein. Small, frequent meals can help when you have poor appetite. Changes in taste and smell during treatment will also impact food choices.

Talk to medical professionals if you are having difficulty eating or getting enough calories. Ask about balanced nutrition. Nutrition is an important part of your treatment.

Be sure to check with your doctor before you eat grapefruit or drink grapefruit juice when you are under treatment. A 1997 study at the University of Michigan discovered that chemicals called furanocoumarins, which are unique to grapefruit, could be potentially harmful if taken with certain drugs such as blood pressure medicines and antihistamines.[1] (Furanocoumarins can boost the potency of some such drugs.) Similarly, a more recent study at University of California, San Francisco shows that grapefruit juice can inhibit absorption of drugs that treat cancer, heart failure, allergies, and high blood pressure. Researchers explained that grapefruit juice releases a compound at the cellular level that can expel medications from the body before they reach the bloodstream.[2]

Vitamin therapy and complementary medicine

For years the popular press, supplement manufacturers, and certain health enthusiasts have claimed that it is wise to take vitamins and melatonin for cancer. Research casts serious doubt on this premise and indicates that taking supplements might even help the cancer.

New research has come out that says large doses of vitamins C, E, and A may help cancerous cells resist chemotherapy and radiotherapy.[3, 4] They block the natural housecleaning process known as apoptosis, programmed cell death. It is also believed that leukemic cells have nutritional needs that are fulfilled by vitamins C, E, and A. While the studies, done at Memorial Sloan-Kettering Cancer Center and published in the September 15, 1999, issue of *Cancer Research*, applied to mice—and the findings may not apply to humans—there is further evidence that antioxidant vitamins may not be all-purpose cancer slayers.

Doctors recommend that cancer patients avoid massive doses of these vitamins during active cancer treatment. Echinacea, another herbal supplement sometimes highly touted for affecting cancer, has been found by various studies to have some immunoenhancing qualities, but it has not been studied for leukemia patients.[5] Transplant patients are usually asked to stop using vitamin supplements during treatment because they could interfere with immunosuppressive drugs. Studies have produced conflicting research about this as well.

Exactly which vitamins are helpful and which are hurtful (and in what magnitude) is still unknown. For now, getting those vitamins in their natural state through food is the official recommendation of the American Association of Clinical Oncology.

For helpful information, contact the National Institutes of Health, The National Center for Complementary and Alternative Medicine, at (888) 644-6226, or visit *http://nccam.nih.gov*.

Physical activity

Physical indolence appears to be another possible risk for leukemia. Therefore, health and fitness are not simply for somebody else; they must be a part of your life.

Just as important as proper diet, keeping active and exercising can be most beneficial. If you are used to a high level of exercise but now fight fatigue, it is smart to cut back, but not eliminate, your daily exercise routine. More and more studies are showing that exercise is beneficial in overcoming fatigue and encouraging the body to heal itself. If you have been sedentary, now is a good time to add moderate activity to your weekly routine to build strength that will help get you through treatment. Proper professional help is recommended so that you don't try to do too much, too soon.

Keeping active is not only good for body strength. It is known to assist in maintaining good mental health as well. If you are active and feel well, your emotional responses are normal and focused. Mind-body exercise programs such as yoga and tai chi are helpful in managing stress. Mind-body exercises couple muscular activity with internally directed focus. The participant enters a temporary self-contemplative mental state, resulting in a feeling of well-being, free of stress.

CHAPTER 7

Treatment Options

After you are diagnosed, there will come a point at which you will need treatment. If the leukemia is acute, you need treatment immediately. For other types of leukemia, treatment may not be necessary for months or years.

This chapter gives you an overview of the standard treatment options for leukemia. We will include the theories behind treatment possibilities that are current at time of publication, including chemotherapy, biological treatments, radiation therapy, and bone marrow transplantation. We will explain what you can expect from chemotherapy and biological therapies—the two major treatment modalities.

This chapter is intended only as a starting point for discovering more about the treatments that your doctor may recommend for you. No book can dictate what treatment is best for you. That is something that should be determined by you and your family, after discussions with your own medical professionals. The standard treatment options described here are used in the US, Canada, Australia, and the United Kingdom. Since research is ongoing, there will be new treatments available by the time you are reading this book.

The range of treatment theories

There is a wide range of possible treatment options. Specific treatment depends upon the kind of leukemia, the possible subtype that has been diagnosed, the nature of the cell patterns shown by the blood evaluations, and the signs and symptoms the patient is experiencing. Treatment recommendations are based upon the age and health of the patient, willingness to undergo certain treatment options, and the spectrum of treatment choices currently available.

The doctor will suggest therapy options but, as the patient, you make the final decision. You should clearly understand your options and the reasoning behind your doctor's recommendations. At times you may wish to broaden your options. For example, the doctor might recommend a standard chemotherapy regimen as a curative measure. You'll want to know its "track record" for curing the type of leukemia you have and what other considerations, such as side effects, the doctor is taking into account. If the doctor is recommending a therapy that is intended to bring about a temporary remission, rather than being curative, you'll want to know that, as well as how long the expected remission might be and how the therapy will impact your life. You may want to try another therapy, look into new treatments in clinical trials, forego the therapy, or use the recommended therapy only so long as it is working for you and not significantly affecting your quality of life.

Standard therapies

Standard therapies include chemotherapy, biological therapies, surgery, radiotherapy, and combinations of those treatment methods. Many cancer treatments today are based on what has been learned about chromosome abnormalities and cell markers. Treatments take advantage of the vulnerability of cancer cells, which replicate rapidly. The following list describes common treatments:

- **Chemotherapy.** This is still the first treatment option of choice for most leukemias. Chemotherapy works against leukemia by using chemicals to interfere with the leukemic cell's ability to sustain itself and reproduce. Various kinds of chemotherapy regimens are used to stop the uncontrolled cell reproduction.

- **Biological therapies.** Biological therapies are man-made copies of biological proteins found in the body, that function as protection in immune responses. These therapies work in a variety of ways. In general they involve man-made copies of natural body substances that enhance the action of the natural substances themselves. Other biological therapies are biological response modifiers that change the way the cell responds. Interferons, interleukins, and tumor necrosis factors are examples of biological therapies. They are taken by injection with varying side effects. An oral interferon was tested in clinical trials but has not been approved at this time.

- **Surgery.** Surgery is sometimes used to remove large, painful nodes, or to remove an organ, such as the spleen, that is causing severely decreased platelets in the bone marrow and blood stream. Surgery is seldom used in leukemia therapy unless the patient is having the spleen or nodes removed.

- **Radiotherapy.** This is another way to kill off leukemia cells and slow disease progression. It is usually used to shrink painful, enlarged nodes and to kill off the patient's own bone marrow during a bone marrow transplant.

- **Radiation and chemotherapy.** These two therapies are combined in some standard treatments, and they may also be used as part of the cell killing procedures in transplantation. Chemotherapy may come before or after radiation or be used independently, and can be used as individual substances or in combinations. There are also times when radiation is used as a single resource to shrink or eliminate bulky tumors or enlarged organs.

- **Transplantation.** Bone marrow, peripheral blood stem cell, and cord blood transplantation are often used successfully in leukemia therapy. Transplants are discussed in greater detail in Chapter 9, *Transplantation*.

Chemotherapy

There are six categories of chemotherapy drugs used for leukemias: alkylating agents, antimetabolites, antitumor antibiotics, immune suppressants, topoisomerase inhibitors, and tubulin binding agents. These drugs fight cancer cells in different ways. Sometimes drugs are combined, either within or between categories. There are also rescue drugs used to offset the dangerous effects of chemotherapy. Each category of drug is described in the following sections.

Alkylating agents

Alkylating agents form new bonds within the twisted DNA strands. This disrupts the normal functions of DNA, especially its ability to divide. Alkylating agents are able to affect a cancer cell even when the DNA is not uncoiled and separated, which may explain their relatively high activity against many cancers. Examples of alkylating agents used against leukemias include busulfan, chlorambucil (Leukeran), cyclophosphamide (Cytoxan), ifosfamide, pipobroman, and nitrogen mustard (mechlorethamine).

Antimetabolites

Antimetabolites impede any cell's metabolism—its building up and breaking down of cell parts. Each of the antimetabolites used against leukemia acts in a different manner. The following list does not include all the antimetabolites used in leukemia therapy, but it does describe several that act differently:

- **L-asparaginase.** An enzyme that deprives the cell of the amino acid asparagine needed for protein synthesis.

- **Cytosine arabinoside (cytarabine, Ara-C).** A close copy of deoxycytidine, a natural body substance that lengthens a DNA strands as it is being copied. Ara-C substitutes in deoxycytidine's place so the DNA cannot reproduce.

- **Fludarabine, cladribine (2CdA), and pentostatin (2-deoxycoformycin).** Appear to interfere with certain enzymes that aid in copying, lengthening, or repairing DNA and RNA, although their exact mechanisms of action are still unknown. Fludarabine and 2CdA are purine analogues, a special kind of antimetabolite. Purine analogues are anticancer drugs that replace purines and/or pyrimidines, substances that are the building blocks of the DNA and RNA. The replacement forces the cell to go through programmed cell death (PCD or apoptosis). They do not appear to cause secondary malignancies.

- **Hydroxyurea.** Blocks ribonucleotide reductase, without which DNA synthesis is impaired.

- **Methotrexate.** A folate agonist. It blocks the action of an enzyme needed for the metabolism of folate. Folate (folic acid), a B vitamin found in many green vegetables, is needed to make the building blocks of DNA. Without these building blocks, new copies of DNA cannot be made.

- **Mercaptopurine.** Can be substituted in DNA in place of adenine, leading to a misreading of the DNA message. It also can be converted to a substance called a nucleotide that inhibits manufacture of the DNA building blocks called purines, needed for synthesis of DNA and RNA.

Antitumor antibiotics

Antibiotics constitute another important group of antileukemic drugs. These are antibiotic chemotherapy agents, as opposed to antibiotics that work against bacteria. When first introduced to the idea, most people believe that antibiotics cannot be chemotherapy. However the idea of using antibiotics makes sense when you think that the aim of antibiotics is to stop bacteria growth. In the case of cancer, they work to stop cancer cells growing.

Antitumor antibiotics owe their cytotoxic action to their interaction with DNA. These drugs are antineoplastic substances made from natural microorganisms. They insert themselves between chromosome base pairs. Some antitumor antibiotics interact with DNA by inhibiting topoisomerase enzymes that break and reseal DNA strands; others change cell membranes.

The anthracycline antibiotics daunorubicin and doxorubicin are widely used in the treatment of acute leukemia. Other antibiotic cytotoxic agents are bleomycin and mitomycin.

Immune suppressants

Immune suppressants such as dexamethasone (Decadron), prednisone, and methylprednisolone are man-made copies of the human corticosteroid hydrocortisone normally produced by the adrenal glands. They are used against hematological cancers to suppress the rampant growth of cancerous white blood cells. They also stimulate the erythroid cells (red cells) of bone marrow and lengthen the survival time of erythrocytes and platelets.

Topoisomerase inhibitors

Topoisomerase inhibitors are enzymes used by cells to break DNA bonds before replication and to repair breaks after. Topoisomerase inhibitors interfere with DNA repair, causing cancer cells to die. Cells die because damaged DNA cannot be translated into proteins that the cells needs to breathe or eat. Examples of topoisomerase inhibitors used against leukemias include: amsacrine, doxorubicin, daunorubicin, etoposide, idarubicin, and mitoxantrone (Novantrone).

Tubulin binding agents

When a cell has made a copy of all of its chromosomes and is ready to divide, spindles made of tubulin form to pull the two copies of each chromosome apart into two identical clusters of 46 chromosomes each. Tubulin binding agents stop spindles from forming, thus stopping the cell from dividing. Vincristine, vinblastine, vindestine, and paclitaxel are examples of tubulin binding agents.

Rescue drugs

Rescue drugs offset certain dangerous effects of chemotherapy. They include:

- **Leucovorin.** A form of folinic acid, one of the B vitamins. It is used several days after taking methotrexate to offset the toxicity of this folate antagonist and to allow the building of DNA to resume in healthy cells.

- **Allopurinol.** Used to protect the kidneys from toxicity associated with the purine analogues. Because purine analogues can bond securely with body tissues, they must be completely eliminated by the kidneys—allopurinol accomplishes that. Purine analogues have an elimination half-life of ten to twenty minutes. This drug may be given before treatment and at the time of chemotherapy as well.

- **Mesna.** Protects the bladder by offsetting the negative effects of cyclophosphamide metabolites, which are excreted in urine and can cause a severe form of hemorrhagic cystitis. It is given just prior to chemotherapy as an intravenous drip.

Biological therapies

Biological therapy (biotherapy) uses protein or cells that are involved in the body's natural defense mechanism. Biotherapy has developed as a result of scientists' understanding of the body's defense mechanisms and of recent developments in the genetic engineering of molecules. Rapid progress in biotherapy has resulted in the discovery of natural agents and genetically engineered variants of the natural agents. Attempts are being made to couple natural substances with toxins, drugs, and isotopes. The field of biotherapy is still in its infancy, but it has already produced biologic agents that have demonstrated antileukemic activity in animals and humans.

There are a number of biological therapies in use and they each work differently. Biotherapy for leukemia includes antibodies, cytokines, and such growth factors and cells as T-lymphocytes and natural killer cells.

Monoclonal antibodies (MoAbs or Mabs)

Monoclonal antibodies (MoAbs) are man-made copies of proteins—antibodies—that our white blood cells secrete. Because a particular cell surface protein, or antigen, attracts a particular antibody, natural antibodies are responsible for attaching to foreign substances in the body and for initiating attacks against invaders such as viruses and bacteria. Man-made copies can be used to boost the natural immune response to cancer.

When mass-produced in the laboratory, antibodies can be made all of one type (monoclonal) to target only a certain kind of invader. Cancer cells are different from normal cells in some ways, such as in the proteins that mark their surfaces. Therefore, man-made MoAbs can be created to aim only for cancer cells by sensing these surface proteins. MoAbs may be used alone ("naked") or may be coupled or conjugated with another substance called a payload. The payload is a toxic substance such as ricin or a radioactive substance (radioisotope) such as iodine-131 or yttrium-90. When the conjugated MoAb attaches to the cancer cell's surface protein, the proximity of the toxic substance damages or kills the cancer cell.

Naked monoclonal antibodies attach themselves to leukemia cells in the body, keeping them from reproducing, and ultimately killing them. Thus, naked MoAbs are used to purge quantities of blood cells that have been removed from the patient in order that non-leukemic cells can be returned to the patient with the comforting assurance that this marrow is cancer free. This process is used in an autologous bone marrow transplant—where the replacement cells come from the patient's own blood.

Each monoclonal antibody is a bit different from the next, because each cell surface protein to which it binds plays a slightly different role in the cell's life. For example, Rituxan (rituximab), a naked antibody, couples with cancer cell surface antigen CD20, causing the cell to die. Rituxan has also been shown to resensitize drug-resistant B-cell leukemia to chemotherapy.

Another advantage of MoAbs is their tendency to target a specific cell surface antigen and cause whatever attaches to it to be carried inside the cell. Scientists take advantage of this by having the antibody deliver selected cytotoxic molecules to leukemia cells. This type of procedure may ultimately assist in different kinds of genetic therapy as well.

Three more monoclonal antibodies currently in use to treat leukemias are the CD19+ MoAb called B43-Genistein; Campath-1H (tested in Europe as a mouse antibody, LDP-03) a humanized antibody that binds to the antigen CD52; and Bexxar (iodine I 131 tositumomab), which has been more effective in non-Hodgkin's lymphomas, but is being tried with leukemias as well. All three of these are presently in clinical trials.

The Food and Drug Administration (FDA) has just approved Mylotarg, a CD33 monoclonal antibody, for use with acute myelogenous leukemias. This MoAb looks extremely promising for those with AML at this time.

Cellular biotherapy

Cells with antitumor activity may be found in animals and humans. Both T cells and natural killer (NK) cells have been shown to have antileukemic activity. Cytokines, like interleukin-2 may activate both T-cells and NK cells to become lymphokine-activated killer cells (LAK).

Cytokines

Cytokines are substances that the body uses to trigger other immunologic events. As such, Cytokines can be used to fight leukemia. Examples are:

- **Interferons.** Inteferon-alfa-2B, the interferon most often used in leukemia therapy, halts proliferative growth, forces cells to maturity, and interrupts cell motility. It stabilizes some leukemias and keeps them from progressing.

- **Interleukins (IL).** There are several interleukins. The one best studied for use against cancer is interleukin-2 (IL-2). Interleukin-2 stimulates development and maturation of white blood cells (lymphocytes) and can direct lymphocytes to attack tumors.

- **Tumor necrosis factor (TNF).** This is a biologic protein mediator, or cytokine, that helps regulate the immune response and some hematopoietic functions. It appears to have a role in killing both healthy and cancerous cells when the body feels it is being invaded and needs protection. TNF appears to induce both apoptosis (programmed cell death) and growth stimulation for those with myeloid leukemia cells, depending upon which action appears to be needed.

Several hematopoietic cytokines are being evaluated for their enhancing effects on marrow recovery after chemotherapy or after transplant. This would definitely have an effect in reduction of morbidity, mortality, and hospitalization costs.

Colony stimulating factors

Colony stimulating factors are substances that stimulate and encourage the growth of new cells. For those undergoing leukemia therapy, they can be used to help grow new white blood cells or platelets. All are injected under the skin (subcutaneously).

- **Granulocyte colony stimulating factor (G-CSF).** A man-made copy of a protein that causes bone marrow to grow new white blood cells (neutrophils). Neupogen is the trade name. It is also known as filgrastim, the generic name for G-CSF.

- **Granulocyte-macrophage colony stimulating factor (GM-CSF).** Like G-CSF, this is a man-made copy of a protein that causes bone marrow to grow new white blood cells, called neutrophils, and new monocytes. It is known generically as sargramostim and its trade name is Leukine.

- **Erythropoietin (EPO).** Like the previously listed colony stimulating factors, this is a man-made copy of a substance made by the kidneys, and in lesser quantities, by the other organs like the liver and adrenal glands. EPO causes bone marrow to produce new red blood cells. It is also known as epoietin alfa, and its trade names are Epogen and Procrit.

- **Thrombopoietin (TPO).** Like the others listed, this is a man-made copy of a body protein that causes bone marrow to grow new platelets. It was also known as pegylated megakaryocyte growth and development factor. Neumega (Oprelvekin) is another platelet growth factor.

Choosing the best treatment option

Making a choice of treatment is usually very difficult, especially if there are several possibilities that are considered standard therapy. Many patients are faced with several types of treatment that offer varying ability to control the leukemic cells. Even if the doctor has given as much information as possible, there are choices the patient must make and things that must be considered.

Gains to be expected

When looking at any treatment option the patient needs to know what gains are to be expected as a result of treatment. Is the treatment to control cell proliferation? Is it curative in intent? Is it meant to get the patient into a remission and moving toward further treatment? Is it to lower counts or prevent complications until a particular clinical trial reopens? Is it to shrink a particularly painful node that is enlarged? Is it to extend life? Each of these is a goal of treatment and you need to have firmly in mind what outcome you expect from therapy. In some cases treatments will be chosen with an end in view—for instance, ensuring that a treatment option used first will not hinder the patient from having a bone marrow transplant later.

In order to clarify treatment options and goals, the patient should ask the following of the doctor:

- Considering the type and extent of leukemia I have, as well as my age, lifestyle, physical condition, and other factors, what treatment options are available to me?
- Looking at all the options, which would you recommend and why?
- What is the treatment supposed to do?
- What are the short-term and long-term risks?
- How can we tell if it is working?
- How long after treatment will you know if it is working?
- Will the blood work show improvement?
- Will enlarged nodes shrink?
- Are there other gains that should occur within the bone marrow?
- Will flow cytometry be used to determine improvement?
- If not, how long after treatment will a bone marrow biopsy be needed?
- If this treatment is given, what will my quality of life be like during and after treatment?
- Are there viable alternatives to this treatment?

Side effects to anticipate

Most cancer treatments have side effects, as discussed in Chapter 12, *Side Effects of Treatment*. Some are more difficult to live with than others. Some are permanent, and some just temporary. Some are life-threatening and some are simply annoying. In any event, they affect the patient's quality of life and ability to function in family and work situations. Therefore, questions that need to be considered are:

- What are the side effects that you have seen in patients using this treatment option?

- Are side effects known to be temporary, long-term, and/or delayed?

- What symptoms or side effects should I watch for and report to you during treatment (fever, muscle aches, nausea)?

- Will it be helpful for me to take specific medication before treatment to mitigate side effects? How about after treatment?

- Is there another technique that can successfully prevent or minimize temporary side effects of this treatment? Will meditation, visualization, prayer, or self-hypnosis be helpful?

- Shall I change my diet or drinking habits during this treatment?

- How will this treatment option affect my other medical problems (heart disease, arthritis, high blood pressure) or the medications I am taking for them?

- What are possible complications that could result during the treatment?

- How will I recognize them and what shall I do about them?

- How will treatment affect my ability to work or take care of my family responsibilities?

- Will the treatment affect me emotionally or sexually?

- Will the results of treatment affect my ability to have children? If so, how? What recommendations do you have for me before treatment begins?

Sexuality and fertility

Unfortunately, the treatments for leukemia in use today may affect male and female sexual functioning, fertility, and libido. For some of us, sexuality takes a back seat during the diagnosis and treatment phases of the cancer experience. For others these are very emotional issues—almost as emotionally charged as the cancer itself.

Psychological distress related to sexuality, after treatment for leukemia, has been documented. Often, sexual problems relate to fatigue and discomfort and other stress related concerns. Physical problems include inability to have and maintain an erection, or inability to ejaculate for males, and vaginal pain and/or dryness for women. In cases of physical problems, there are usually medical solutions, but since much of sexuality lies in the libido, some survivors find that they need counseling to help with the emotional issues. It is important for partners to communicate about sex, and to cuddle, touch, and be affectionate, even if you're not up to having sex as you once knew it. Many partners report that sexual pleasure does not require penetration with an erect penis. Sex can be very good after cancer, but it may not be exactly the same as it was before cancer.

Be sure to bring fertility issues to your oncologist's attention if you want to have children. Do not permit your doctor's assumptions about your age, family planning, or sexuality to place your fertility and sexual function at risk. If you are thinking of having children, even in the distant future, it makes sense to harvest sperm or ova before undergoing chemotherapy or radiotherapy. Even if you think you will never want children, it is wise to take the precaution of preparing for future fertility possibilities. A diagnosis of cancer can cause profound changes in outlook for most survivors, and your decision about whether or not to have children may well change as your cancer experience plays out.

Leukemia patients who later want to have children sometimes come in to family doctors, oncologists, or fertility specialists. However, if they have already had chemotherapy with no sperm or ova collected, it can be too late to address fertility concerns. Doctors and families become very frustrated when faced with this impasse.

For females, having been treated with chemotherapy for leukemia appears to present some risk for subsequent infertility. However, there have been reports of studies about women becoming pregnant after having chemotherapy. Another likely possibility for women having had chemotherapy is that they prematurely enter menopause. Alkylating agents, such as cyclophosphamide, have been shown to damage ovarian function, but less severely than they damage the testes in males. For males, chemotherapy with alkylating agents, like cyclophosphamide, may affect fertility permanently. However, some studies show a very slow return of male fertility over a span of years after chemotherapy. Radiotherapy is also known to cause loss of fertility.

If a woman becomes pregnant following chemotherapy there is the possibility of partial inability to carry a child to term. However, some studies show that after conception, it is likely that a woman will carry to term and give birth to a healthy child. In such cases, there appears to be no increase in cancer or other health related problems, or in cognitive problems, among children of leukemia survivors who were treated with chemotherapy.

This leukemia survivor talks about what she experienced preparing for treatment while she was still in childbearing years:

> I heard my doctor begin to talk about the aftereffects of therapy, and the words "You may be left infertile" screamed in my skull. I definitely want a child if there is any possibility that I will be in permanent or long-term remission.
>
> "How do I ensure that I may have the option to have a child," I asked the doctor.
>
> He answered, "Many of my patients go to have their eggs harvested and saved until they are ready to think about childbearing. That would be a good option for you."
>
> I was embarrassed just thinking about it, but I did talk about it with my husband that evening, and indeed, that is what we did. Knowing that I had ova stored was a very reassuring thing for me and I'm so glad I thought about it early enough to make that choice.

Pregnancy and leukemia

Nature's cruelest trick is to allow a pregnant woman to develop cancer. The mother-to-be is terrified for her unborn child and gravely concerned for her own health as well. Talk with your oncologist at once if you even suspect that you may be pregnant. Discuss how treatment options may affect the unborn child and what options are available to you. If the patient has a chronic form of leukemia, she may choose to defer treatment until after the child is delivered. An early, induced delivery may also be possible if the pregnancy is sufficiently advanced and the mother needs more immediate treatment. It might be wise to prepare for the possibility that some oncologists may well suggest terminating the pregnancy to save the mother's life. There is little information available about using chemotherapy or monoclonal antibody therapy for a pregnant woman because the largest numbers of cases of leukemia still are found in the over-60-year-old population, which is beyond childbearing years.

Emotional concerns

No two people go into the treatment situation with the same emotions and no two people respond to treatment in the same way, but we all feel fear, hope, and concern as this new phase of the cancer story plays out. Our family situations differ, and our support systems vary, but we all need to deal with our emotions as we undergo treatment.

As we encounter new situations in our cancer journey, we come face to face with our own mortality again and again. We identify with our diagnosis and tend to forget that much of our body functions normally while battling this disease. Really, our emotions, our inner resources, and our determination to control this dragon of ours comes to the fore during treatment. We are not our cancer! We are fighting for our eventual health and for our lives. We can't let others define how we feel or how we will react. This is the time when we reach bedrock, and we use everything within ourselves to meet cancer's challenge.

Starting and undergoing treatment makes you recognize that your life is in danger, that saving your life may require treatments that are more severe than the symptoms of your leukemia. You recognize that you have lost physical integrity, that you are facing rapid changes in your work and relationships, and that you face the possibility of a long period of rehabilitation. That is a huge pill to swallow at one time.

When you talk with long-time leukemia survivors, universally they say that they have made peace with the cancer and are now moving on to do whatever it takes to get on with life. Some call this "having a positive attitude," some call it giving their problems to the Lord, some just say, "OK, I'll do what I must, but I'm going to beat this thing." It doesn't matter how you do it or what you call it, what matters is that you feel that you are in control and you are moving in a positive way toward overcome the disease.

What to expect during treatment

Leukemia patients spend a great deal of time discussing treatment options and what is best for them. Many patients and their families are quite fearful of these treatments because they truly don't know what to expect and they have heard some real horror stories. In this section we will talk about what it is like to undergo chemotherapy, so you know what you may be facing in the days ahead.

Research indicates that some chemotherapy drugs work better when combined with others, or with a biological therapy. Treatment plans exist for many of these combinations. Responses are assessed based on accumulated data from many patients.

Some treatment plans, known as protocols, are standard for a disease and are given routinely with dosages based upon the patient's age, weight, and disease status. There is usually more than one possible treatment option for a given leukemia, and the doctor needs to determine which will be best for the patient. The reports about cell structure, morphology, and CD markings help the doctor to make staging and treatment decisions specifically for the patient.

Other therapies are new, perhaps being tried for the first time, or are being tried for a new disease after having been previously approved for a different disease. Doctors are continuing to learn how best to use the treatment. This process of learning how to use a drug, and what the best dosage will be for an individual, usually takes place by means of clinical trials. These are experimental treatment protocols that assess the safety, efficacy, and dosage of new treatments to see if they will work successfully against the disease for which they are being tested. Clinical trials will be discussed more fully in Chapter 10, *Clinical Trials and Beyond*.

The information provided in this chapter is not a substitute for your doctor's expertise. Always ask your doctor when any aspect of your treatment is unclear, or when you have questions about it. Report immediately to your doctor any adverse reactions that arise during or after treatment.

Treatment protocols

Treatment protocols are often used so that results from the chemotherapy that a doctor gives one patient can be compared with the same therapy given by another doctor to another patient. In this way, dosage and methods for administration of the therapy become consistent. Many treatments are given using protocols. Don't get upset, however, if no protocol is presented. You may receive standard treatment for your disease that is based upon many years of testing dosing and treatment schedules, so a protocol becomes largely unnecessary. There is complete information about protocols in Chapter 8, *Treatments for Individual Leukemias*.

After being informed as to procedure, what to expect, and risks involved, the patient will be asked to sign a paper indicating that this information has been shared. The patient has the right to request the official copy of the protocol that is being used by the doctor, in addition to the patient information copy. If you like to know everything that is going on, it is wise to have the copy of the full protocol in hand before you sign the informed consent form.

Preparation

Chemotherapy and biological therapies are administered in much the same manner. Some require a hospital stay, some are given in a treatment room at the doctor's office or the hospital, and some are taken orally or injected at home. It is not unusual for your doctor to ask you to come in to take the first treatment so that your reactions may be monitored, even if the drug you will be receiving is normally given on an outpatient basis or taken at home.

Patients respond differently to chemotherapy even when they are receiving the same drug in the same dosage. No one knows for certain how you will respond. The drug may make you sleepy, nauseated, or weak. It may affect your ability to drive or to concentrate, or it may have none of these effects.

You may be sitting in a treatment room that is too warm or too cold for several hours, so dress accordingly. Don't hesitate to ask for a warm blanket if you are chilly. Wear comfortable clothing with sleeves that can be rolled up and out of the way if you'll be getting therapy intravenously.

Treatment can take a half-hour or several hours. Bring along something to read or to do. Puzzles, books, knitting, needlework, and battery-operated laptop computers are all part of the scenery in a chemotherapy treatment center. Often, individual televisions are available, but ask before you assume they will be provided. Unless you have been told not to eat, make it a point to have something light in your stomach up to two hours before treatment.

Certain chemotherapy treatments cause you to react differently if you've been eating certain foods. Ask the oncology nurse or your doctor if there are certain foods, supplements, or vitamins that you should avoid during treatment. Be careful about grapefruit juice, which is known to enhance liver metabolic responses to several common chemotherapy drugs. It may make your body react almost as if the drug dosage has been increased. Smoked cheeses and smoked meats that contain tyramines have also been reported to change chemotherapy responses. Overdoing potassium supplements may trigger a metabolic imbalance in people with bulky disease, where there is lots of lymphatic tissue involvement. Make sure the medical team knows what you are eating and taking so that you don't inadvertently make things harder on yourself and on them.

Chemotherapy makes some people unusually sensitive to the sun so it might be wise to stay out of it or use heavy sun blocks if you must be out. Wide brimmed hats are sensible to wear as well. Chemotherapy drugs affect blood counts, which fall rapidly when you are responsive to treatment. About two weeks after treatment with many of these drugs, your counts reach their nadir (lowest level). At that time you may not have enough neutrophils to fight off infection; therefore, it is wise to avoid crowded places and people who are ill.

Do get to know the oncology nurses who will be working with you. They have lots of helpful information to share with you and they are some of the most caring people you'll ever meet. If they know you're concerned about something, they'll go out of their way to ease things for you.

It may be wise to have someone go to your initial chemotherapy treatment with you. You may want that person with you for moral support—beginning chemotherapy treatments are not as easy to cope with as they may seem at the start. You may be given verbal instructions about what and when to eat and information about aftercare of the site where a catheter may have been inserted. Questions about aftereffects of treatment undoubtedly will arise. Prescriptions for antinausea medicines, antidiarrhea medicines, or stool softeners may need to be filled. You may need to schedule appointments for subsequent treatments and to keep track of those dates. These demands on your attention all happen when you are not feeling very well. This is when it is wonderful to have a friend available: to get a glass of water or hard candy for you to suck on so your mouth won't be so dry, to make purchases at the pharmacy for you, to keep track of details and get them all recorded, and to drive you home after treatment.

Although the antinausea drugs used today are excellent, it is a good idea to have a bucket in the car just in case there are problems during the ride home. Ask the oncology nurse or your doctor, in advance, about preferred nausea medications. Have them on hand and take them as instructed. Ask for suppositories if oral medicine won't stay in your stomach. Don't try to be a superhero! Even though you may feel perfectly fine when you leave the doctor's office, the possibility of experiencing nausea later is real. Discuss antinausea medicine possibilities with your doctor before starting treatment.

Scheduling

The schedule for the administering of chemotherapy is based on years of research that determine a drug's effectiveness at a certain dose and interval. That information is found in the protocol. Some chemotherapies and biological therapies are given as daily outpatient care for a few days to a week, with a period of rest (no treatment) for several weeks in between. This pattern may be repeated for several courses until the entire series of treatments has been given. Some regimens require a hospital stay because the patient's reactions must be closely monitored or because several treatments must be done in a certain order. High-dose cytoxan, for example, is best given in the hospital because it is known to harm the bladder, and is best administered after mesna and heavy amounts of intravenous fluids.

Other treatments are given once a month for many months. Some are done as outpatient treatments using hospital facilities. In this instance, drugs are dripped into the vein overnight so that the patient can get a bit of sleep and be ready for work the next morning. If you find that you don't have major side effects from the chemotherapy and you wish to try this kind of set-up, speak with your doctor and the nursing staff to see how it can be arranged. Another way to handle working and chemotherapy is to schedule your treatments just before a weekend break so that you can take some time to recover and adjust before you must return to the stress of the workplace.

Here's an example of creative scheduling one person used to make a difficult situation practical:

> I was bound and determined that I wasn't going to miss any more work because of the treatment situation. Even though my employer had been very cooperative about the time I'd taken off, I knew it looked as if I wasn't trying very hard to work with him. I talked at length with the nurses in the treatment center, explaining my dilemma, and they arranged for me to come to the hospital Wednesday, Thursday, and Friday after work for outpatient intravenous treatment.
>
> For some reason I could handle treatment on Wednesday and Thursday evenings and still get to work the next day, but by Friday night I

would be zonked and I'd come home, fall into bed, and sleep away the entire weekend. My husband was a real dear and foraged for meals by himself, just pushing fluids at me whenever I surfaced. It sure kept the nausea at bay!

By Monday, or sometimes on Tuesday at bad times, I was ready to return to work as usual. That was a really effective way for me to handle things, and my boss really appreciated it also.

No two patients have the same schedule for therapy, even if they are on the same drug. You may be unable to tolerate the full dose and be on a dosage schedule that lets you get the same amount of the drug over a few more days or hours. You may be on a drug that is known to be toxic to the heart, but you may be on a less condensed schedule that is intended to lessen the potential heart problems.

The timing of subsequent therapy may be influenced by the blood counts that are seen in the weeks following therapy. Your treatment is monitored using blood counts scheduled to follow your progress and to ensure that you are able to go on with therapy. It is not unusual, if your counts are lower than anticipated, for the doctor to suggest that therapy be delayed for a week or even two.

One patient, whose treatment has been ongoing, describes what he has been through. Notice that he describes both the normal method of giving this chemotherapy drug and the changed treatment plan that has been individualized for him by his doctor:

I have been doing fludarabine most of this year, off and on, for my chronic lymphocytic leukemia. Off-times being due to infections or hospitalizations that have been interfering with my treatments!

This current session has been pretty free of side effects. I do weekly IV treatments (50 mg fludarabine). This is in contrast to the normal five days in a row, once a month protocol. I don't seem to do things "normally," so my oncologist decided at the beginning of this round of therapy to do this weekly treatment.

Administering therapies

Different chemotherapy or biological agents will require different methods of administration, some of which are discussed in this section.

IV infusion

In the most common scenario for IV infusion of chemotherapy, a needle is inserted in your arm, hand, or wrist vein to allow intravenous delivery of the drug or biological therapy. This is called using a peripheral IV. If you are scheduled to have more than one treatment during the day, the insertion may be more permanent than if you are only having one treatment. If you are allergic to tape, band aids, or other such supplies, it is important that you inform the person who is inserting the needle. Request that an antiallergenic dressing or paper tape be used to hold the needle in place during therapy.

Perhaps you will have a central venous catheter or a port inserted into a large vein in your chest to facilitate chemotherapy and to save you from constant needle sticks. Although cleaning the dressings can be annoying, most people really appreciate not feeling like a pincushion during therapy. Other chemotherapies are delivered by way of portable pumps that provide a constant infusion of the drug throughout the day. Some drugs are injected directly into your IV line from a large syringe. This method is called a bolus push. Still others will be given orally at home, on schedules that may require you to take pills several times a day, or on a tapered dose over several days.

If you have had much chemotherapy, you know that your veins will hide, roll, close, or blow when the phlebotomist is attempting to insert the needle. If this is happening to you, remember the advice about blood tests given in Chapter 4, *Tests and Procedures*, and ask for the smallest possible needle to be used, a butterfly needle. Sometimes a butterfly needle is too small to allow the free flow of the drugs you must receive, but the rest of the time it is a very helpful solution to the problem. You may feel a warm flush when certain drugs are administered. Verify with the medical staff whether this is normal for the drug you are receiving. Many chemotherapy drugs are damaging if they come in contact with the skin. Notify the staff immediately if you feel any pain or burning, or if you see swelling or redness at the site of the needle in the vein.

You are now about to make the acquaintance of the IV pole, the bane of many a chemotherapy patient. More patient humor has been created about IV poles than any other single part of cancer therapy. Drugs are prepared in plastic bags with tubes coming from them and the bags are hung on the IV pole. If you are having combination therapy, involving several drugs administered at the same time, you might have an interesting collection of bags of varying sizes, shapes, and colors hanging from the pole. As the drugs drip through the plastic tubes and into your vein, the machine on the IV pole monitors them. They may be mixed with other drugs and with saline solution to dilute them and keep you hydrated. Some of them are brightly colored and some of them are clear. The brightly colored ones may be responsible for color changes in your urine after treatment. Don't panic. That's perfectly normal.

One patient describes using the bathroom while attached to IVs:

> You are attached to the IV pole by the tubes running into the needle and catheter arrangement in your veins. Once the connection is made, you and your pole are married and inseparable until therapy is completed.
>
> If you need to go to the bathroom, your pole will be your intimate companion. You will push it along with you to the facilities, maneuver it into the bathroom, and turn it so that you have enough slack in the tubes to get to the toilet, which means untwisting the pole. After taking care of business, you then must repeat the process as you return to the chair or bed you have left.
>
> Things are fine if your IV pole cooperates, but if you happen to get stuck with one that hasn't a sense of direction, or that has uneven rollers, or that simply doesn't want to move, you are in quite a pickle.

The machine on the IV pole is monitoring the rate at which the drugs are dripping into you. If you move your arm inadvertently and a tube kinks, or if an air bubble forms, or one solution runs out, the machine beeps and keeps on beeping until a nurse comes in to check the apparatus and ensure the even flow of the treatment once more. That's not too bad with one monitor. But if several of the machines sing out at once, and the nurses are busy with other patients, the beep, beep, beep can begin to drive you wild. This is when you must plumb the depths of your soul to find the hidden cache of humor hiding below the surface. Patients report that after hospitalization, they hear the beep, beep, beep of the machines in their dreams and wake up to reassure themselves that they are only dreaming.

Oral therapy regimens

Oral therapy regimens may include oral medication in conjunction with or in place of intravenous administration. You also may be given oral antinausea medicines. Although oral medication is easy compared to other means of administration, you need to be aware of some issues.

Chemotherapy drugs can occasionally cause pill-swallowing problems. After several days or weeks of treatment, you may experience dry mouth, caused by the death of rapidly dividing cells in your mouth. Cultivate the habit of wetting your mouth before you attempt to swallow tablets. It is advisable to keep a supply of sugarless hard candy nearby because some chemotherapy drugs dry your mouth out so much that your lips curl back from your teeth temporarily until you moisten the area again.

Keeping track of when you should be taking pills, especially if you have several to take at different times, is not easy even when you're well. When you're not feeling your best, it's even harder. It's helpful to use a plastic pill organizer to ensure that all doses are taken. Another successful method is to make a list of what needs to be taken each day, and at what time. Then cross off what you are taking as you swallow the pills.

If you are taking steroids, like prednisone or dexamethasone, it is imperative that they be taken as prescribed. They are known to cause spurts of energy, emotional overreaction, and fluid retention in some people. When the time comes to stop taking these drugs after you have been on them for a while, if your doctor has not recommended tapering your dose, ask why. Stopping such drugs abruptly can cause severe physical and emotional side effects.

Leukapheresis

Leukapheresis is the term for circulating blood through a machine that filters out white cells showing specific CD markers. The rest of the blood is then recirculated back into the body. Since the cells removed are the white cells, which are at dangerously high levels, the patient's white blood count drops after leukapheresis. Leukapheresis is used to keep white counts below dangerous levels while the patient awaits treatment with another agent. The same process is used to remove selected stem cells from the bloodstream for stem cell transplants, and it is very similar to what you have experienced if you have ever donated platelets.

Here is a patient describing her experiences undergoing leukapheresis:

> Today was my first leukapheresis treatment and it went extremely
> well. Of course, there was pain with the insertion of the needles in both
> arms, but after that, it was smooth sailing. I was in a private room in the
> blood donor section of the hospital. I was in a bed with heated blankets, a
> VCR, and an RN who stayed with me the entire time. Pretty nice, huh?
>
> And best of all were the results of this initial treatment! They took lab
> values immediately before and after the leukapheresis. My WBC went
> from 230,000 to 90,000! I am thrilled! I know there will be some rebound
> in the next week, but I can't imagine that it will return to its prior level.
> So, I am eager to do the second treatment a week from now. Hopefully,
> my insurance company will be impressed with the results and authorize
> further treatments.
>
> Psychologically, it was wonderful to see the bag of leukemic white
> cells removed from my body and thrown away!

Subcutaneous injection

If counts become really low, the doctor may suggest that you be injected
subcutaneously (under the skin) with the growth stimulating factors
described earlier: G-CSF to raise white counts, GM-CSF to raise neutrophils
and monocytes, epoetin (EPO) to raise red counts, or thrombopoietin to
raise platelet counts. Inteferon-alfa-2B and interleukin-2 are given by injection as well.

Any of these treatments may be given at the doctor's office or self-injected at
home once you are, or someone else is, trained to do it. Your insurance company's reimbursement policy will determine where the treatments are given.

Injections can be painful. A trick to use when receiving growth factors is to
have the RN or doctor warm the substance before injecting it. Each patient
has a favorite procedure after inserting the needle. Some inject the medication slowly and some do it quickly. Whichever way, the patient is usually
convinced that the selected method is the one and only way to make it less
painful.

Here is how one patient made the injection of G-CSF easier:

> I warm the Leukine before I use it. Room temperature is great. I
> warm it by holding the vial in my hand. I make sure to change the needle
> after drawing up the solution into the syringe. That way I'm using a
> sharp, new needle that will go in easily. I found that injecting slowly is
> easier on me than going fast, so I took the task over from the nurses and
> did it my way. I didn't hesitate to play around with the way I injected it
> until I found something that worked for me. I also chose to have the shots
> in the thigh, because my arms were sore enough from peripheral IVs. My
> Hickman got infected at day twenty, and I was without a central venous
> catheter thereafter, so my arms were black and blue. I sure wasn't about
> to let them inject me there.

Other considerations

Before leaving the treatment center, be sure you have received any pertinent
written instructions regarding dietary or behavioral requirements. Be sure
that you are feeling well enough to leave. Be aware of side effects you need to
watch for, and have the doctor's emergency numbers handy. Don't forget to
use the rest room before you leave if you've been treated with something
diluted with saline solution. You'll be amazed at how much fluid you've
absorbed, and you don't want to be caught with a sense of urgency halfway
home.

Remember to hang on to your sense of humor as you go through this therapy. If you lose your hair, there are wonderful T-shirts with messages like:
"I'm having a no hair day," "Bald is beautiful," or "I'm too sexy for my hair.
That's why it isn't there." Do wear hats, especially in cool weather. You'll be
amazed at how cold your bare head can become and how sunburned it can
get in summer.

For many patients, a good wig is a worthwhile investment. You can have it
set to match your present hairstyle. Check with your insurance plan and see
if they will pay for what insurers call a "cranial prosthesis." If they will, ask
your doctor to write a prescription for one.

There will be days when you will simply feel awful. Sleep it off if you possibly can! You need that rest, and you're less likely to feel nauseated if you're sleeping. On better days get up, get dressed, and go about your business, even if that's just taking a walk at an easy pace. The important thing is to try to keep some semblance of normal life.

During the period of nadir, when your counts are at their lowest and you're most susceptible to infections, avoid crowds. If you are neutropenic and have few good white cells to battle germs, stay away from other people. You really can't afford to catch cold or pick up the latest virus that's making the rounds. You need your immune system to fight the cancer—not bacterial or viral infections.

CHAPTER 8

Treatments for Individual Leukemias

Treatment options vary significantly according to the type of leukemia you have, its stage, and other characteristics, such as subtype or genetic markers. Treatment recommendations may change over time as new standard treatments evolve to improve chances for remission, increase long-term survival rates, and decrease side effects that can adversely affect your quality of life.

This chapter gives an overview of standard treatments according to diagnosis and stage or subtype. It is limited to general information rather than specific cases, since every situation is unique. Standard treatment recommendations (and some promising treatment directions still under study) are provided first for acute leukemias: acute lymphocytic leukemia and acute myelogenous leukemia. Next come chronic leukemias: chronic myelogenous leukemia and chronic lymphocytic leukemia. Then we discuss hairy cell leukemia, prolymphocytic leukemia, splenic lymphoma with villous lymphocytes, and finally, acute T-cell leukemia. You may wish to read only the section that applies to your disease.

The specifics given in this chapter about drugs, protocols, and dosages are not meant to indicate that those specifics apply in your case. Your doctor is the one who knows the specifics of your situation and is the one to ask about the best treatment for you. The information given here, however, provides background information on common treatments. This background can help you better understand the reasoning behind recommended treatments. The material can also help you formulate questions for your doctor, such as why a standard treatment is not recommended in your case, and give you the names of therapies that you might research further.

The information in this chapter comes from the National Cancer Institute's *Physician's Data Query (PDQ) Treatment Information* for professionals; from

Henderson, Lister, and Greaves, *Leukemia*, sixth edition; Whittaker and Holmes, *Leukemia and other Related Disorders*; Wintrobe, *Clinical Oncology*, tenth edition; and from many research papers found in professional journals. Much that is presently being published in the professional literature is still too experimental to be used in treatment plans. But some have entered human trials in which patients are participating as part of a formal clinical trial protocol (plan).

For more information about clinical trials, see Chapter 10, *Clinical Trials and Beyond*, and Chapter 19, *Researching Your Leukemia*. Appendix A, *Resources*, includes treatment resources to permit more detailed follow-up on options of interest to patients and their families. Many drugs used in treating leukemias are listed and classified in Appendix G, *Leukemia Drugs*. If the one you are seeking is not included, go to one of the pharmacy sites on the World Wide Web and look for it there. Helpful web sites for finding pharmaceutical drug information include: *http://www.pharminfo.com* and *http://www.druginfonet.com*. The other places to look are *http://cancertrials.nci.nih.gov* or *http://www.fda.gov*. Use the search engine on the FDA site to find the name of the drug you're looking for.

Treatment protocols

A treatment protocol is a complete plan for a specific group of patients receiving a particular therapy. Institutions engaged in specific research studies use protocols to delineate explicitly what happens. For example, your protocol will tell you:

- The person(s) in charge of the trial
- Eligibility requirements to participate
- A clear statement of the objectives of the protocol so you know what they hope to discover
- Background information that makes this study logical, and information about the drug(s) to be used
- The exact treatment plan:
  - Procedures to be done
  - Drugs to be administered

- How, when, in what order, and where treatment drugs will be given
- All other drugs to be administered including pre-medications, anti-emetics, preventive medicines, antibiotics, etc.

- Evaluation criteria for patients: clinical information and/or tests to be required before, during, and after participation

- Statistical objectives: the number of institutions participating, the number of patients participating, and the duration of the trial

- All possible side effects and problems that the researchers can imagine and suggestions for ways to deal with them

New protocols are constantly tested and treatment plans are constantly refined. Some involve single chemotherapy agents and some involve combinations of drugs and therapies.

Research into chemotherapy regimens (referred to by patients and professionals alike as "chemo") has indicated that often combinations of drugs are more successful in treating leukemias than single drugs alone. Sometimes, however, the opposite proves true and the combination of two active drugs may be more toxic. For example, fludarabine and chlorambucil, combined at dosages that were perfectly tolerable for each drug individually, were proven to be too toxic a regimen for most patients. Research shows what dosages and what different ways of using chemotherapy work best. Since research is going on constantly, new and better ways of combining drugs can change the treatment protocols fairly often.

It is important for you to learn your treatment protocol. Learn which drugs will be given in which order. Ask the oncology nurse to explain the sequence and the time span for receiving your chemotherapy. She can also explain the reason why there may be rest periods between the treatments.

Your doctor selects dosages for your chemotherapy regimen according to your body surface and age. See Appendix C, *Body Surface Area in Square Meters*, for a dosage chart. Your dosage may be different from that of the patient next to you in the treatment center, who may be on the same or a similar protocol. Your doctor may alter your dosages if your blood counts have not returned fully to normal by the time you are due your next treatment or delay treatment until counts improve. It is wise to learn and document dosages of the drugs you receive so that you or your caregiver can verify that you are receiving the proper drugs and dosage.

Acute leukemias

Major advances in the diagnosis, classification, and treatment of acute leukemias have resulted in significant increases in the number of complete remissions and long-term survivors. Proper diagnosis of acute leukemias is critical because there are great differences in prognoses and treatments for ALL and AML. Both types of acute leukemia require immediate treatment.

Acute lymphocytic leukemia (ALL)

Pre–B-cell ALL is the most common malignancy in children. In this patient population, combination chemotherapy is very successful and more than 80 percent of children are cured. The outcome for adults with this disease is not as good. However, major advances in the treatment of adult ALL have occurred in the past few years. Therefore, the prognosis for ALL patients has improved due to the use of more intensive treatment strategies. The treatment objective is to eradicate the leukemia cell population from the bone marrow and other sites. At present, 80 percent of adult patients can expect to achieve a complete remission for a period of time, but just over one-third of them become long-term disease-free survivors living normal lives.

There is no staging system for ALL. Doctors speak of untreated, newly diagnosed patients, and those who are in remission. Remission is defined as having bone marrow showing normal cells with less than 5 percent blasts, and laboratory tests showing normal white blood counts, differential, hematocrit, hemoglobin, and platelet values. In addition, there should be no signs and symptoms of the disease or of central nervous system involvement.

Standard treatment for ALL is divided into three phases: remission induction, central nervous system (CNS) prophylaxis, and remission consolidation or maintenance.

An important prognostic indicator, known as the Philadelphia chromosome, occurs in 20 percent of people with adult ALL. Patients whose blood samples show indications of the Philadelphia chromosome are referred to as having positive or Ph+ ALL. Patients who show no indication of the chromosome are referred to as negative or Ph– ALL. The Philadelphia chromosome transformation is discussed in detail in Chapter 5, *Subtype, Staging, and Prognosis*, under "CML."

In more than half the adults having Ph+ ALL, the molecular abnormality appears slightly different from that in Ph+ CML. Unfortunately, the prognosis for Ph+ ALL is worse than for other types of ALL. These patients are often candidates for bone marrow transplants in first remission if a suitable donor is available since their remissions are usually short when using the standard chemotherapy regimens.

The following account comes from Jenny, a leukemia survivor with ALL who has been through all phases of treatment. She has survived by keeping her sense of humor intact, and having knowledgeable doctors with whom she works well:

> I was diagnosed in December 1996 at age 23. I was just finishing my student teaching, and was working long hours into the night to keep up with the mountains of paperwork required by the supervising teacher. I was fatigued and my body was bruising easily. Two weeks before diagnosis, I had astronomically huge hematomas from head to foot and no idea of where they were coming from. Other than the bruises, I was white as a sheet. I went in to the gynecologist, who took a CBC the minute he saw me. He said, 'If this is what I think it is, it's bad.' My white cells were 180,000 and platelets were at 10,000.
>
> He sent me to a hematologist right from his office, and diagnosis came that afternoon. The hematologist did a bone marrow biopsy, found 95 percent blasts, and had me in the intensive care unit immediately. The next week he told my parents, who fortunately had come to that meeting with me, that I wouldn't make it through the week. His bedside manner was not his strong suit.
>
> I had a large central venous catheter inserted in my groin area and went through pheresis that evening, bringing my white counts down to 80,000. The hematologist on call that night told us what to expect. This caring, considerate man sat with my family and me, and explained the two-year protocol I'd be starting. He consoled us, eased our fears, and held me while I cried. I was going to have chemotherapy with cytoxan, daunorubicin, vincristine, L-asparaginase, prednisone, and Ara-C. Amazingly, I was in remission in three to five weeks. I was out of the hospital the third week in January.

Then this ALL survivor continued treatment and began preparing for a bone marrow transplant:

> By this time I had gotten rid of the catheter and had a port inserted for induction therapy. I went for treatment twice a week in the treatment room of the doctor's office. Course two of the chemotherapy, also called early intensification, was repeated twice. It included intrathecal methotrexate, cytoxan, 6-MP (mercaptopurine), and Ara-C. The second round included vincristine and L-asparaginase. You will notice that they were treating for central nervous system involvement, even though at this point I didn't have that problem to worry about.
>
> In April I started seeing a transplant specialist because they found that I had a chromosomal translocation, 4;11, which made me a candidate for transplant. I changed oncologists at that point, because I couldn't communicate well with the one I had been seeing and this was a logical time to change. In April, also, the National Bone Marrow Donor program was contacted to seek a donor immediately. Chemotherapy continued for CNS prophylaxis, which was supposed to last for twelve weeks. No brain radiation was done, because I was going to have total body irradiation as part of my transplant, but the intrathecal methotrexate, 6MP, and oral methotrexate were used until September 1997.

Looking ahead to long-term survival issues, she had ovarian tissue removed before the transplant:

> At age 23, I was too young to be willing to accept a life of sterility, and the BMT was likely to make me sterile, so I was the first woman in this area to have ovarian tissue freezing done. Support came from the BMT doctor and my gynecologist. The surgeon removed my right ovary and I kept the left one. The ovary was sliced into millimeter slivers so everything would freeze at once. It was cryogenically frozen, and will be reconnected onto my left ovary, which has the blood supply, when I am ready to have a child. They believe I will be able to conceive naturally.

Remission induction for ALL

The first phase of standard treatment for ALL is remission induction. Appropriate initial treatment, which may include a combination of drugs added to vincristine and/or prednisone, delivers complete remission in 60 to 90 percent of patients.

The well-known standard induction treatment protocols for treating ALL include: vincristine, prednisone, and anthracycline, with or without L-asparaginase or cyclophosphamide. Examples of specific protocol drug combinations are:

- Daunorubicin (DNR), vincristine (Oncovin), prednisone, and L-asparaginase

- Mitoxantrone, cytarabine, vincristine, and prednisone

- Cyclophosphamide (Cytoxan), daunorubicin, vincristine, prednisone, and L-asparaginase

- Cytarabine, mitoxantrone, etoposide, and prednisone

All possible treatment options cannot be included here, since therapies change rapidly according to the results of the latest research. Your doctor and the treatment center you go to may have a different preferred combination of drugs in use for ALL induction therapy.

The protocols listed above are often not used against B-cell and T-cell ALL. Patients having B-cell ALL that expresses surface immunoglobulins and certain cytogenetic transformations are not usually cured by standard ALL regimens. Aggressive cyclophosphamide-based regimens have shown higher response rates for these patients and for those having T-cell ALL. Often, ifosfamide and methotrexate will be included. It is highly recommended that these patients enroll in clinical trials designed to improve treatment outcomes.

Myelosuppression (inhibition of bone marrow function) is an expected consequence of both the leukemia and its treatment with chemotherapy. Patients must be closely monitored during remission induction treatment. Hematological support and treatment of infections will be required for these patients. This may involve red blood cell and platelet transfusions as well as hematopoietic growth factors G-CSF or GM-CSF and antibiotics.

Treatment options for CNS prophylaxis

At the same time patients receive remission induction treatment, they may be at risk for ALL spreading to the central nervous system (CNS). The central nervous system includes the brain and spinal cord. Treatment prevents ALL cells from infiltrating the central nervous system, the lining of the spinal cord, and brain (the meninges). Not all patients have CNS involvement, but enough do that CNS treatment is often automatically included as part of induction therapy. Leukemic cells can escape from chemotherapy when they hide in the meninges and inevitably cause relapse (meningeal leukemia). Treatment strategies, therefore, consist of systematically administered combination chemotherapy with CNS preventive therapy.

CNS preventive therapy may include:

- Cranial irradiation plus intrathecal methotrexate (injected through the sheath of the spinal cord into the subarachnoid space)

- High-dose systemic methotrexate and intrathecal methotrexate without cranial irradiation

- Intrathecal chemotherapy alone

Consolidation and remission maintenance

Even when a patient is in remission, leukemia cells may still be present in small numbers. Optimal treatment of ALL includes maintenance chemotherapy—which may involve drugs not used in the original remission induction therapy.

Current approaches to post-remission therapy for ALL include:

- Short-term, relatively intensive chemotherapy treatments followed by long-term therapy at lower doses (maintenance).

- High-dose bone marrow–killing chemotherapy.

- Allogeneic (using a donor's cells) bone marrow or stem cell transplantation with high-dose chemotherapy and radiotherapy. This results in the lowest incidence of leukemic relapse for high-risk ALL patients and has led to the theory of graft-versus-leukemia (GVL) effect. In essence, patients who develop a mild form of GVL as a result of allogeneic transplant have a better chance of staying disease free. The complications of allogeneic bone marrow transplant can be graft-versus-host disease that may be chronic, veno-occlusive disease of the liver, failure to engraft, or graft rejection. Any of these may cause significant long-term discomfort and can occasionally be fatal.

Standard drug combination protocols used for consolidation therapy may include:

- Dexamethasone, vincristine, doxorubicin, cyclophosphamide, cytarabine (Ara-C), and thioguanine

- Ara-C, methotrexate, thioguanine, vincristine, prednisone, L-asparaginase, and cyclophosphamide
- Vincristine, prednisone, daunorubicin, Ara-C, teniposide (VM26), and methotrexate
- Cyclophosphamide, Ara-C, 6-mercaptopurine, vincristine, L-asparaginase, doxorubicin, dexamethasone, and thioguanine

Maintenance combinations may include:

- 6-mercaptopurine and methotrexate
- Vincristine, prednisone, doxorubicin, 6-mercaptopurine, methotrexate, carmustine, dactinomycin, and cyclophosphamide
- 6-mercaptopurine, methotrexate, vincristine, and prednisone

Relapsed refractory ALL

More than half of all adult patients with ALL relapse within two years. The primary site for relapse is in the bone marrow, but many relapses involve the central nervous system.

Several protocols have been used to treat relapsed ALL patients. High-dose Ara-C alone or with other chemotherapy agents results in complete remissions in 50 percent of these patients. Unfortunately, the response may not last very long, so if patients are young or strong enough to be able to withstand high-dose therapy, they are also candidates for allogeneic bone marrow or stem cell transplants when they are in second remission.

Autologous (using one's own cells) bone marrow transplants (ABMT) or peripheral blood stem cell transplants (PSCT) have been used for patients who do not have a suitable donor or who are considered too old to tolerate an allogeneic PSCT. The age question is diminishing, however, as stem cell transplants replace bone marrow transplants. As techniques for transplantation improve, older individuals in good health are increasingly being considered for PSCT. One problem with this method is the inability to eradicate minimal residual disease effectively at the time of marrow harvest. Use of a variety of techniques to purge the marrow cells has helped to alleviate, but not totally surmount, this problem.

Acute myeloid leukemia (AML)

Advances in the treatment of AML have resulted in substantially improved complete remission rates. Approximately 60 to 70 percent of adults attain complete remission following appropriate induction therapy. Remission rates for adult AML are inversely related to age, with better results in younger patients.

Treatment for AML is generally divided into two stages: remission induction and consolidation.

Remission induction for AML

Despite the complicated subtyping of AML, with its subtle prognostic and treatment implications, antileukemic therapy is similar for many of the subtypes. There is no clear staging system for AML. Untreated, newly diagnosed patients are treated with induction therapy. Patients in remission are given consolidation therapy. Patients are considered to be in remission when they show normal peripheral blood counts, normal cellular marrow—with less than 5 percent blasts in the marrow—and no signs or symptoms of the disease.

Here, a patient describes his AML induction chemotherapy experience:

> In the evening, I started chemotherapy. This was really scary. I wondered if I would throw up constantly. Would it be painful? It was less traumatic than I thought, only because I had imagined the worst. There was little nausea and no pain. The chemotherapy was the fairly standard AML induction therapy of seven days of continuous Ara-C with three days of daunorubicin. The next day was April 1st, April Fool's Day. Perhaps someone would come to my room, tell us it was all a joke, and let us go home. No one ever came.

The patient describes feeling better quickly after induction therapy:

> After spending 24 days in the hospital, I got out. I had lost most of my hair and about 25 pounds (11 kg) as I had not been eating much. My doctor said that I should soon start to feel better than I had for a long time. He was right. I began to feel a lot better very quickly. My appetite came back and I started eating as much as I could. I figured that the next chemotherapy session would be like the first, and I would again lose a lot of weight.

Consolidation for AML

Successful treatment of AML requires control of bone marrow and systemic disease, including treatment of central nervous system involvement if it is present. The standard treatment strategy involves systematic administration of combination chemotherapy. Only 5 percent of patients with AML develop CNS involvement, so CNS prophylaxis is not normally part of the treatment plan. Consolidation therapy, so successful for ALL, has not proven itself to be beneficial for AML. Most AML patients are given intensive consolidation therapy over a short period of time, after which treatment is discontinued. Consolidation therapy appears to be effective when given immediately after remission is achieved, or when delayed for nine months.

Here, a patient describes undergoing AML consolidation chemotherapy:

> I started consolidation chemo, consisting of four days of high-dose Ara-C again, twice a day, twelve hours apart, with mitoxantrone on the first three days. Initially the doctor had told us that I would have to be hospitalized to get the chemo. However, after we questioned him a bit, he said it would be possible to do it as an outpatient. For four days, I went into the doctor's office for Ara-C and mitoxantrone (the first three days), as well as hydration and Zofran for nausea.

> In the evening, a home health nurse would come to administer more Ara-C and Zofran. I also had a syringe of Zofran to mix in juice to take during the day. Zofran was not available in tablet form at the time. I thought I might be able to work during treatment, but I was mistaken. Although I was able to eat this time, the chemo wore me out so much that most of the time, when I was not actually receiving medication, I was sleeping.

After treatment, this patient was able to return to work and received welcome news:

> I was anxious to be finished with chemotherapy and get back to work, not so much because I had really important things to do at work, but because I wanted to get my life back to the way it was before I had been diagnosed.

> A bone marrow biopsy, done after the chemotherapy was finished, had shown no sign of leukemia or of the inversion in chromosome 16. As my doctor so dryly remarked, "This was better than the alternative."

The anticipated result of leukemia and its treatment is myelosuppression (inhibition of the bone marrow); so patients undergoing chemotherapy must be closely monitored during therapy. It is not unusual for patients to require platelet and blood transfusions and treatment with antibiotics for various infections. G-CSF and GM-CSF, the white cell growth factors, are often administered following chemotherapy to ensure that counts return to normal as rapidly as possible. Growth factors are especially helpful in older patients. Clinical trials are still ongoing to determine the best use of G-CSF and GM-CSF.

The two-drug regimen of cytarabine (Ara-C) in conjunction with daunorubicin results in 65 percent of patients having a complete response, e.g., going into some degree of remission. Sometimes thioguanine is added for a three-drug combination. Studies have also implied that adding etoposide to the two-drug Ara-C and daunorubicin combination may improve remission duration. In some studies, idarubicin appears to be as effective as daunorubicin, although the doses of the two have not been equivalent. The addition of mitoxantrone, amsacrine, and higher doses of cytarabine are under study. There is much interest in the possibility that higher doses of cytarabine, administered during induction therapy, may have a significant impact on disease-free survival. Another combination, VAPA, includes vincristine, doxorubicin, prednisone, and cytarabine.

Treatments for AML continue to evolve. In January 2000, Maxamine, an immunotherapeutic drug, was approved as an orphan drug for treating AML. Study results, presented at the American Society of Hematology 1999 conference, show that Maxamine produces encouraging increases in leukemia-free survival in patients with AML who are treated in remission. Maxamine therapy for AML patients in remission combines Maxamine and low dose interleukin-2 (IL-2). The objective is to prevent relapse, prolong leukemia-free survival, and maintain a good quality of life.

Recurrent or refractory AML generally does not respond as well to chemotherapy as does newly diagnosed AML. Patients with recurrent or refractory AML can be effectively treated with mitoxantrone and intermediate-dose cytarabine (Ara-C), according to new research.[1] A very small subset of AML patients develop central nervous system involvement. Chemotherapy for central nervous system involvement may include cranial irradiation, and/or cytarabine administered into the spinal fluid.

AML treatments by karyotype

AML is not treated by stage. Tests that examine characteristics of the leukemic cells, called cytogenetic analysis, provide doctors with prognostic information for AML patients, especially in those newly diagnosed. Treatment decisions usually are based upon chromosome patterns. It is important to remember that because granulocytes are the cells involved in AML, there are no clusters of differentiation on the leukemic cells. Only lymphocytes have CD antigens. AML patients reading this should obtain a copy of their cytogenetic report results to help them understand treatment options. The karyotype profiles are listed on the report so that the information following will make sense. Karyotypes are described in greater detail in Chapter 3, *Diagnosis*.

The following table translates abbreviations used in cytogenetic report notations:

Abbreviation	Meaning
t(x)	Translocation of the chromosomes at the points listed in parentheses
inv(x)	Inversion of the chromosomes at the points listed in the parentheses
del(x)	Deletion of the chromosomes at the points listed in the parentheses
p(x)	The short arm of the chromosome
q(x)	The long arm of the chromosome

The most favorable AML cytogenetic profiles include t(8;21), inv(16), and t(15;17). Normal cytogenetics imply average-risk AML.

Unfortunately, patients with AML characterized by deletions of the long arms of chromosomes 5 or 7, by translocations or inversions of chromosome 3, t(6;9), t(9;22), or by abnormalities of chromosome 11q23, have particularly poor prognoses for chemotherapy. Bone marrow transplantation is often used for these patients.

Treatment by karyotype is the usual pattern, and some, but not all possible examples are included here:

- In patients with karyotype t(8;21), the complete remission rate usually will be high and its duration will be long, using standard induction and consolidation chemotherapy alone.

- In patients with karyotype inv(16)(p13q22), t(16;16), or t(15;17), the complete remission rate usually will be high and duration likely will be intermediate to long, using standard induction with an anthracycline and intensive consolidation chemotherapy with high-dose cytarabine.

Transretinoic acid given prior to chemotherapy for t(15;17) is still being tested. See the section "Acute promyelocytic leukemia."

- In patients with karyotype t(9;11) the complete remission rate can be expected to be high, but its duration will be short using standard induction.

- In patients with karyotype del(5q), +13, +8, inv(3), del(12p) the complete remission rate usually will be low and its duration will be short using standard induction. New induction regimens including the use of growth factors during chemotherapy or modulators of drug resistance may be recommended by your doctor. A peripheral blood stem cell transplant is often considered during first remission.

Acute promyelocytic leukemia (APL) or M3 APL

Promyelocytic leukemia (APL) patients have benefited from recent treatment advances. Formerly one of the major risks of treatment of APL was that it triggered diffuse intravascular coagulation (DIC), or blood clotting, within the veins. This often caused fatal bleeding complications. The treatment of APL has been revolutionized by all-trans-retinoic acid (ATRA, tretinoin, Vesanoid), an oral, biologic derivative of vitamin A. It is now an essential component of first-line therapy for APL, replacing standard intravenous chemotherapy induction regimens. It can induce remission in 70 to 90 percent of APL patients according to various research studies. Importantly, the use of ATRA has greatly decreased the incidence of bleeding complications. ATRA also kills leukemic cells, so normal blood cells mature.

Nevertheless, ATRA is not effective in patients with AML that resembles the APL subtype (M3) and who do not have the PML-RAR alfa gene rearrangement typical of APL. More is being learned as clinical trials continue and oncologists work to discover why some patients on ATRA develop hyperleukocytosis (extreme destruction of leukocytes) and a syndrome of respiratory distress known as retinoic acid syndrome. Treatment with dexamethasone is usually successful in dealing with this problem.

Research into other effective treatment continues. Recently, investigators have reported major activity of arsenic trioxide in APL.[2] Over 80 percent of patients with relapsed APL in clinical trials with arsenic trioxide achieved complete remission. Arsenic trioxide has now been approved by the FDA for the treatment of patients with APL who have failed both chemotherapy and ATRA.[3]

Secondary AML

Some cases of AML are secondary, arising out of conditions other than an original diagnosis. Patients with AML arising from myelodysplasia, or secondary to previous cytotoxic chemotherapy, have a lower rate of remission than those initially diagnosed with AML. Patients with secondary leukemia may be candidates for allogeneic bone marrow transplants if their overall status is adequate, potentially sparing them the additional toxicity of the standard induction chemotherapy.

Refractory AML

Monoclonal antibody–based therapies are beginning to show the promise that was predicted with the advent of the core technology more than 20 years ago. Antibody-based therapies targeting tumor cell surface antigens on B cells, CD20 on malignant B cells, and CD33 on leukemic blasts have been effective in clinical trials. Combinations composed of anti-CD33 antibodies and the chemotherapy agent calicheamicin show promising activity in patients with relapsed or refractory acute myelogenous leukemia.

In May 2000, the Federal Drug Administration approved Mylotarg (gemtuzumab ozogamicin), a monoclonal antibody for the treatment of patients aged 60 or older with CD33 positive relapsed AML. Currently, this is the only medication approved for the treatment of relapsed AML patients. It acts on the monocytes in patients with AML. Mylotarg carries a drug on the antibody that gets into the cell and causes cell lysis or destruction of the cell. Mylotarg is in a new class of anticancer therapy called antibody-targeted chemotherapy, which is based on a "linker" technology that combines a potent antitumor antibiotic with an antibody that binds to the CD33 antigen commonly found on leukemic cells. This antigen is also found on other bone marrow hematopoietic cells, but not on pluripotent progenitor cells (cells capable of developing into any blood cell).

Check the National Cancer Institute clinical trials registry for additional ongoing clinical trials recommended for refractory AML patients. See Chapter 19, *Researching Your Leukemia*, for specific information.

Chronic leukemias

Chronic leukemias usually follow a slower course than the acute leukemias. The bone marrow cells involved in chronic leukemias mature farther and are able to perform their necessary functions longer than those involved in acute leukemias. Some subtypes have been known for centuries, while others have only been identified as distinct clinical entities in the past few years. The clinical manifestations of chronic leukemias are diverse, as are the treatment approaches.

Chronic myelogenous leukemia (CML)

CML is the most common of the myeloprolific disorders (disorders of stem cells). It is not now curable. Treatment usually starts with chemotherapy and moves to interferon-alfa or some form of bone marrow transplant. Patients usually stay in the chronic stage for four or five years before the disease progresses into the accelerated and then blastic (acute) stages. The blood cells of most patients display the Philadelphia chromosome (Ph+), and if they don't, molecular techniques will usually show the chromosome 9;22 translocation even without a visible Ph+.

About 5 percent of all CML patients do not show the Philadelphia chromosome transformation (Ph−). Those patients showing Ph− have a poorer prognosis than those showing Ph+. We do not yet know why some patients show the Philadelphia chromosome and some do not. Oncologists are discussing whether CML without this marker is a different disease from CML with Ph+. As we learn more about the human genome, we will discover more about this as well.

Standard treatment for chronic phase CML

There are many different approaches to treatment for chronic-phase CML, depending on individual circumstances. Among them are: busulfan, hydroxyurea, interferon-alfa (IFN-alfa), PSCT, and splenectomy.

Busulfan (Myleran). One of the first chemotherapy agents for CML was busulfan, an alkylator that is usually given orally. It occasionally results in unpredictable, prolonged myelosuppression—inhibition of the bone marrow. Other side effects of busulfan include pulmonary fibrosis (scarring of the lung tissue) and symptoms similar to Addison's disease (deficiency in the secretion of the adrenal cortical hormones). It can also result in secondary acute leukemias when given over a long period. Although busulfan is somewhat effective in chronic-phase CML, newer options are proving more desirable. It is still being used, but the present gold standard for non-transplant treatment of patients is interferon-alfa and Ara-C. Busulfan is used as a conditioner for transplants (to get rid of enough leukemic cells that the patient can undergo transplant).

Hydroxyurea. Hydroxyurea is currently used in the treatment of chronic-phase CML. It is generally preferred to busulfan because it provides a significantly longer median survival and fewer severe side effects. (However, busulfan still has its uses. For some people who don't respond to hydroxyurea, doctors can then go to busulfan. For some other leukemias, busulfan is preferred to hydroxyurea.)

Hydroxyurea is usually given daily by mouth, 1 to 3 grams per day as a single dose on an empty stomach. A dose of 40 milligrams per kilogram per day is often used initially in patients with very high white blood counts (WBC) and frequently results in rapid reduction of the count. When the WBC drops below 20,000 per cubic millimeter, the dosage of hydroxyurea is often reduced until the blood count levels even out.

As one CML patient recounts:

> My WBC counts were controlled with hydroxyurea. They were hard to control for a while, swinging too far either way from normal. I finally helped my doctor find a dose that kept them stable, in a normal range, by tracking counts on a computer spreadsheet. It worked perfectly and I went into my BMT with normal counts.

Interferon alfa (IFN-alfa). Interferon alfa is the latest treatment used for chronic CML. IFN-alfa is composed of approximately 150 amino acids. It is a natural protein with the ability to modulate the immune response, and it is not considered chemotherapy. There are several different forms of interferon, but IFN-alfa 2a and 2b are the types normally used for CML. IFN-alfa produces complete hematological remission (where no cancer cells are found in the blood) in around 70 to 80 percent of patients and reduces the number of cells containing the Philadelphia chromosome in about 50 percent of patients. For some patients this remission is only temporary and delays the onset of blastic transformation. New research is suggesting that INF-alfa treatment be considered for newly diagnosed patients.

Compared to hydroxyurea and busulfan, some researchers report that interferon regresses patients to an earlier stage of disease (according to the blood work), delays disease progression, and prolongs overall survival. It appears to be most effective when combined with other drugs and when given in the earliest stages of the chronic phase. Adding cytarabine (Ara-C) to IFN-alfa increases the survival benefit, but also increases toxicity.

In trials at M. D. Anderson Cancer Center, the combination of IFN-alfa plus cytarabine resulted in a positive response rate in 90 percent of patients.[4] Patients need to know, however, that a history of neurological or psychiatric illness increases the risk of developing severe side effects when treated with this combination.

IFN-alfa is given subcutaneously daily, and has significant toxic effects that may require dosage modification or, in some cases, discontinuation of therapy. Side effects are flu-like symptoms, especially with the initial dose. Nausea, anorexia, and weight loss may also occur. Other immune system complications may be seen after long-term use.

Bone marrow transplant (BMT) or peripheral blood stem cell transplant (PSCT). At initial AML diagnosis, patients younger than age 60 should be considered for treatment with transplantation. Allogeneic transplantation from related or matched unrelated donors during the chronic phase offers a chance for cure. The key is to find an appropriate donor.

Survival curves for BMT/PSCT show at least half the patients are alive five to ten years post-transplant. Patients taking IFN-alfa show relapses after about seven to eight years. The survival benefit with transplantation must be weighed against the potential serious harm and mortality rates that may accompany the procedure. The risk of relapse is less when transplantation is done early and when patients develop at least some graft-versus-host disease. This permits graft-versus-leukemia effect and improves chances for longer remissions. Patients should be offered information about the tradeoffs of the various treatment options and given the opportunity to share in the treatment option decision. See Chapter 9, *Transplantation*.

Splenectomy. Removal of the spleen may be required for patients experiencing platelet destruction or physical discomfort if the spleen is enlarged. Although removing the spleen may increase patient comfort, removal has not improved patient survival statistics.

CML treatments in trials

The following drugs are currently in clinical trials, being considered as effective treatments for CML.

Homoharringtonine (HHT). Homoharringtonine is a plant alkaloid, an extract of tree bark. It is being used in clinical trials with INF-alfa and/or Ara-C for CML. HHT alone induces remission in 72 percent of patients in late chronic-phase CML. It also induces genetic responses in 30 percent of the patients. About 5 percent have a complete response. Combinations of HHT plus Ara-C, and HHT plus IFN-alfa were given to patients who were intensively treated and unresponsive to IFN-alfa alone. The resulting response rate was about 65 percent.[5]

Tyrosine kinase inhibitor. Tyrosine kinase inhibitors, another new treatment option for CML, offer a less toxic approach for those who do not respond well to IFN-alfa. The Philadelphia chromosome, so often found in CML patients, involves the fusion of the ABL oncogene to the BCR gene, producing tyrosine kinase. That kinase is capable of inducing leukemia in mice, which implicates this protein as the cause of CML. The hypothesis is that inhibiting BCR/ABL kinase will most likely prevent the growth of leukemic cells during the chronic phase of CML.

STI571. STI571, an experimental drug, produced a 100 percent remission rate in advanced CML patients in Phase I trials. STI571 inhibits a specific protein necessary for growth of Philadelphia chromosome leukemia cells. All of the 31 patients taking STI571 saw their white blood counts return to normal levels, according to researchers reporting at the 91st annual meeting of the American Association for Cancer Research (AACR).

Treatment for accelerated phase of CML

Autologous bone marrow or stem cell transplantation (ABMT), using the patient's own cells, may return the patient to the chronic phase with the possibility of a durable remission. One problem with ABMT is that malignant cells may be reinfused. In addition, there is no graft-versus-leukemia effect (the graft cells from the donor fighting the leukemic cells of the patient or host), so remission time is shorter. ABMT is most successful in the chronic phase and less successful in the accelerated and blastic phases.

While a third of CML patients are candidates for bone marrow transplants, the rest have to rely on interferon-alfa. IFN-alfa treatment provides a lower response rate than bone marrow transplants, but durable responses and suppression of leukemic cells have occasionally been reported. Chemotherapy treatments normally used for acute leukemias have also been used with inconsistent results. Continued treatment with hydroxyurea and/or busulfan may also be used along with supportive transfusions of blood and platelets.

Treatment for the blastic phase of CML

The blastic phase of CML is acute leukemia. It may be lymphoid or myeloid. Patients with lymphoid blast crisis (about one-fourth of the cases) have a higher response rate to treatment, although the responses tend to be short-term.

When blast crisis occurs (often accompanied by fever, enlarged spleen, and increased blast cells in the peripheral blood), treatment is usually unsuccessful. Treatment with vincristine and prednisone can work with some patients (about 25 percent of CML patients) whose lymphoblastic cells are positive to the enzyme terminal deoxynucleotidyl transferase (TdT). Sometimes an anthracycline, such as daunorubicin, is added to the therapy combination to improve response.

Clinical trials are ongoing for the use of 5-azacitidine and mitoxantrone alone or in combination to treat CML. STI571 is also in trials for patients in blastic as well as in chronic stages. Patients in accelerated and blastic phases of CML are encouraged to participate in clinical trials since the existing treatments are usually unsuccessful. See Chapter 10 for new possibilities.

Meningeal CML

Meningeal CML is diagnosed when the CML cells have infiltrated the spinal fluid and the brain. Treatment options for meningeal CML include intrathecal (within the spinal canal) methotrexate, intrathecal cytarabine, or cranial irradiation.

Relapsing CML post BMT

CML relapse, following allogeneic BMT, sometimes can be reversed by discontinuing graft-versus-host (GVH) therapy. When GVH therapy is stopped, graft-versus-leukemia effects can combat the relapse because the donor's cells are able to battle the host's leukemic cells, causing the relapse.

Treatment with interferon alfa, performance of a second bone marrow transplant, or infusion of leukocytes that come from the original transplant donor are other methods of fighting relapse. Leukocyte infusion, without additional chemotherapy, works well with about three-quarters of the patients who experience molecular remission during the chronic phase. The infusion of lymphocytes from the original marrow donor (donor lymphocyte infusion) often reinduces complete remission in a high percentage of BMT patients. Unfortunately, this treatment is far less effective with advanced blastic disease.

Refractory CML

Many individual and combination chemotherapy treatments have been used unsuccessfully for refractory CML. But don't give up hope because there are new clinical trials underway that may help give you a new lease on life. See Chapter 10 for more information.

Chronic lymphocytic leukemia (CLL)

Chronic lymphocytic leukemia is the most common form of adult leukemia in the western world. It is considered a disease of older men, but more young people and women have been diagnosed with CLL in recent years. Nevertheless, most cases involve people over 55. CLL is different from other leukemias in that it does not generally turn into an acute leukemia. However, it can transform into a lymphoma, and it permits the longest period of watchful waiting as standard treatment. Watchful waiting means that blood counts are tracked and symptoms watched for, but there is no other treatment until the patient is showing annoying symptoms. While watchful waiting may not feel like much of a "treatment" to some newly diagnosed patients, it has been used because it is better (in terms of survival time and quality of life) than beginning treatment earlier. Presently, there is discussion among leading practitioners treating CLL to consider earlier treatment. The situation at present is still tilted toward the watchful waiting protocol.

CLL patients are very likely to be plagued by infections that tend to hang on. They often have compromised immune systems, so treatment of anything they catch or that develops, such as an infection, can last longer. Early recognition of infections and proper treatment are keys to patient survival.

Acute hemolytic anemia, immune thrombocytopenia (abnormally low platelets), and depressed immunoglobulin may occur in patients at any stage of

CLL. Some patients report recurring sinus infections, and some report bone and joint pain. Treatment may include corticosteroids such as prednisone or dexamethasone to control the autoimmune destruction of the blood prior to chemotherapy. Such patients may be difficult to transfuse with red blood cells or platelets. Alternate therapy procedures include high-dose immune globulin, cyclosporine, low-dose radiation of the spleen, or removal of the spleen. Tumor lysis syndrome, often seen in non-Hodgkin's lymphoma following chemotherapy, is uncommon in CLL. There are, however, early reports of fludarabine and Rituxan causing tumor lysis syndrome (characterized by symptoms of kidney failure) in a minute number of patients with extremely high white counts.

Herpes zoster viral infection (shingles) is associated in CLL patients with a lack of gammaglobulin and the inability to defend against bacterial or viral agents. Pneumonia caused by *Pneumocystis carinii*, a protozoan, and fungal infections caused by *Candida albicans* are often problems. Treatment with IV immunoglobulins in patients who have compromised immune systems is sometimes effective. Currently, the supply of IV immunoglobulin is scarce and is hard to obtain in the United States and Canada. Although this expensive treatment helps control the infections, it does not improve survival.

Treatment options range from early stage "watch and wait" and treatment of infections and immunologic complications to a constantly evolving variety of experimental therapies. CLL is normally slow to progress, and is not officially curable (although we know of one young CLL patient, ten years post autologous bone marrow transplant, who was tentatively declared "cured" in October, 1999). Treatment used to be conservative, done only to control symptoms, but recently it has become more aggressive and varied, looking toward cure.

First-line treatments include the chemotherapy drugs classified as purine analogues and alkylating agents. Research has shown fludarabine phosphate (Fludara) to be as effective alone, in untreated patients, as when combined with other drugs. Fludarabine is combined with the alkylator cyclophosphamide (Cytoxan) for therapy once patients relapse after previous treatment, or it can be combined with the antitumor antibiotic, mitoxantrone (Novantrone). The purine analogue 2-CdA (cladribine, Leustatin) is also used, and so is pentostatin (2-deoxycoformycin). The long-time standard drug is chlorambucil (Leukeran), an alkylator that has been used for at least 30 years. It may be combined with prednisone. None of these drugs are curative.

Other combinations of chemotherapy are also used with CLL.

The anthracyclines, such as doxorubicin (Adriamycin), are used in combination with drugs such as cyclophosphamide (Cytoxan) and prednisone, creating the combination called CAP; but less than 45 percent of patients using this treatment achieve complete remission and they require continued therapy with cyclophosphamide and prednisone to maintain the remission. The drug combination called CHOP (for cyclophosphamide, doxorubicin, vincristine [Oncovin], and prednisone) is often used in the later stages. Other combinations less frequently used are ESHAP (etoposide, methylprednisolone, with high-dose cytarabine/cisplatin) and BEAM (carmustine, etoposide/cytarabine, and melphalan). All three of these combinations are frequently used for non-Hodgkin's lymphoma as well. Secondary malignancies, and treatment-induced acute leukemias, occur in a small percentage of cases. Development of PLL or transformation of CLL to diffuse, large cell lymphoma, known as Richter's syndrome, carries a poorer prognosis, but with today's aggressive combination chemotherapy regimens, some patients live for five years or more after transformation.

Treatment recommendations and patient experiences can vary widely for CLL, depending on the stage, precise diagnosis, and a host of individual factors. The only consistent thing one can say about CLL is that it is a most inconsistent disease. The following stories illustrate some of the variations in recommended treatment options that CLL patients may be offered by their doctors. In each case other CLL patients have echoed the information provided.

A wife describes the arduous course of her husband's CLL treatment:

> James is 56 years old and was diagnosed with the presence of swollen nodes. He was first treated with chlorambucil and prednisone and then with fludarabine. His platelet counts continued to fall following one treatment of fludarabine.
>
> His local oncologist recommended removing his spleen. So we did it. His platelet count rebounded and was over 400,000 before he left the hospital, but unfortunately, the white count also shot up. James then headed to the cancer center, M. D. Anderson, where he was started on fludarabine and cyclophosphamide, followed by a daily shot of GM-CSF. His counts responded well. The cancer in his marrow was reduced from 96 percent to 50 percent.

He had six months off treatment, and then his doctor wanted him to try the Campath clinical trial to try to knock out what was left. He was treated with Campath from July to the first part of August. He started with a 3-mg dose and then was bumped to 10 mg, three times a week. His counts held very well, but in September of this year he noticed a lymph node growing in his neck again. It was biopsied in October, and the biopsy revealed that his CLL had transformed into Richter's syndrome. Now his doctor says he is going to treat James as if he had acute leukemia. He is hoping for some good results this time in Houston—something long lasting.

Beth's treatment experience with CLL was different:

I was given a standard dose of fludarabine (25 mg/m2) administered intravenously, via a central venous catheter, for five consecutive days, over a total of eight 28-day cycles (September to April). Side effects were minimal, and I was able to continue my normal teaching and research schedule at the university. I did experience some uncomfortable, but bearable, headaches during the week of treatment and arranged for my treatments to be administered in the late afternoon after my classes were over so that I could go straight home. I also had a nasty bout of shingles following six cycles of treatment, but experienced no other viral, bacterial, or fungal infections.

This treatment was followed in June by four standard Rituxan infusions (375 mg/m2) administered over five to six hours one day a week for four consecutive weeks. My only negative response to this was a slight fever that lasted several weeks.

Linda was diagnosed with CLL/SLL. CLL/SLL is a very common diagnosis at first until the oncologist sees which way it goes. Some patients never lose the CLL/SLL diagnosis. SLL is small lymphocytic lymphoma and the big difference between the two diagnoses is that CLL remains mostly in the bone marrow, while SLL is mostly in the lymph system. Linda describes her understanding of CLL/SLL and the watch-and-wait treatment recommended for her at this time.

I was diagnosed yesterday with CLL/SLL as a result of four blood tests over a period of two months and a recent bone marrow biopsy. I'm a "very healthy" 55-year-old—no symptoms, caught only because of my routine annual exam. Originally the doctor thought it was probably CLL, though there were a few weird blood results that made him do the bone marrow biopsy. So this is a new wrinkle, so to speak, and I can find far less information on the Internet on CLL/SLL.

The doctor was very positive about prognosis. However, he did say that he wants to see me every three months with the SLL addition instead of only every six months with "classic" CLL. That way he can see which direction it goes clinically over the years: SLL or CLL. He says, "Great drugs to treat/control when needed, so don't worry, just continue your healthy lifestyle and live as if you were well." I like that!

Hub Kennedy tells of the watch-and-wait treatment recommendation for his wife's diagnosis of smoldering CLL.

When we returned from vacation, on about June 23rd, Monta (age 41) had scheduled a removal of what we thought was a cyst—a 1 1/2 centimeter node under her arm. Much to our dismay, and what has been an earth-shattering event, she was diagnosed June 28th with SLL.

Her blood work was within normal limits. Then, the flow cytometry said CLL.

We went to M. D. Anderson yesterday to meet with Dr. Susan O'Brien. After a day of testing, and looking at the B2M markers, Dr. O'Brien told us to go home. She said, "I know you don't want to hear this—but ignore this for now." She further told us that Monta's level of 1.6 on the Beta 2 Micro-globulin test was among the lowest she had ever seen, and that as a prog-nosticator, it told her that Monta's presentation was that of a smoldering CLL. It may be five or ten years before treatment.

Apparently, Dr. O'Brien is also doing a chromosome prognosticator check.

Karin Laasko credits removal of her spleen after an automobile accident with why she is still alive fourteen years after a diagnosis with aggressive CLL:

I was diagnosed with aggressive CLL fourteen years ago. That I'm still around is considered quite a mystery. (One that I'll gladly accept.) I am now in Stage II, although I no longer have an enlarged spleen to prove it.

I was in a severe auto accident five years ago, lacerating my spleen. (When you hear the surgeon say, "I don't think we can save her," it's not

reassuring!) Losing my spleen at that time has been something of a bless-
ing in disguise. I had been about to start chemotherapy for low counts.

Splenectomy is known to help low counts temporarily. But, no one
has heard of five years. It's not a cure, but has bought me some time.

Currently my white count is about 100,000 (once 280,000) and I
have never had chemotherapy. My hematocrit and platelets are back up
within normal limits.

I have never had more than the smallest lymph nodes palpable. I do
have a poor immune system. I am actually immunocompromised on three
fronts: CLL, congenital immune deficiency and, of course, no spleen. I
noticed problems six months before diagnosis. My IgG level was below
normal at diagnosis. I am maintained using intravenous immunoglobulin
every four weeks.

Remission criteria for CLL

According to the NCI-sponsored Working Group Guidelines for Response
Criteria in CLL, complete remission requires all of the following for a period
of at least two months:

- Absence of enlarged lymph nodes
- Absence of enlarged spleen and liver
- Absence of constitutional symptoms
- Normal complete blood count (CBC) as exhibited by:
  - Neutrophils greater than or equal to 1,500 per microliter of blood
  - Platelets greater than 100,000 per microliter of blood
  - Hemoglobin greater than 11 grams per 100 milliliters of blood

Bone marrow aspirate and biopsy should be performed two months after all
of the previously listed requirements have been met. Less than 30 percent of
the nucleated cells in the marrow sample must be lymphocytes. Lymphoid
nodules should be absent.

Treatment based upon CLL staging systems

Treatment for CLL is based upon the stage at which one is diagnosed. The
stages listed here include the combined Rai and Binet systems.

Stage 0 CLL. Stage 0 CLL is usually not treated. The patient is watched to see how the disease progresses. Doctors call this the "watch and wait" stage, but some patients, call it "watch and worry." Studies show that there is no survival advantage for starting therapy before it is needed.

Stage I CLL. In some situations, Stage I CLL will be treated by chemotherapy. Or it may require no treatment yet.

Primary treatment options include the purine analogues fludarabine phosphate (Fludara) and 2-chlorodeoxyadenosine (2-CdA, cladribine) or 2-deoxycoformycin (pentostatin, Nipent).

Other possibilities include treatment with alkylating agents such as chlorambucil (Leukeran) or cyclophosphamide (Cytoxan) in standard doses with or without corticosteroids (prednisone or prednisolone).

When treating patients with large lymph node masses, saline solution and allopurinol are suggested before therapy to protect the kidneys.

Some patients benefit from field-radiation therapy, receiving relatively low doses of radiation therapy to organs like an enlarged spleen or swollen lymph nodes.

Stage II CLL. Stage II CLL may still include watch and wait in asymptomatic patients.

Combination therapy using fludarabine and cyclophosphamide has been used successfully. The synergy in this combination appears to be more effective than treatment with either drug alone in previously treated patients. Fludarabine has also been used in combination with mitoxantrone (Novantrone); that combination is known for turning urine bright blue for a few hours following therapy.

Fludarabine combined with biological response modifiers such as filgrastim (G-CSF) and sargramostim (GM-CSF) has been used. Combination therapy with fludarabine and the monoclonal antibodies (MoAbs) Rituxan and Campath-1H has undergone trials for leukemias. The FDA has approved Rituxan for use with NHL, and Campath is awaiting approval. Rituxan, given alone, shows some activity in CLL, and used in combination with other drugs, may be more promising. Other biological therapies are also under clinical evaluation. Patients with Stage II to Stage IV CLL may wish to consider participating in clinical trials.

Stage III and IV CLL. Stages III and IV usually require treatment, although some patients attempt to put off starting therapy by using leukapheresis (removal of selected white blood cells) to reduce very high white counts.

Any of the previously listed therapies for Stage II may be employed for Stage III and IV patients as well. CHOP (cyclophosphamide, doxorubicin, vincristine, and prednisone) is also part of the anti-CLL arsenal, although analysis shows no benefit from CHOP when there is bulky disease. Stem cell transplantation, autologous or allogeneic, is sometimes considered at this stage. Various treatment centers are reporting encouraging results with all types of transplants, bone marrow and peripheral blood stem cell, and cord blood as well. See Chapter 9 for more complete information.

Refractory CLL

With refractory CLL, clinical trials should be considered where possible. Bone marrow transplantation may also be considered.

The following patient story describes use of high-dose methyl prednisone (HDMP) to treat refractory CLL. The drug is given "pulsed," which means it is given rapidly for several days to a week, followed by a rest period of several weeks. This is not chemotherapy *per se*, but it is used to control the growth of leukemia cells:

> About five months ago I started my first ever treatment with a steroid. The treatment was "pulsed" high dose methyl prednisolone (HDMP) (IV) at 1 gm/m2. For me, it worked out at 2 grams per day, which is a lot. It was given for 5 days, and was repeated at intervals of 28 days. After five courses and some good results we decided to stop. My bone marrow infiltration went down from 68 percent to 18 percent and my extensive abdominal lymphadenopathy has all but disappeared. Luckily, the side effects were temporary and did not trouble me to any extent.

> According to my information, HDMP has only been tried in advanced and end-stage CLL. It is a harsh treatment and the patient needs to be closely monitored. The attraction for me was the HDMP's reputation in dealing with lymph nodes and I am more than pleased with the results in that department. Before the treatment started we established that my CLL was sensitive to it by using a special test called DiSC assay. I would not have gone ahead if I weren't likely to benefit.

The DiSC assay (differential staining cytotoxicity) is described in Chapter 4, *Tests and Procedures*.

Adult T-cell leukemia (ATL)

ATL is a newly classified, separate disease with several phases. It is a rare disorder, but treatment options are growing. This disease is caused by exposure to the human T-cell lymphotropic virus type 1 (HTLV-1) and transmitted during birth from mother to child. The disease is also passed along by blood transfusions or blood exposure.

Acute T-cell leukemia

Acute T-cell leukemia is generally treated with combination chemotherapy. Complete remission rates have risen from 16 percent with a four-drug combination to 43 percent with an eight-drug combination. Survival rates have not increased, however, with median survival time still at eight months at time of writing.

Smoldering or chronic ATL

The smoldering or chronic form of ATL has a longer natural course and may be negatively impacted by aggressive chemotherapy. Alternative strategies are needed for these patients. Regardless of the specific chemotherapy used, the inevitable impairment of T-cell function places the patient at high risk for infections.

Most ATL patients have been treated with CHOP (cyclophosphamide, doxorubicin, Oncovin [vincristine] and prednisone). Although ATL in the acute stage often is not responsive to this combination chemotherapy, smoldering and lymphoma types respond better. Studies appear to show that sometimes, higher doses, given more frequently in the acute stage, are better. Treatment protocols often include VEPA (vincristine, doxorubicin, prednisone, and cyclophosphamide).

Potential treatment possibilities for ATL

Treatments for ATL continue to evolve. Other treatments presently in clinical trials include the adenosine deaminase inhibitor pentostatin (2-deoxycoformycin) and the monoclonal antibody anti-Tac. Two patients treated only with etoposide showed complete remissions lasting three and twelve months. Recent reports of the presence of interleukin-2 receptors in ATL cell samples, have encouraged treatment with interleukin-2. Another possibility is the use of diphtheria toxin, which appears to be very lethal to ATL cells. Promising results of clinical trials with interferon-alfa and zidovudine are encouraging to researchers at this time as well.[6] For further information, see the references listed in the "Notes" section at the end of this book.

Prolymphocytic leukemia (PLL)

Prolymphocytic leukemia (PLL) is a rare lymphoproliferative disorder that takes a rapidly progressive course. Therapeutic interventions are often unsuccessful. Treatment for prolymphocytic leukemia is generally the same as for CLL.

There are B-PLL and T-PLL subtypes. Less than 20 percent of patients with B-PLL respond to treatment with chlorambucil or COP (cyclophosphamide, vincristine and prednisone). About 50 percent respond to treatment with CHOP (cyclophosphamide, doxorubicin, vincristine, and prednisone), but remissions are short lived. Low-dose splenic irradiation has proven effective with some patients. The purine analogues, cladribine (2-deoxycoformycin), fludarabine and pentostatin, have been used with better success.

Possible future treatments for PLL

Promising responses to Campath-1H have been described for those with T-PLL, whose median prognosis for survival is only seven months at present. An effective schedule for treatment of T-PLL may well be Cladribine (2CdA), followed by Campath-1H in patients who achieve only partial responses or whose leukemia does not respond to 2-CdA. An alternate approach may include Campath-1H as first-line therapy. A stem cell transplant in young adult patients may offer the possibility of cure.

Richter's transformation

Richter's transformation is characterized by a change in the leukemic cells to large cell lymphoma, which is aggressive and difficult to treat. Treatment for Richter's transformation is basically the same as for non-Hodgkin's lymphoma. The combination of drugs known as CHOP (cyclophospha-mide, doxorubicin, vincristine, and prednisone) has been used with some success. Most patients with Richter's fail to respond to standard therapy used for large granulocytic leukemia and acute myelogenous leukemia.

Hairy cell leukemia (HCL)

Highly effective treatments have been developed in the last ten years for hairy cell leukemia (HCL). The accepted indications for treatment are signifi-cant deficiency of various types of blood cells, life-threatening infections, and symptomatic enlargement of the spleen. At present, asymptomatic patients with mild cell deficiencies and minimal spleen enlargement may be watched, but not treated immediately. Treatment for HCL is sometimes offered to asymptomatic patients with few cancer cells present.

Splenectomy for HCL

Since an enlarged spleen is one of the major concerns in HCL, splenectomy (the removal of the spleen) was originally the first treatment for this disease. Splenectomy can result in improvement in up to 90 percent of patients. Nor-malization of the blood counts occurs after splenectomy in 40 to 77 percent of patients, and has been shown to prolong survival. Nevertheless, new and improved treatments have made splenectomy almost obsolete.

Chemotherapy for HCL

The most successful treatments for hairy cell leukemia today are the purine nucleoside analogues. Cladribine (2-chlorodeoxyadenosine, 2-CdA) or Pen-tostatin (2-deoxycoformycin or DCF), are the most effective of these. Cladribine is given intravenously for five days in an outpatient setting. Pen-tostatin is given weekly by IV bolus, or as an IV infusion over a twenty-minute period. Both are well tolerated by patients, with no nausea, vomit-ing, hair loss, renal dysfunction, or neurotoxicity. A single course of either drug induces complete remission in the majority of patients with HCL. Pen-tostatin and 2-CdA have become the first-line treatments of choice for HCL. Testing is being done to create an oral form of these drugs. Relapsing patients may be given another course of the same treatment after a single treatment if the initial remission has been long.

The following patient talks about a typically positive response to 2-CdA for his HCL:

> Once the diagnosis was definite, and we knew that treatment was required, my doctor suggested that I be treated with Cladribine. He said it was a drug that was showing almost curative results with this disease. Who could resist such a wonderful possibility when treatment was inevitable anyhow?
>
> On Monday afternoon I went into the treatment room in the doctor's office and the nurse hooked me up to the battery-operated pump. There was no nausea at all, and once I became used to it, no real problems either. I didn't lose any more hair—my male pattern baldness doesn't count here. I stayed home from work the first time, just to make sure things would go well, but there were no side effects, although I had been warned to expect that my cell counts might drop suddenly, and I'd feel fatigued.
>
> Today I'm feeling wonderful and showing no signs of HCL. I sure hope that it stays that way.

Fludarabine phosphate, another purine analogue, has proven effective for CLL but has not been well tested for HCL. There are also some patients who do well with interferon alfa treatment. Multiple trials have shown the effectiveness of interferon alfa in creating partial remissions, but it is not as effective at this time as the purine analogues.

Splenic lymphoma with villous lymphocytes (SLVL)

Splenic lymphoma with villous lymphocytes (SLVL) is an indolent (slowly developing) disorder with survival rates of seven to ten years. It is considered a lymphoma variant of CLL and hairy cell leukemia. SLVL has a chronic course, which, in a minority (10 percent of patients) does not require any therapeutic intervention. Rarely, slow regression of the splenomegaly (abnormal enlargement of the spleen) may occur. Treatment is indicated when there are symptoms of anemia or, occasionally, sweating, excessive fatigue, or progressive lymphocytosis (increase of lymphocytes in the blood).

Splenectomy (removal of the spleen) is the treatment of choice in this disease unless surgery is prohibited by other health considerations. Splenectomy results in correction of the large spleen problem, reduction of the lymphocyte count, and improvement in well-being in the majority of patients.

The effects of splenectomy are often long-term, ranging from six months to more than ten years. When splenectomy is contraindicated for clinical reasons, low-dose irradiation of the spleen may give good responses. Single agent chemotherapy is not usually effective, although some responses may be observed. Chemotherapy with fludarabine may also be useful. Because the survival of patients with SLVL may be very prolonged, one needs to be cautious about initiating therapy. The median survival can be greater than 6 years.[6]

Some patients with SLVL respond well to alkylators (a type of chemotherapy drug) such as chlorambucil and/or cyclophosphamide, with or without steroids like prednisone. Interferon alfa also has been used to treat this disease. Recent reports indicate good responses for some patients taking fludarabine. However, some SLVL patients are resistant to interferon alfa and chlorambucil.

CHAPTER 9

Transplantation

Having a marrow or stem cell transplant is one of the riskiest and most intense forms of treatment for leukemia. Being knowledgeable and well prepared makes the journey much easier and less frightening.

Chemotherapy treatments control some leukemias, but many patients cannot be cured by chemotherapy alone. After a while, the positive results of chemotherapy begin to fade and symptoms reappear. For some patients, this is the time to look into the possibility of a bone marrow transplant. Other patients know from the beginning that they will soon need a bone marrow transplant. For these patients, chemotherapy represents a holding pattern until they can reduce the tumor burden and become eligible for transplantation.

Most leukemia patients must be put into remission before bone marrow transplantation can go forward. However, some centers will transplant a patient who is not in remission if there is need for it and if the patient meets established criteria.

A bone marrow transplantation procedure is not the answer for every patient due to age, other complicating medical conditions, general state of health, or lack of donor match for those using donor cells. But for many patients, transplantation offers the best possibility of a cure. It is also a rather daunting treatment, and many are unwilling to consider it because they do not understand it.

This chapter explains the many facets of bone marrow transplants. We first describe several basics: why transplants are done, how transplants originated, why results are improving, and what the terminology means. We next look at the various types of transplants used for leukemia, along with the potential benefits and problems associated with each. We then look at the total experience of transplantation: considerations for patients thinking about a transplant and the general steps of treatment including, what you might expect. We describe what life may be like post-transplant, and discuss follow-up care, length of recovery, and possible long-term effects. The chapter ends with a description of becoming a donor.

Bone marrow transplant basics

Bone marrow transplantation uses high doses of chemotherapy, sometimes in combination with total body irradiation, to kill off diseased cells. Unfortunately, a major side effect of such high-dose therapy is that the normal stem cells in the bone marrow—the cells that produce most of the body's normal blood cells—are also destroyed. Without adequate supplies of healthy blood cells, the body cannot fight infection, supply tissues with oxygen, or control bleeding.

To replace the diseased bone marrow and to give the patient a supply of healthy cells, stem cells are infused through a catheter in a large vein near the chest. The usual source of stem cells is bone marrow, which has a rich supply. Alternatively, stem cells may be coaxed out of the bone marrow into the bloodstream, where they can be collected and used for transplant. In some cases, stem cells from an umbilical cord are used.

Cancer cells divide constantly. High-dose chemotherapy kills off these rapidly dividing cells. When bone marrow is affected, the patient is unable to produce the normal cells needed to keep the body functioning. Bone marrow and stem cell transplants replace damaged cells with healthy stem cells that can produce normal blood cells. Not all leukemia patients undergo transplant using donor cells. Some undergo transplantation using their own cells.

Background and statistics

Statistics in the US indicate that 20,000 people are currently alive five years after having a bone marrow transplant (BMT) for hematological malignancies. They likely wouldn't be here today if BMT weren't available. In Europe, marrow transplantation has been performed in 24,000 cases of acute leukemia, 9,800 cases of chronic leukemia, 2,700 cases of myelodysplastic syndrome, and 460 cases of chronic lymphocytic leukemia. Results have improved dramatically due to the decrease in treatment-related mortality associated with allogeneic transplantation (transplants from a donor). The treatment-related mortality for allogeneic transplants done prior to 1987 was 40 to 45 percent; since 1987 it has dropped to 20 to 25 percent. These numbers are averages; the risk of mortality varies according to age, stage of disease, general health, and a host of other factors.

The relapse rates following transplantation, by leukemia type, appear to be unchanged over this time period. The five-year leukemia-free survival for acute myelogenous leukemia is more than 60 percent. With allogeneic transplant for acute lymphoblastic leukemia, the leukemia-free survival is 55 percent at five years. The changing trends in transplantation for leukemia, such as the use of low-intensity conditioning regimens (using less high-dose chemotherapy and eliminating total body irradiation) with donor lymphocyte infusions (see the explanation later in this chapter) as part of the protocol, are being studied carefully to see what difference they make in both mortality and survival rates.

While leukemia-free survival numbers are the most encouraging statistic, they can also be misleading. Most patients will assume that a five-year leukemia-free survival of 60 percent means that of 100 patients who were transplanted, 60 were alive and disease-free five years after treatment. This is incorrect. Such a leukemia-free survival number means that of those who were in remission following the transplant, 60 percent remained alive and disease-free five years later. So, if only 60 of the 100 patients transplanted were in remission after transplant, and 60 percent of those were alive and disease-free five years later, that means that only 36 percent of those 100 patients transplanted were alive and disease-free five years later.

Transplantation is most successful when used as a first-line treatment. In the case of some leukemias, chemo is followed by more chemo, and only when that fails does the doctor talk about transplant. While this is certainly true in some instances, it is not true in all. For some patients, transplant is a first line, or near first-line, treatment of choice.

Oncologists have struggled for years with what to do when a leukemia patient does not respond to chemotherapy or other available treatments. Large doses of chemotherapeutic drugs deplete needed normal blood cells as well as cancer cells. Ultimately, the patient becomes anemic, and the blood cells in the bone marrow begin to fail. One response to this is a bone marrow transplant. However, in many cases, patients who reach this stage are very poor candidates for a transplant. Patients with AML, for example, who fail to respond to prior chemotherapy or come out of remission, usually have a poorer prognosis than those who are not heavily pre-treated and who remain in remission. CML patients in blast crisis have a poorer prognosis than those treated earlier in the progression of their disease. (Blast crisis is the phase of chronic myelogenous leukemia in which the number of immature, abnormal white blood cells in the bone marrow and blood is extremely high.)

The technology of bone marrow transplants has evolved over time. In the early 1950s, researchers studying mice discovered that the bone marrow could regenerate itself after a nearly fatal dose of radiation if some of the marrow was saved before treatment and reinjected a few days later. By the end of the 1960s researchers knew more about the importance of white blood cell compatibility and began to use marrow transplantation to treat some leukemias and lymphomas. BMT then was considered the last resort in treating cancers but in the last ten years it has been used more widely to treat many diseases. Protocols have become easier for patients to handle and mortality rates have declined. BMT is now considered a standard treatment for several leukemias and lymphomas, and is used with most forms of leukemia—either as standard, secondary, or experimental treatment.

Transplantation involves potentially serious risks and should be done at established centers. When considering a center, ask how many transplants have been done there and the success rates using the kind of transplant you are considering for your subtype of leukemia.

Donor matching and haplotyping

Most patients with leukemia undergo an allogeneic transplant—a transplant using donor marrow or stem cells. When you receive a donor's bone marrow cells after yours have been killed off by high-dose chemotherapy, the success of the transplant depends in large part on how well those donor cells are matched to yours and how your immune system responds to them. A closer match of white blood cell characteristics is required for marrow or stem cell transplantation than for other organ transplants, because it is the immune system itself that is being transplanted.In order for a graft to be accepted or for graft-versus-host disease (GVHD) not to be serious, the donor and patient must have a closely matched marrow type. Donor tissue must be checked before the transplant. Historically, marrow matches are determined by looking at protein markers on the surface of white blood cells called antigens. There are many antigens on white blood cells, but those critical for matching are HLA-A, HLA-B, HLA-C, and HLA-DR.The HLA antigens will determine acceptance or rejection by recognizing and accepting similar tissue but attacking foreign white blood cells. Too small a dose of infused stem cells may result in graft failure (when new cells don't grow), graft rejection (when the recipient's cells reject the donor's cells), or a serious disease called graft-versus-host disease (GVHD), in which the donor's white blood cells attack the recipient's body organs.

Certain genes on chromosome 6 control the HLA antigens on which donors and recipients are matched. The genes that come together on that one chromosome make a haplotype. Each person has two copies of each of these haplotypes—one copy inherited from each parent. So one haplotype for tissue typing is made of the A, B, and DR HLA antigens from the mother and the other is made up of the A, B, DR HLA antigens from the father. This means that there are double the amount of sites that must match.

Within these haplotypes are subtypes of almost inestimable variation. High-resolution DNA typing shows more subtle differences in genetic makeup. Newer DNA technology has enabled doctors to determine, with even greater accuracy, whether or not a donor is a good match. These newer techniques hopefully will reduce the incidence of GVHD and graft rejection.

Currently, six to ten antigens are tested, depending on the laboratory. An increasing number of antigens will be measured in the future, as other genes are discovered that have a bearing on tissue rejection. You might hear matching success referred to as a 6-out-of-6 match or a 4-out-of-6 match, abbreviated as 6/6 and 4/6. Since you inherit half of your genes from each parent, the most likely person to match you is a sibling who has inherited the same sets of genes. Matching other family members is, to some extent, a roll of Mother Nature's dice. Each sibling has a one in four chance of being HLA identical. Therefore, the odds of having a sibling match increase with the number of siblings you have. Fortunately, on some occasions, a match can be found among first cousins. On rare occasions, extended family members have served as donors, although an unrelated donor is often a better option. If there is not a match available within the family, it may be possible to find an unrelated donor. The number of Caucasians who are matched by the National Marrow Donation Program (NMDP) these days is approximately 85 percent.

Other ethnic groups have a more difficult problem finding matched donors because fewer volunteers sign up. This is partly because the population segment is smaller to begin with, and there is a lower percentage of volunteers within the various ethnic groups. It is important to note that there are fewer possible matches for some ethnic groups because there is not enough awareness of the problem. This means that NMDP's pool of 3 million donors is not equally useful for everyone. It's important to increase awareness of the need for marrow donors among ethnic groups. Friends and loved ones may join the NMDP by calling (800) MARROW-2. A blood sample only—not marrow—is required for donor testing.

Most transplant centers aim for a 6/6 match or better if an unrelated donor is used but will accept a 5/6 match with a related donor. A few centers will do transplantation using partially matched 3/6 or 4/6 related donors, and others are conducting clinical trials to improve partial-mismatch transplants. More detailed discussions of genetic inheritance and the calculation of odds of inheriting genes can be found in any textbook on genetics.

Types of cells transplanted

Progenitor stem cells are the most primitive type of stem cells. They reside in the marrow. They can self-replicate or produce myeloid stem cells and lymphoid stem cells. (This is described briefly in Chapter 1, *What Leukemia Is*. A longer, more technical discussion may be found in Appendix F, *Progression of Cell Development*.) The various types of blood cells evolve from these two kinds of stem cells. The progenitor myeloid and lymphoid stem cells can be moved (mobilized) from the bone marrow into the bloodstream. A few may be found in the bloodstream normally, but not a sufficient quantity for a harvest. Growth factors such as Epogen, Neupogen, and Neumega, whether given alone or with chemotherapy, are used to move the stem cells into the bloodstream.

Transplants can be done with cells from several sources. Replacing leukemic bone marrow with healthy bone marrow is called having a bone marrow transplant (BMT). If stem cells collected from the bloodstream are transplanted, the procedure is called a peripheral blood stem cell transplant (PBSCT). It may also be called a progenitor stem cell transplant (PSCT), a stem cell transplant, or a stem cell rescue. If stem cells from an umbilical cord are used in the transplant, the procedure is called a cord blood transplant or cord blood stem cell transplant.

Medical personnel and patients alike are not precise about terms when speaking of various kinds of transplants. To add to the confusion, all types are sometimes referred to as a bone marrow transplant.

Types of bone marrow transplants

There are different kinds of transplants depending on whose cells will be infused into the patient's body. Generally, if the patient's own stem cells are used in the transplant, the procedure is called an autologous transplant. If the stem cells used in the transplant are from a donor, the transplant is called an allogeneic transplant. However, if the donor is an identical twin, the transplant is called a syngeneic transplant.

Technically, a transplant involves receiving marrow or blood products from a donor. When the patient's own blood products are used, the procedure is more correctly called a marrow or stem cell rescue. It is also called an autograft. Nonetheless, most medical personnel and patients generally refer to both procedures as transplants.

Autologous transplants

An autologous transplant uses the patient's own cells. One may have an autologous bone marrow transplant (ABMT) or an autologous peripheral blood stem cell transplant (AuSCT). Following high-dose chemotherapy used to kill the remaining bone marrow, when the patient is in remission, the patient's own marrow is collected. The patient must have minimal cancer cells in the body for the autologous transplant to be successful. That means patients must first undergo chemotherapy to get into remission—to reduce the number of cancer cells in the blood and marrow. Bone marrow cells, taken from an individual by surgical procedure, are "harvested." Stem cells are apheresed—separated from the rest of the blood. Harvested cells may be used for an immediate transplant or stored for future use when the disease becomes active again. Few institutions have facilities to store cells for any length of time. In the past, bone marrow was the source of stem cells for autologous transplants. Today, however, most autologous transplants use stem cells collected from the bloodstream. However, if insufficient stem cells can be moved to the bloodstream, a bone marrow harvest may be needed.

In order for an autologous transplant to work, some treatment centers believe that the patient's blood cells must be separated, with most or all leukemic cells removed. However, there certainly have been patients who've been transplanted with unpurged bone marrow and have lived to tell about it. In fact, the question of whether to purge or not to purge leukemic cells is a major controversy.

As mentioned earlier, if stem cells are to be used in the transplant, they must be apheresed. Apheresis is a process that separates the blood by selecting out particular cells. In the case of transplants, the apheresis machine examines all the cells in the blood and selects only precursor (immature) cells, which will be given back to the patient later in the transplant process. The rest of the blood is returned unchanged to the patient.

For the process of apheresis, a needle is placed in each arm or in the catheter. Blood is removed from one side and goes through the apheresis equipment; what isn't selected is returned through the other side.

Autologous transplants are done following various protocols. Some protocols require the further process of purging the harvested cells before storing, to remove cancerous or preleukemic cells. How cells are identified to be removed varies by protocol, depending on which cells are suspect. The techniques used for purging also vary by protocol. Purging techniques include destroying cancerous cells (for example, monoclonal antibodies destroying cells expressing certain antigens) or separating and saving healthy cells (such as putting the cells through a CD34+ stem cell separator).

Although it might sound like an excellent idea to purge the collected white blood cells before putting them back into a patient's body, the question of purging is still under study. Lots of centers don't purge because it is not yet clear that purging actually improves survival rates. It may be residual leukemia in the patient—not tumor cells in the marrow—that cause relapse. The vast majority of harvested cells are not manipulated (purged) or treated with anything else.

Whether the collected cells are purged or not, after collection they are frozen at a very low temperature in a preservative, dimethylsulphoxide (DMSO), and stored until needed.

After the marrow/stem cells are harvested, the patient is given either high dose combination chemotherapy, or chemotherapy and radiation. After that the marrow/stem cells are reinfused. Depending on the protocol that is used, not everyone gets radiation

The following patient describes her experience with an autologous bone marrow transplant. Her protocol required high-dose chemotherapy and total body irradiation prior to the restoration of her own purged bone marrow cells:

> *The first two days my protocol called for high-dose Cytoxan to kill off what was left of my bone marrow. Since the next three days required total body irradiation, I was packaged securely into a wheelchair and pushed onto a special elevator to the radiation suite. There I was placed on a sailcloth bed with radiation equipment above and below me. My lungs were shielded, my favorite music was turned on, and I spent twenty minutes morning and afternoon being irradiated. I felt nothing at all. That went on for two-and-a-half days.*

Then the incontinence began and I was truly miserable. In addition, I had mouth sores (mucositis) and couldn't eat. Food had to be cooked until it was dry, and I had no saliva. I lost about 30 pounds, although that wasn't all bad, since I needed to lose it. The quality of nursing care was very high and I owe a great deal to the nurses on the unit.

I don't remember a lot about what went on the next few weeks. I do know that we watched anxiously for the white count to rise and the neutrophils to increase, until I reached the magic numbers that meant release.

I made it through, and now, over three years out, I show no signs of leukemia in my pathology reports. It was a long 25 days, but if I had to, I would do it again.

Autologous transplants are sometimes done on an outpatient basis. The patient is treated for twelve hours or so a day in the outpatient unit, then returns home or to lodging near the hospital to spend the night.

An autologous transplant recipient shares her thoughts looking back at a transplant that happened several years ago:

First, you should understand that everyone's transplant experience is different. For example, while I was in the transplant unit, there was a man in his twenties who was eating three square meals a day. All the rest of us were heaving our guts out.

Second, as transplant hospitals/staff gain more experience, the protocols change—sometimes dramatically. When I was at Dana-Farber, for an autologous transplant, the protocol did not use growth factors such as G-CSF (Granulocyte Colony Stimulating Factor, or "G," as the transplant team calls it). I received a single dose of G, but only because I was progressing slowly after my counts zeroed out. I talked to someone who went through the protocol two years later, and now everybody is getting it. That makes the hospital stay shorter (2 weeks versus my 31 days) and it shortens the recovery time as well.

Allogeneic transplants

When the patient has a donor to provide cells for the transplant it is called an *allogeneic* bone marrow or stem cell transplant. The term BMT means bone marrow transplant using someone else's cells; it is also used generically to mean the process of having the procedure. Allogeneic transplants are also known as allografts. They are the most common type of bone marrow transplant for leukemia in use today.

If the matching cell donor is a relative or a sibling, the transplant is called a matched related transplant. If the matched donor is not related, it is a matched unrelated (MUD) transplant. Sometimes the donor's cells are perfectly matched to the recipient; sometimes the only available donor is not quite a perfect match. Then one has a mismatched transplant or a partially mismatched transplant.

If an unrelated donor is used, white blood cell characteristics must be matched very carefully to reduce the chance of graft failure, graft rejection, or graft-versus-host disease (GVHD), which may result from immune system mismatches.

Given equally matched donors, fewer problems arise with a related donor, although the reasons this occurs are not well understood. Some centers have equal outcomes using matched related and matched unrelated donors. A related donor is a not necessarily superior if he or she is poorer quality match than an unrelated donor.

The preparation regimens for autologous and allogeneic transplants, at least as they pertain to chemotherapy and total body irradiation, are similar. However, for an allogeneic transplant, the patient's immune system is suppressed with immunosuppressant drugs to prevent the development of graft-versus-host disease. The addition of immunosuppressive drugs makes a big difference in patients' experiences.

Bob Farmer is a CML patient whose transplant was done seven years ago. He was fortunate enough to have his brother, John, as a fully matched, related donor (fully matched on those haplotypes which were known and tested for at that time). Still, he went through some difficulties:

> *I started my treatment the last week of August. There was a full week of testing and preparation for my BMT. I went through all the normal stuff, including having a catheter installed. On September 1, I was admitted into the Fred Hutchinson Cancer Research Center. My treatment was high-dose chemotherapy (cyclophosphamide and busulfan) for seven days with no total body irradiation. Then I was allowed a day off and the BMT was done on September 9.*

> I had some problems, but the allograft and the hospital stay went
> well. Then I had a major allergic reaction to the growth factor injection
> (GM-CSF). I felt as if I was going to die.

Gradually, after being taken off the growth factor injections, he began to improve:

> I did my daily exercises and watched TV. I could not read well but I
> tried to play with my laptop computer, write a few things, and track my
> investments and blood work. After a while, I was too shaky to type or think,
> so I didn't play with my laptop much. For a few days I had to use a cane to
> get around. I enjoyed showers. They were the major event of each day.

> The last week before being released as an inpatient, I would go for a
> walk outside and fly my fighter kites from the rooftop parking lots near
> the Hutch. The staff was impressed.

> I was released to my apartment a few blocks away on October 1. My
> wife and brother, Perry, had brought over all my things (computers and
> toys) and prepared the place the day before. I felt so good and strong that
> I went for a three-mile walk that day. A few days later I started to have
> bad stomach problems.

Bob then went through treatment for graft-versus-host disease (GVHD):

> On October 15, an endoscopy showed that I had Grade 2 GVHD of
> the gut. This was the beginning of several therapy cycles to treat GVHD
> using high-dose prednisone and cyclosporine. I was not able to eat or
> drink much, so I was on IVs. I quickly became very weak and could
> hardly walk. No more three-mile walks. I could barely walk the few
> blocks to the outpatient clinic.

> After being released, I spent most of my time trying to eat and drink
> enough to get off the IVs. It took me until October 25 to get off total
> parenteral nutrition IVs. Several times a day, and at night, I would throw
> up. This was the most uncomfortable thing for me after the BMT.

> November 11, after a final discharge conference, I was released to go
> home, taking with me a long list of instructions and medications.

> I spent the night before Thanksgiving in the hospital getting two units
> of blood transfused in order to get me through the holiday. My son, Dan,
> picked me up to bring me home just in time for Thanksgiving dinner. It

was my first visit with him since prior to my BMT. He had just arrived home from a tour of the Orient with his professional music group.

At my 80-day post BMT check-up in December, the bone marrow biopsy showed no Philadelphia chromosome, which was great news. The skin biopsy was GVHD positive. This was predictive of an 85 percent chance of chronic GVHD in the first two years after BMT. To be safe, I was entered into a six-month cyclosporine protocol to prevent GVHD.

Despite some hard times with chronic GVHD, today Bob is back at work, flies his hang glider again, and has good quality of life.

Some allogeneic protocols call for the removal of T cells, the presence of which are believed to cause engraftment problems after transplantation. There are a number of protocols now using selected T-cell depletion. T cells in donor marrow can trigger GVHD but removing them completely and causes an increase in graft rejections. Then it was discovered that T cells also appear to confer a graft-versus-leukemia effect so now they try to deplete only those types of T cells that cause GVHD, without removing those that confer the graft-versus-leukemia effect.

Mini-transplants (Non-myeloablative transplants)

The mini-transplant is a form of allogeneic transplant, although researchers are also evaluating autologous mini-transplants. The mini-transplant uses cells from a matched donor who may be related or unrelated to the patient. In this procedure, the patient's bone marrow is not totally wiped out in preparation for the transplant. Total body irradiation (TBI) is not used for some patients; for other patients, lower dose TBI has been called for in some of the protocols. In addition, the patient may be given just enough chemotherapy to allow the donor's bone marrow or stem cells to engraft in the patient.

If all goes as planned, the donor's T cells recognize the patient's leukemic cells as foreign, and mount a response against the leukemic cells. This is called the graft-versus-leukemia effect. Evidence for a graft-versus-leukemia effect is strong in some diseases—most notably CML, CLL, and myeloma—and weaker in other diseases, such as ALL. Therefore, mini-transplants are offered more for those diseases where there is a chance that the donor cells will create graft-versus-leukemia effect.

While the patient does receive chemotherapy, it is less toxic than the standard transplant regimen. The mini-transplant was devised to allow older patients to have transplants when they are needed. The mini-transplant is still controversial among various medical teams. While the risks in a mini-transplant may be less than in a standard allogeneic transplant, the risk of developing chronic graft-versus-host disease is still significant. For this reason, the mini-transplant is certainly not a minor undertaking as its name might suggest. Indeed, it should be viewed as having the same potential for long-term complications as a standard allogeneic transplant. However, it does allow the patient to go through the transplant with less exposure to high-dose chemotherapy and radiation.

Syngeneic transplants

A syngeneic transplant uses the cells of a perfectly matched identical twin who is willing to provide the donor marrow. For a long time this was considered the ideal transplant situation, because there was little likelihood of rejection and/or graft-versus-host disease. Recent clinical trials, however, show that some patients are more likely to relapse after syngeneic transplants than those who had matched related donor transplants, because there is almost no graft-versus-host effect (graft-versus-leukemia effect). It also appears that the genetic make up of the twins is so close that the host's (patient's) body may provide fertile ground for development of leukemia in the donor's newly infused cells.

Umbilical cord blood transplants

(Umbilical cord blood is rich in stem cells that develop into mature white blood cells, red blood cells, and platelets. More importantly, because a newborn child's white cells are not trained to attack anything including foreign tissue, the naive status of T cells in umbilical cord blood makes them ideal for transplantation) Graft-versus-host disease (GVHD) occurs after many cord blood transplants, and if new techniques for expanding cord blood samples for use in adults succeed, we'll probably see more.

In the last ten years, the public has been encouraged to donate or store umbilical cord blood, which previously was discarded just after childbirth. Storage for one's own use or donation to a cord blood bank make these products available for future use by you, your family, or others who need it. This is controversial. Most BMT experts *discourage* banking for one's own use, unless there is a family history of transplantable genetic disorders or an immediate need for the product. The odds of ever being able to use it for your own use are miniscule, and most doctors view the practice of pressuring parents to bank umbilical cord blood as panic peddling. Unfortunately, facilities that accept samples for public use are still limited, but hopefully will grow. See Appendix A, *Resources*, for resources for donor registries.

Cord blood from a single umbilical cord contains only enough material to transplant children or small adults. Research is underway to find safe ways of combining cord blood from several donors and to multiply cord blood stem cells to provide a larger volume for transplantation.

Donor leukocyte infusion (adoptive immunotherapy, buffy-coat infusion)

Donor leukocyte infusion (DLI) is also called adoptive immunotherapy or buffy-coat infusion. Mature white blood cells are collected from the donor in the same way stem cells or platelets are collected—several hours of apheresis, using two arm veins—and are then infused into the leukemia survivor. Donor leukocyte infusion is usually done following an allogeneic transplant if marrow fails to engraft. It may also be used after a relapse of leukemia following allogeneic transplantation or as part of a clinical trial to measure the added success of following marrow infusion with leukocyte infusion.

Sometimes this boost of donor material will trigger engraftment; it may, however, put the patient back into remission. Donor material can also increase the likelihood of graft-versus-host attacks against body organs, which can cause serious illness but may also trigger a graft-versus-leukemia effect, which can fight the leukemia.

A number of transplant processes are being closely examined, to see which give the best results under which circumstances. Modifications of DLI are also being studied. For example, there are some studies underway to test the effect of chimerism—a mixture of donor marrow and residual patient marrow—on leukemia. This is one form of mini-transplant. Other researchers are testing the feasibility of converting the patient's marrow to donor marrow slowly, via repeated donor leukocyte infusions, without first destroying all of the patient's marrow. This is another form of mini-transplant. Nevertheless, donor leukocyte infusion is very much in use with leukemia patients today.

Stephen Addison tells the story of relapsing four months after his transplant and how he was treated with donor leukocyte infusion:

> My wife and I were gaining confidence and slowly returning our lives to normal. I decided it was time to go into the hospital for my weekly blood work and check-up by myself, without my wife at my side, so she wouldn't have to miss any more work.
>
> The doctor came into the room and said, "Steve, I am sorry to say we have some abnormal blood activity. Let's take a bone marrow biopsy. You may have relapsed."
>
> Compared to this news, what I felt when I first heard that I had been diagnosed with leukemia was just a stroll in the park. Memories of the all-too-frequent and painful spinal taps, hours and hours of receiving blood products, vomiting, pain, loss of my hair, and the loss of my dignity all filled my head. This news put the fear of God in me instantly. It was an overwhelming fear, and it was terrifying. Suddenly my whole life changed for the second time
>
> I was told I must go through another round of chemotherapy and, once I was in remission, they would try a relatively new procedure called a donor leukocyte infusion. This procedure had previously shown very good results, but it, too, had its dangers. My doctor informed me that almost all his recipients of donor leukocyte infusion were still living, but his most recent patient died because of uncontrolled graft-versus-host disease. However, he said, all the leukemia had disappeared.
>
> Receiving leukocytes for the infusion was much more dramatic than actually receiving stem cells during my transplant. The bag of blood containing the leukocytes, which my sister had just donated, was brought into the room while still warm. No time was wasted hooking it up to my Hickman catheter and infusing it directly into my bloodstream. We all knew my treatment options were depleted after this.
>
> One more donor leukocyte infusion finally brought on some graft-versus-host disease. We celebrated when I was given the word. That's what we wanted, graft-versus-host disease, or did we? Having GVHD for a period of time would greatly increase my chances of survival as long as it didn't get out of hand and we could control it.

Eight months after my second and final donor leukocyte infusion, I still show signs of the Philadelphia chromosome. I still have leukemia. We suspect that the donor leukocyte infusion is doing its job, keeping me from relapse, but it needs a jump-start to blow the disease away.

Considerations for patients and families

A bone marrow transplant is a major step in treatment and cannot be taken lightly. Many people are frightened but know they have no choice if they want to live a full life. No one goes into this procedure thinking it will be an easy experience, and there are many things to consider before you have one. Among them are the type of leukemia, your age and general health, the availability of transplant centers doing protocols into which you fit, plus the willingness of your insurance company to pay.

When to transplant

Bone marrow transplant (BMT) is a treatment option for most forms of leukemia. The timing, however, varies according to the type of leukemia, age of the patient, stage of the disease, response to prior treatment, and donor availability. In some cases, the optimal time to transplant may be as soon as the patient is diagnosed and gets into a first remission. In other cases, patients may be able to delay a BMT and use other therapies to keep the disease under control. Patients with early-stage CML, for example, may choose to delay transplantation until their disease progresses to a more advanced stage. In some cases, optimal timing remains controversial.

Type of transplant

If BMT or PSCT is recommended, an allogeneic (rather than an autologous) transplant is usually the treatment of choice since it is considered curative. However, allogeneic transplants involve more complications—GVHD and a prolonged risk of infection due to the immunosuppressive drugs that accompany it. Older patients as well as those with pre-existing medical problems aside from the leukemia, such as lung or heart problems, may not be good candidates for allogeneic transplants. In these cases, doctors may recommend an autologous transplant instead. An autologous transplant may also be recommended for a patient who is unable to find a suitable marrow donor.

Age

Age is a relevant factor when considering a transplant. Younger patients tend to want, and are often better able to withstand, aggressive treatment. In some cases, aggressive treatment also seems to be more effective in younger patients. Older patients frequently don't want, or choose not to deal with, aggressive therapy to avoid all the potential side effects. The ability to rebound from high-dose chemotherapy diminishes with age, and the risk of graft-versus-host disease increases with advancing years.

In the past, allogeneic transplantation was usually not an option after a patient reached age 60, and autologous transplantation was usually ruled out after age 65. Many centers now do autologous transplants for patients who are up to 70 years old or even older, and mini transplants are specifically designed to accommodate older patients. The overall fitness of the patient can be an overriding factor.

Transplant may not be considered in early stages of disease if the patient may reasonably expect to have many more quality years of life ahead without treatment. Treatment decisions must be made on an individual basis. Some patients may have five or more years of quality life, relapse or progress, be unable to get into remission, and therefore, not be eligible for a transplant that could cure. Some people decide for earlier intervention, banking on a cure.

Which is better: Autologous or allogeneic?

In general, mortality rates are lower for autologous transplants and there is no risk of GVHD. Allogeneic transplants are more curative for leukemia, however, and may be more effective in protecting against relapse, but do entail higher risk of treatment-associated mortality.

Currently, the mortality rate associated with high-dose, transplant-related treatment procedures alone, as opposed to death from leukemia, is on average about 5 percent for autologous transplantation and about 20 to 30 percent for allogeneic transplantation. The risk becomes higher as the degree of mismatch increases. Mortality rate really varies depending on the type of leukemia, age of the patient, and the way the patient responds.

One patient describes the reasons for deciding on an autologous transplant:

> My leukemia was active again. The remission was over! We all
> agreed that I was facing an autologous transplant, because there were no

related donors, and at 65, I was too old for an unrelated match. The mortality rates were just too high.

Availability of donors

Even if your doctor believes that your leukemia type is best treated with an allogeneic transplant, the lack of a suitable and willing donor may leave autologous transplant as the only choice. When your health team determines that your leukemia is best treated with an allogeneic transplant, the search for a donor begins. In some cases, if the leukemia is transforming to a more aggressive type, the search must move quickly.

The best place to start is within your own family because of the higher likelihood of finding a very good match. In many of today's smaller families, however, a good match might not be found and it may be necessary to search for unrelated donors.

The transplant physician communicates with the National Marrow Donor Program about the patient in need of a transplant. They reply within 24 hours as to whether or not anyone in the database is a preliminary match. The preliminary search returns those who are identical and partially matched donors. Based on this data, the transplant doctor may request further testing on that potential donor. If so, the donor is contacted by a local donor center, educated about the process of donating marrow, and asked to undergo further testing. The patient isn't even supposed to know which local donor center is communicating with a donor.

Your transplant doctor's request for further testing on a subset of the preliminarily matched donors initiates the formal search. Additional HLA typing may need to be done on the donors at this time. To start the formal search, you must be working with a doctor from a National Marrow Donor approved transplant center. The average (median) time from formal search to transplant takes approximately four months. Because of the possibility of needing four months, the National Marrow Donor Program recommends starting the preliminary search process early in the course of investigating treatment options.

If you know your ethnic heritage, consider publicizing your need for donor testing in your community, or in similar ethnic communities around the country. Ask ethnic associations to spread the word to other cities and states. You might also go to local radio and TV stations. Most stations have a consumer advocate or goodwill officer who might help. Though the likelihood of finding a donor by this method is miniscule, the more patients that promote donor drives, the more likely it will be that someone will find a match as a result. Then someone else's donor drive may find a match for you.

You should also make sure all donor registries are contacted. There are international and national registries in many countries that work together to find donors. See Appendix A for a list of registries.

Choosing a transplant center

Bone marrow or stem cell transplantation is an expensive, lengthy, complex, and serious procedure. It demands state-of-the-art medical expertise, and caregivers with experience dealing with your type of leukemia and the kind of transplant being planned. It also requires a willingness and ability on the transplant center's part to assist or guide your local doctor in providing appropriate follow-up care.

Your medical insurance carrier may restrict your ability to choose a transplant center; it might have a contract with a particular center. You can make a case for having a transplant elsewhere if you can prove that another center will be better at handling your particular circumstances.

The Foundation for Accreditation of Hematopoietic Cell Therapy (FAHCT) gives accreditation to transplant centers. Two leading scientific groups in the field of transplantation, the American Society of Blood and Marrow Transplantation and the International Society for Hematology and Graft Engineering, created FAHCT in 1996. The foundation has developed quality standards for stem cell and bone marrow transplant programs. Accreditation requires the transplant team to include licensed and board-certified transplant physicians and other licensed specialists, including registered nurses with oncology/hematology certification. FAHCT also tracks the number and kinds of transplants done at each center. Although this will change over time, a lot of places are not yet accredited simply because FAHCT has not had sufficient time to do the site review, etc. You are advised to ask if the center you are planning to use is accredited or has sought FAHCT accreditation. However, at this time, lack of accreditation is not necessarily associated with poor quality.

Some transplant centers specialize in transplantation from unrelated donors. Others prefer to transplant only patients who have a related donor. A few centers specialize in doing mismatched transplants. Still others specialize in treating children.

You also need to check out more practical aspects, such as nearby housing and psychological, emotional, and educational support for your family. A center with a lengthy waiting list, for instance, will not be a good choice if your leukemia is transforming to a more aggressive stage.

See Appendix A for resources to help choose a transplant center.

Questions to ask the transplant team

Before you enter a transplant program, you will usually meet with the cancer center transplant team. They will listen to and answer questions about what to expect. It is a good idea that the patient's closest personal caregiver be present at that meeting so that this hardworking individual will also be informed and aware.

Every bone marrow or stem cell transplant is done according to a protocol. The informed consent document you will be offered doesn't spell out all the possibilities you may encounter, but the formal protocol will. Get a copy of the entire protocol and have it explained so you know what is coming.

Other questions to ask the transplant team:

- How many transplants have you done for my particular disease? BMTs? PSCTs?

- How many transplants were autologous and how many allogeneic? What are the statistics (complete remissions, partial remissions, mortality, etc.)?

- Will I receive inpatient treatment in an isolation unit? (If so, ask to see the isolation unit and learn about arrangements for visitors and your family. Not all transplant centers have isolation units. For autologous transplants particularly, it's controversial whether strict isolation really is needed. The trend is toward less isolation, not more.)

- Will I be seen only by RNs, or will there be LPNs too? How are their duties divided? How much oncology training have they had, and how much experience with transplants? What is the RN/patient ratio?

- If I'm to receive outpatient treatment, what precautions must I take in my home or apartment to ensure that I don't pick up infections? Will I need to be masked at all times around people? Can I have visitors? What precautions must be taken?

- What kind of psychosocial support services are available for me and my family members?

- What kind of home help will be provided in case of emergency, and what are the emergency procedures to follow?

- What kind of central venous catheter will you insert into my body? (You'll want to know how and when the catheter will be inserted, how long the catheter will be left in place, and all about the care and cleaning of the catheter.)

- What kind of chemotherapy will I have? What are the possible side effects? What can I expect after treatment?

- Will I be given radiation? If so, how much? How often will it be given? How long will each session be? What side effects are possible?

- Can I listen to music while undergoing radiation therapy to soothe and calm me? What effects will I encounter immediately afterwards? What are the long-term effects that I need to watch for?

- If I'm having an allogeneic transplant (using a donor), what about graft-versus-leukemia effect and graft-versus-host disease? How do you treat it? How many cases of chronic GVHD do you have each year and what kinds of problems can I expect to encounter?

- How should my diet and eating habits change during and after treatment? (For example, if you are neutropenic and cannot fight off infections, you may not eat raw fruits or vegetables; they must be cooked. No raw or rare fish, meat, or poultry may be eaten. You may be told not to eat anything that hasn't been prepared at home under hygienic conditions. You may not eat at a restaurant or buy prepared food. As your counts improve you may add raw fruits that require peeling, such as bananas and melons. You will be told to avoid eating from salad bars and buffets for up to a year after treatment, although the rules relax once you are no longer neutropenic.)

- What sort of support will be available from the transplant center for local doctors who will take care of me once I return home? (This is particularly important if you live far from your treatment center.)

Getting insurance company approval

In 1999, the average cost of a transplant was $160,000. Prices ranged from $75,000 to $200,000. Costs for long-term follow-up care over the years can easily approach $500,000 or more.

Some insurance companies closely scrutinize any medical plan that involves a marrow transplant because of this extraordinary expense. Staff, with little or no medical training, may arbitrarily deny approval, claiming that transplantation for your disease is an experimental procedure and not covered by your policy.

If your employer offers an annual open enrollment period—a period during which no previously existing medical conditions can be held against you—use this opportunity to upgrade your policy to the most liberal one offered.

Until legislation provides cancer survivors with fully reimbursed access to clinical trials, this battle is in your court. To overrule insurance company denials, you need to be familiar with state-of-the-art treatment for your subtype of leukemia. See Chapter 19, *Researching Your Leukemia,* for help in finding the latest and most reliable information about leukemia transplants.

If you're not satisfied with your insurance company's decision, challenge it. Ask your oncologist for a "letter of necessity," and ask your employer to intervene, a tactic that is surprisingly successful, especially for those working for companies that are self-insured.

Self-insured companies often have their plans administered by an independent health insurance firm, but always pay the cost of your treatment from their own pocket. This means that, if you're working for a self-insured company, your employer, not the insurance company, is denying you payment. This is a sensitive situation that you can turn to your benefit by arguing that it's in the company's best interest to keep you healthy or, more frankly, to avoid you embarrassing them.

Only a fraction of an insurance company's clients ever challenge the company's decisions. The money saved on the silent majority easily covers the costs of the few who challenge these rulings. The Blood and Marrow Transplant Information Network has a list of lawyers who specialize in transplant approval problems. Contact the network at (847) 433-3313 or visit *http://www.bmtinfonet.org.*

There is a specific legal process for challenging denial of coverage. If you (or the hospital) do not follow it exactly, you may not have legal recourse later on. For example, if you or the doctors haphazardly submit documentation to the insurance company about why the procedure is a reasonable, medically necessary, accepted practice, etc., during the appeals process, you will be precluded from presenting this information later on to a judge should you decide to take legal action. Similarly, if you don't submit your appeal within a certain time frame, you may lose your right to appeal.

Some people go ahead and pay for the transplant, assuming they can go back and fight the good fight later. It doesn't work that way.

Patients are often reluctant to involve an attorney when there are problems because they assume it will delay the process. Patients think there may have to be a big court battle before they get treated. That's wrong. Challenging a denial of coverage expedites the process in many cases. Sometimes what works is simply a letter from an attorney that rings the wake-up bells at the insurance company and causes them to agree to pay. If not, the lawyers can file for a temporary restraining order, which essentially requires the insurance company to pay now and argue about it later. This should be one of the things patients ask their transplant center about—how successful and experienced are they in persuading insurers to pay. Some centers are marvelous, others are not very helpful.

You might want to consider using a facility that has few or no charges. Free treatment is provided at the National Cancer Institute in Bethesda, Maryland, but for clinical trials only. The issue is whether or not you qualify for the trial. The same thing is true of the BMT program at the National Institutes of Health. Some transplant centers will work out a financial repayment agreement with you if you are left with an unusually high bill after health insurance reimbursement. In some states, state-funded hospitals must provide you with care if you are unable to pay.

There is an extensive, and extremely helpful, chapter on insurance reimbursement in Susan K. Stewart's book, *Autologous Stem Cell Transplants: A Handbook for Patients*, distributed by the Blood and Marrow Transplant Information Network.

Where transplants are done

Traditionally, transplants are inpatient procedures. The patient is kept in the hospital from the period before transplant when chemotherapy and/or radiation are given to kill the patient's marrow, through the infusion of donor marrow or reinfusion of the patient's own marrow, until the cells have engrafted and the patient's immune system has become usable again. Some inpatient centers place the patients in carefully air-conditioned rooms with special air filters. Some keep patients in virtual isolation, while others allow visitors in the room when they have washed hands and donned masks and gloves. Still others have even less stringent rules as more is learned about how patients do in the less sterile environment. The hospital staff provides all patient care, day and night. The whole procedure is expensive and staff-intensive.

Today, many people undergo outpatient transplants. They stay in lodgings near their transplant center and travel to the centers daily, usually wearing masks. They spend nights at home with their caregivers; that way they avoid isolation and the high cost of hospital beds. The caregivers take care of the medical procedures that would have been done in the hospital. Patients are very dependent on their caregivers, who may be really stressed doing a job that was once done entirely by hospital personnel.

For outpatient transplants, most of the heavy-duty medical procedures are done during the day while the patient camps out at the outpatient clinic. Evening procedures are usually limited to monitoring temperature, giving medications, etc. These procedures can be done with the help of a nurse or caregiver. A bonus of outpatient transplant is that you're home without the annoyance of interruptions for hospital procedures, and you're eating foods you like, cooked in familiar ways.

Problems of outpatient transplants include the need for extra cleanliness to minimize the risk of infections and the need to care for the catheter site. Caregivers must keep IV medicines going and see that medicines are given on time. Many patients say that this is harder on the caregivers than on themselves. The overall cost of the transplant is cheaper, but it's much more harrowing for the poor caregiver who feels that the patient's life is in his or her hands.

How transplants are done

When you are considering whether to have a transplant or preparing to have one, it is very helpful to have an idea of what it will entail. Although each protocol and each experience is different—whether inpatient or outpatient, whether chemotherapy or total body irradiation are used, the length of time needed to engraft, side effects, results, etc.—there are general steps which are the same. The transplantation process generally includes:

- Preparation for transplant
- Induction therapy to achieve remission
- Harvest of marrow or stem cells
- In some cases of autologous transplants, purging marrow or stem cells
- Consolidation
  - For AML, CML, and ALL, there is usually, but not always, consolidation chemotherapy (which is low-dose chemotherapy followed by high-dose chemotherapy), with or without radiation (called conditioning).
  - For CLL patients there is high-dose chemotherapy with or without total body irradiation.
- Infusion or reinfusion of marrow, stem cells, or cord blood
- Engraftment

After the procedure is completed, the patient is discharged and follow-up care begins.

Preparation

Before you can undergo the high doses of chemotherapy and radiation used in some transplantation protocols, you must be tested to determine if you're healthy enough to withstand this treatment and to establish base lines against which organ functions can be measured later. In an outpatient setting, your heart, lungs, kidneys, liver, and pulmonary function will be assessed, and a dental examination will be done. Anything that needs to be removed, fixed, or filled should be done before transplant.

A central venous catheter (CVC) will be inserted under your skin, most likely in your upper chest, to deliver chemotherapy directly into the large veins near your heart. Among the benefits of having a catheter are:

- It spares you from repeated punctures with IVs and needles.
- It can save your arm veins from damage.
- The catheter's location near the heart assures that drugs are pumped evenly and quickly to all parts of the body.

- Apheresis, the collection of various blood cells such as platelets and stem cells from blood, is easier and more comfortable when a catheter is used.

- It can be used to access the vein to measure important body functions such as central venous pressure (CVP). This helps your doctor determine the amount of IV fluids you need.

- If mouth sores become severe and you cannot eat, you'll need parenteral nutrition. These thick feeding solutions can cause terribly sore arm veins, so the catheter is really helpful.

This patient describes her experience upon entering the hospital for an autologous transplant:

> It was beautiful weather in Boston that June day when I entered the bone marrow transplant unit. My husband and I walked through one set of double doors, waited until they closed, and then through the second set of doors. That was to keep unfiltered air out of the isolation unit. Normally patients arrived on a stretcher after surgery to have a Hickman catheter inserted, but I was a day ahead on that procedure, so I walked into the unit that was to be my home for the next month.
>
> The nurses were predictably busy, so we waited to be told where I was to stay until my nurse finished caring for her current patient. Knowing I was going to need that nursing care myself shortly, I wasn't upset at the delay. Finally, I was shown to a room about fifteen feet square that was to be my home away from home. Construction of another building was going on outside my window, and watching the workmen doing the construction became a very integral part of each day in the unit.

Tom Storer wrote to his support group about his preparation for a bone marrow transplant at the Dana-Farber Cancer Institute:

> I'm happy to report that after just two rounds of treatment with the Fludara/Cytoxan combination, my bone marrow involvement was well below the magical 10 percent threshold!
>
> Things have moved quickly since then. Over the course of three weeks, I managed a swift turnover of my work responsibilities while undergoing a large number of tests and orientations for the BMT program. (Luckily, Dana-Farber Cancer Institute and its affiliated institutions are just about a fifteen- to twenty-minute drive from my home and from my work.)

I had my bone marrow harvest yesterday with reportedly good results. (I chose to do it with general anesthetic, which I had for the second time in my life; it was an intriguing experience and, I think, the right choice.)

I report in tomorrow for admission and placement of the Hickman line, with chemotherapy scheduled for Saturday and Sunday and seven sessions of total body irradiation, two a day from Monday through midday Thursday, and reinfusion of my bone marrow next Friday. Seems like a lot of action in a very short time. Total inpatient stay is projected at four to six weeks.

I was pleased to learn that I will be able to see visitors (as long as they're healthy, wear masks and gloves, and don't touch anything I use). I am taking them up on their suggestion that I could bring in a small stereo system to keep me going with my favorite CDs during the treatment and recovery period.

Induction therapy

An induction phase may be used before transplantation for leukemia to try to induce a remission or limit leukemic cell involvement in the blood and marrow. Induction is standard chemotherapy, although the doses may be somewhat higher than you've had in the past and the drugs may be different. Because it's so much like first-line chemotherapy, the induction phase may be done in your home town by your local oncologist, even if your transplant will be done out of town. If a second round of chemotherapy is given to increase the likelihood of a cure, it's called consolidation chemotherapy. The higher dosage given before transplant is the preparative, or conditioning, regimen.

Some people do not achieve remission in the induction phase before transplant. This is a big concern. For some, if not most leukemias, not being in remission prior to transplant significantly reduces the likelihood that the transplant will cure. Some cancer centers won't even transplant if the patient is not in remission. Keep in mind, however, that prognoses and survival are very much a function of the stage and type of disease, prior treatment, age and health of patient, and that new treatments are always being devised.

Harvest

Harvesting bone marrow is gathering the cells needed for transplant. If you're having an autologous transplant, the harvest will be done before high-dose chemotherapy starts, and the harvested cells will be kept frozen (cryo-preserved) until the day of transplant. If you're donating marrow or stem cells for someone else, the marrow is usually not frozen. It is collected and used immediately. If the donor is an unrelated donor found through the NMDP, the marrow is collected locally, then chilled and flown directly to the transplant center.

It is not required that an unrelated donor actually be at the transplant center. However, related donors are often asked to be present at the transplant center, if possible, so that they can donate platelets and other blood products to the patient after transplant. Minimizing the number of persons who donate blood products to the patient reduces the likelihood of certain blood product-related complications.

Harvest of the bone marrow

If stem cells from marrow will be used, you'll be given a general anesthetic for the procedure, which may require an overnight stay in the hospital. Four to six very small punctures that will not require stitches are made in the skin, usually over your rear hipbones. Dozens of punctures are made in the bone to withdraw about a quart of marrow.

You may be sore for a few days to a week after this procedure. You will feel as if you slipped on ice and landed on your bottom. You may also feel tired and lightheaded for a day or two. Anesthesia alone can cause the fatigue. In the vast majority of cases, these are the only side effects. However, some patients do experience pain that is not controllable with simple Tylenol, and some experience pain longer than two weeks.

This patient describes the experience of having bone marrow cells harvested for an autologous transplant. This is the same experience that a donor would have providing marrow for a recipient:

> The day I was to have my bone marrow cells harvested, they told me I'd have to be at the hospital at 5:00 a.m. I am not a morning person, so it was very hard indeed to drag myself out of bed at that unreal hour. My husband is an early bird, but even he felt sorry for me as I groaned and rolled out of bed.

Paperwork completed, I was taken to the anesthesia staging area and gowned. The anesthesiologist was very careful to make sure I knew what he was going to do. The doctors had already explained the procedure to be followed, so I felt pretty confident. Once I was asleep, two surgeons worked over me and made a total of six holes in my hips. They told me afterwards that they sucked out enough marrow cells to do the job twice over. The cells were taken for purging with a combination of monoclonal antibodies, and then cryogenically stored while I healed, ready for BMT.

They kept me overnight in the hospital so that I could recover, but aside from a slightly sore posterior for a few days when I had to get in and out of cabs, I wasn't in any real pain, just some discomfort.

Harvest of peripheral stem cells

Many transplant centers now use stem cells collected from the bloodstream instead of cells from the bone marrow. Stem cells from the blood stream are collected (harvested) by inserting a needle into one arm vein or one lumen on your catheter, extracting blood, and passing it through an apheresis machine that will separate out stem cells. The remaining blood product is returned to you through a needle inserted into your other arm or catheter lumen.

When patients look at the bag of white cells being selected and removed from their body, they are sometimes surprised to see that the removed "white" cells look red. This is normal.

There are fewer stem cells in the bloodstream than in marrow, but the number of stem cells in the bloodstream can be boosted if drugs known as colony stimulating factors (natural body products replicated in pharmaceutical laboratories) are administered first. Granulocyte colony stimulating factor (G-CSF), or granulocyte-macrophage colony stimulating factor (GM-CSF), is administered under the skin by injection (subcutaneously) several times the week before harvesting. These substances may make your bones and joints feel sore. Ice packs and Tylenol should relieve this pain. GM-CSF may also cause fever or lung or heart inflammation. Call your doctor if you have fever, chest pain, or difficulty breathing.

The harvest (apheresis) will typically take two to six hours over a one- to five-day period. The nursing staff will provide blankets to warm you because you may be temporarily anemic, and you may feel chilled.

Very rarely, patients have an allergic reaction to the anticlotting agent used in apheresis. If you feel shortness of breath or break out in hives inform the nurse. Generally, nurses are at your side throughout the entire procedure.

The anticlotting agent may reduce the calcium supply in your blood. If you sense an unusual heartbeat or feel tingling sensations, weakness, or numbness around the mouth, tell the nursing staff immediately. You will be given intravenous or oral calcium.

It's not unusual to have to undergo repeated harvests, perhaps up to six times, until enough stem cells are collected. If sufficient stem cells can't be harvested from the bloodstream, the patient may be to asked undergo harvest of bone marrow in addition to, or instead of, stem cells.

Leukemia itself, or its previous treatment, sometimes compromises the marrow's ability to produce stem cells. Healthy donors usually undergo fewer sessions. The donor's body will replace marrow and stem cells in three to four weeks. Donor side effects are fewer and recovery time is shorter.

The following patient, who underwent an autologous transplant, describes her experience with apheresis:

> The doctors decided to take peripheral blood stem cells, select out the ones expressing CD34, and purge them using a CD19 reactive monoclonal antibody. I had been heavily treated with Fludara in the past, and they were concerned about my ability to provide enough stem cells. For four days I was given subcutaneous injections of white cell growth factor, G-CSF, and finally the blood work showed that I was more or less ready. It appeared to be a good possibility, though not a certainty, that I could provide enough cells for transplant.

> They inserted a Groshong catheter in a vein in my upper chest. That was an eerie experience for me because I had never had a catheter before. I definitely hated seeing it protrude from my chest. It had two tubes sticking out called lumens, but they looked like antennae. The next day they drew the blood out via one lumen, while the blood that wasn't selected was returned to me through the other lumen. Finally I understood why they wanted such a large catheter with double lumens.

> Before apheresis I made sure to go to the bathroom. They told me I would be hooked up to the machine for four hours, and I don't work with bedpans at all. I lay flat on a bed while I was attached to the apheresis

machine. There was no pain. It was just boring. I had been warned, so I
had brought a book to read. Other patients were watching TV on the sets
that were provided, but I just find that a noisy distraction. At one point I
became chilly, and the nurses brought me a blanket that had been kept in
a warming bin of some kind. I really appreciated that.

After four hours I was unhooked for the day, and you've never seen
anyone move so fast toward a bathroom. It took three days of apheresis to
collect enough cells for a stem cell transplant, but by then they had two
bags full. They purged one, and stored them both for the time in the future
when I would be ready to use them.

Purging marrow or stem cells

As previously described in "Autologous transplants," the protocols of some autologous transplants call for purging of the patient's harvested white blood cells before they are infused back into the patient's body, after any therapy.

Research is still continuing to find the best ways to separate healthy cells from cancerous cells, which currently include the following:

- Two types of purging are now in use—one using monoclonal antibodies and the other using chemicals (pharmacological). Monoclonal antibodies are special proteins that react with specific cells. They are often selected for the purging process, since they will kill off cells expressing specific CD markers. When cleaned of all collected cells showing suspect CD markers, the remaining cells are ready to be reinfused into the patient's body.

- A process of separating and saving healthy stem cells is called CD34 positive, or CD34+, selection. Although its end goal is similar to purging, it is called selection of cells rather than purging cells. Much research is underway on selecting only healthy cells. Healthy stem cells, for instance, express a surface antigen identified as CD34 that cancerous cells do not express. Antigen CD34+ selection techniques also permit a one-step method to separate stem cells from mature white blood cells.

The difference between purging and CD34+ selection is that purging kills diseased cells while CD34+ selection separates out the healthy cells and the rest of the sample is discarded. Since any purging or CD34+ selection would happen to cells after they were harvested from your body, you will only know about what kind of purging, if any, is used on your cells from discussing the protocol with your transplant team. Your doctor can also explain the thinking behind the protocol: why purging was/wasn't included in your protocol.

Consolidation, high-dose therapy, conditioning

For a traditional autologous transplant, high-dose chemotherapy follows the harvesting of marrow or stem cells. If donor marrow is to be used, the harvest occurs just after the patient undergoes high-dose chemotherapy treatment. The high-dose chemotherapy is called the conditioning, or preparative, regimen. Consolidation, if there is any, is lower-dose chemotherapy and occurs prior to the conditioning or preparative regimen.

Many different chemotherapeutic regimens are used for high-dose treatment of leukemia, and new combinations are always being tested. Your oncology team will select one of the standard protocols they use, or a new one being testing. They will take measures to protect against known possible complications, while still following the protocol. Some drugs being used in various combinations include: cyclophosphamide, busulfan (Myleran), etoposide, carmustine, cytarabine, melphalan, and cisplatin. Other drugs and new combinations are always being assessed for superiority. Usually, high-dose chemotherapy is administered over a two- to ten-day period.

In some cases, total body irradiation (TBI) is used in addition to high-dose chemotherapy to destroy leukemic cells. When TBI is used as part of consolidation, the dosage is spread over several days. This spreading, called fractionating the dose, permits more radiation to be given than the body would be able to withstand if it were given in one large dose. In recent literature, however, there is discussion of ways to decrease or eliminate TBI in a procedure called a mini-transplant. TBI is not a standard part of all conditioning regimens.

Infusion of marrow

Infusion of donor cells or your own cells, done through your catheter, takes about 30 minutes. Marrow and stem cells are infused using an IV line, as with any IV drug. Although the marrow is warmed before it's given to you, you may still feel chilled as it is being infused. Some patients look upon the reinfusion of marrow as an anticlimax after high-dose treatment. Others celebrate, especially if they have searched long and hard for a donor.

Marrow or stem cells are not presently infused until one or two days after high-dose consolidation treatment has ended. This allows chemotherapy and/or radiotherapy sufficient time to have the maximum effect against cancer, and permits toxins to exit the body. Infused marrow takes 10 to 21 days to engraft. During this period the patient must be protected, because the immune system will be unable to fight infection.

During infusion, there may be fever, chills, hives, shortness of breath, or chest pains. If so, tell the nursing staff immediately. They will provide antihistamines to curb any allergic reactions.

Isolation

Within five to ten days following your high-dose therapy, regardless of whether you are having an inpatient or outpatient transplant, you will experience a profound drop in white blood cell counts as your marrow dies. At this point, you have insufficient immune system power to protect you from bacteria, fungi, or viral agents until the infused marrow engrafts and begins producing new white blood cells. This engraftment process takes from two to three weeks or, in rare instances, longer.

You will only go into isolation if you are having a full-scale bone marrow or stem cell transplant. If you are having your transplant on an inpatient basis, special precautions will be taken to guard against infection. It may include restricting visitors, or having them wear gloves and masks when in your room. In this instance, isolation means that you use special precautions so as not to become infected during the time your immune system is not operating at all.

Nowadays, many transplants are done on an outpatient basis. If you are not scheduled for an inpatient transplant according to your protocol, the only time you might find yourself in the isolation unit is if there are problems and the medical team feels that isolation will give you a better chance of a successful transplant.

To avoid infection, you will be kept in isolation until your new marrow engrafts and becomes productive. Some autologous transplantation protocols require administration of colony stimulating factors after infusion to encourage the new marrow to produce white cells more quickly.

Isolation requirements differ among transplant centers. Some rigorously curtail visitors and confine patients in rooms with special air filtering systems.

Others simply require visitors to wear masks and wash hands upon entry. Many require only hand washing. Check with your treatment center about visitor policy, and about which gifts you can and cannot receive. If you are having a transplant done on an outpatient basis, there will also be restrictions; these restrictions also vary.

In general, you'll feel best if your room is homelike and if you have your own comfortable clothing to wear. Transplant unit staffs sometimes limit the kinds of things, including gifts, that may enter your room. Some allow only what can be sterilized in a device called an autoclave: cotton clothing, books, and so on. These rules are made to prevent infection when you have no functioning white blood cells, when you are neutropenic. No fresh plant material of any kind, including dried flowers, and no gifts of food will be permitted. Everything you eat must be cooked under sterile conditions while you are neutropenic.

You may have lost your hair because of chemotherapy. The air filtering systems of many isolation rooms blow down upon the bed, and you might be cold. Since you won't have hair on your head to keep you warm, you will need a substitute. Soft hats, scarves, or turbans work well to keep you warm. Wigs are a nuisance in bed, however—they shift constantly and they get itchy. On the other hand, warm sweatshirts that zip all the way down are helpful. Pullovers aren't convenient. It's not easy get them on and off with the IV hook-ups in the way.

A patient who lost her hair describes how cold her room got and how she appreciated a warm, soft hat and other clothing:

> I had lost my hair from the chemotherapy needed to get me into remission for the transplant. In this room, all the fans and the air filtering system converged, blowing down on the bed. My head was freezing and I knew I'd be wearing turbans and hats all the time just to keep warm. Fortunately, a friend had crocheted a hat for me out of baby wool, and I was really grateful for the warmth and softness it provided.
>
> I also learned to wear a hospital gown tied in the back, with an additional one over it tied in the front, which I covered with a hospital robe. Sometimes I still needed extra clothing because I was constantly cold, but my poor husband was really hot and uncomfortable since he had to be masked and gloved while in my room.

Common side effects

Most side effects of high-dose chemotherapy begin to appear several days after treatment ends. You're still feeling awful from the chemotherapy, are zonked out on pain medications, and in general, feel like a washed-out dishrag.

Allogeneic and autologous transplants have similar common side effects. Generally, those receiving allogeneic transplants are likely to feel worse and to have a longer recovery period than those receiving autologous transplants, especially if an acute case of graft-versus-host disease develops. In allogeneic transplants, patients' immune systems need to be suppressed to control GVHD. This means that they are much more likely to contract infections than patients who are treated with regular chemotherapy. Sometimes drugs are given prophylactically to prevent infections.

One autologous transplant recipient describes feeling sicker as the transplantation process proceeded:

> One issue is the state you're in when you leave the hospital. In non-transplant situations, you are hospitalized when you are quite sick, and you feel better each subsequent day as you recover, or you're hospitalized for surgery and you begin feeling better after a few days.
>
> In transplant, it's just the opposite. You go in feeling quite well. Each day after the first few, you feel weaker and sicker. And that's true even after your counts begin coming back from zero. The transplant nurses tell me that most people feel so wretched the night before discharge that they have serious doubts about their ability to cope when they leave—even with help from family and friends. That group included me.

Many of the side effects experienced during and after transplantation resemble those of standard-dose treatment, and can be found in Chapter 12, *Side Effects of Treatment*. Described here are the side effects specific to transplant recipients, along with information as to how they are managed:

- **Drowsiness, mental confusion.** Many transplant recipients report undesirable cognitive effects, particularly from total body irradiation or cranial irradiation. This condition cannot be treated directly, but good nutrition, rest, and time may improve cognitive skills within a few weeks, although some transplant recipients report lingering effects years afterward. The main complaints are memory problems and associative skills.

- **Fungal infections.** Although neutropenia and infection are discussed in Chapter 12, fungal infections are of enough concern to transplant recipients to mention here. These infections can spread widely through-out the body and can be difficult to eradicate. If your transplant team suspects a fungal infection, cultures will be done to confirm this, and you may be placed on antifungal medication, such as amphotericin.

- **Pneumonia, pneumonitis, adult respiratory distress syndrome (ARDS).** If you develop a dry cough or difficult, painful, rapid breathing within about two months after your transplant, you may have pneumonia, pneumonitis, or ARDS. Viruses such as cytomegalovirus (CMV) can cause pneumonia. Radiation therapy can cause pneumonitis or pulmonary fibrosis. Some chemotherapy can also cause pneumonitis. Treatment depends on diagnosis.

- **Viral hepatitis.** Many viruses that are always present in the body are able to take advantage of immune-suppression, and can settle in the liver. There is no cure for such a viral infection except time and good, supportive care. The use of immunoglobulins and antiviral drugs can shorten the duration of some infections if they're given soon enough.

- **Clostridium difficile-associated disease (CDAD).** While this occurs in few patients, the FDA has confirmed that not only is recurrent CDAD a serious, life-threatening disease, but that there is no satisfactory treatment for it. As of January 2000, however, the FDA has granted fast-track designation to Synsorb Cd, used to prevent recurrence of CDAD. It is estimated that patients suffering from recurrent CDAD remain hospitalized up to 26 days longer than comparable patients, and the fatality rate for untreated patients is between 27 and 44 percent.

- **Acute graft-versus-host disease.** If you receive donor marrow, you may develop acute graft-versus-host disease (GVHD). Caused by white blood cells attacking liver, blood vessels, skin, gastrointestinal tract, and other tissues, it can be controlled by immunosuppressive drugs. In early stages, GVHD usually appears as a rash or peeling on the skin of the hands and feet. At its most severe, GVHD can be fatal if it is not controlled. Acute GVHD occurs only after the white counts start coming back after transplant, within the first 100 days post-transplant.

- **Veno-occlusive disease (VOD).** The high-dose treatment you're given may cause blood vessels in your liver to swell shut, a potentially fatal reaction. There is a higher risk of VOD if you first develop a fever or are receiving an allogeneic transplant or a second transplant. If VOD develops, it's most likely to happen one to four weeks after the transplant. You may have pain in the upper right abdomen, swelling, jaundice, or fluid in the chest or abdomen. Supportive care is given for VOD, which may go away on its own. However, it is a very serious complication and can cause death. Cessation of drugs that stress the liver helps ease the condition.

Engraftment

Everyone eagerly awaits engraftment. As time passes, and the wait seems prolonged, many transplant recipients begin to worry a bit. It ordinarily takes about 14 to 28 days for marrow to engraft. It can be as short as 10 days in autologous transplants, but sometimes the wait is longer.

Patients count the days. In fact, they can be downright competitive about how long they take to engraft and be ready for discharge. Tom Storer inquired about the fastest discharge time when he went in for a bone marrow transplant at the Dana-Farber Cancer Institute:

> Discharge time is based on progress in recovery of blood counts. I asked what the record was for speed of discharge and was told two weeks after reinfusion. I've set myself a goal of at least matching that. (I won't be too disappointed if I miss it.)

Engraftment is presumed to have occurred when the patient's absolute neutrophil count or ANC—the number of mature white blood cells—begins to rise, as tracked by daily blood tests. Sometimes the rise is not steady. The counts may waiver back and forth over several days, but the overall trend should be upward. It may be months before the new marrow produces enough cells to equal the normal range.

In general, stem cells will engraft more quickly than marrow cells. Those who have received an autologous transplant will engraft more quickly and produce adequate numbers of cells sooner than those who have received an allogeneic transplant because they are given growth factors.

Marrow sometimes fails to engraft well or at all. This can be detected in several ways:

- For an allogeneic transplant, genetic testing reveals that the marrow being produced is still the patient's own marrow, not the donor's. This may pose a risk of relapse since the patient's marrow still contained leukemic cells before the transplant.

- For an allogeneic transplant, the marrow is chimeric: a mixture of donor and patient marrow. This phenomenon is not well understood, but it is thought that a risk of relapse may be present.

- For either an allogeneic or autologous transplant, the numbers of cells produced never reach normal levels. This is a poor engraftment rather than a failure to engraft.

A failure to engraft can be addressed with a second transplant, an infusion of additional donor white blood cells, a second infusion of more of the patient's own saved marrow or stem cells, or time. Sometimes, very late engraftments occur. Failure to engraft is seen more often with marrow or stem cells purged of all leukemic cells than with unpurged products.

After treatment

When you are discharged, you will have a follow-up schedule for medical care and instructions about a variety of topics, from food to pets.

Outpatient follow-up

Many transplant centers are shifting their aftercare procedures to the outpatient setting. You may be released from the inpatient unit when your absolute neutrophil count in blood exceeds 500 on two consecutive days. If so, you may be expected to stay nearby for several weeks to facilitate care during possible medical emergencies, and for blood testing several times a week. Other tests will be performed from time to time, such as bone marrow biopsies to verify the productivity of marrow and the continued absence of leukemia. You will likely be placed temporarily on antibiotic, antifungal, and/or antiviral medications as a precaution if your white blood counts remain low.

The high-dose drugs used during a transplant can cause a form of depression known as chemical depression. Antidepressants are recommended, if needed.

Length of recovery

It will take several months or more—perhaps up to a year—to recover from a transplant; there is tremendous variability in individual recovery times. With allogeneic transplants, recovery can take more than a year if chronic

GVHD develops. You may need to stay away from work for most or all of this time, depending on the health risks your job poses. Contact with small children or performing hard manual labor might be considered risky.

Outward appearances may be deceptive. Cancer patients may feel much better than they look. Or they may look much better than they feel. Others may not realize or believe the discrepancy. One autologous transplant recipient describes how perception of recovery can contrast with outward appearance and how others perceive the recovery:

> There is what I'd call "perceived recovery." You come out of a transplant looking like Hell on wheels—no hair, so pallid that a corpse looks healthy next to you, dry as dust from the radiation, probably thin and debilitated, profoundly weak, and, perhaps, with some other obvious physical problems.
>
> But the visible problems are among the first to clear up. Hair and normal coloring return surprisingly quickly. Once you are allowed to resume a normal diet, and once your sense of taste recovers, you'll probably regain lost weight.
>
> So it looks like you're well. But at your core—your literal core in the middle of your body—it will take months until you have recovered and really feel recovered. A significant amount of strength returns early, probably in the first 30 days. Seventy percent of recovery occurs in the first month. The last 30 percent could take six months. It's very difficult for the people close to you to understand why you're still dragging at times, when, to outward appearances, you're back to normal. Their expectations can have an impact on your expectations for yourself.

Pets after transplant

Transplant centers differ in their recommendations about being near family pets after transplantation. Some recommend complete avoidance. Others recommend that the patient and the pets stay in separate parts of the house for the first few months. Still others say you should avoid handling the pet's bedding, kissing the pet, or allowing the pet to lick or scratch you. You should ask the discharge staff and your doctor what they recommend. The issue is not which diseases can be communicated, but whether any can. If the answer is yes, and the patient is immunocompromised, there is a risk.

Some transplant centers will recommend removing pets from the home until the patient's immune system is functioning normally. Cats, in particular, can pose a problem since they can transmit toxoplasmosis. Information is less clear about dogs. This does not mean that you have to get rid of your pet permanently, but do arrange for temporary lodging.

Once the pet returns home, wash your hands after handling it and delegate the task of cleaning its waste to someone else. For people who are emotionally attached to their pets and find great comfort in their presence, any restrictions on contact with their pets can be very difficult. However, if your immune system is compromised, you may not be able to fight off an infection transmitted by your pet. It's less of an issue for autologous transplant patients than for allogeneic patients who may be on immunosuppressive drugs long term.

Long-term effects

Long-term effects specific to transplantation are discussed here. Most long-term effects of treatment in general are discussed in Chapter 16, *After Treatment*.

Sterility

The high-dose chemotherapy and total body irradiation that some patients are subjected to during transplant typically causes sterility and infertility. Sexual function isn't *necessarily* impaired, though it is for many patients. Pain during intercourse, dry vaginal tissues, and decreased libido (for both males and females) are important issues. Talk with your partner about what effects treatment has had for you. Partners may assume that your lack of interest in sexuality is a mental, rather than a physical problem.

Men may want to consider sperm banking shortly after diagnosis, since chemotherapy may impact the quality or viability of the sperm. Some chemotherapy drugs reportedly cause chromosome damage. However, children born to transplant survivors are as normal as those born to the general population. Women can have ova stored before therapy is over, but the likelihood that the ova will be viable is low. Also, those with acute leukemias don't have the time to go through the various medical procedures required to produce viable ova. Fertilized ova can be stored more successfully than unfertilized ova. Donor sperm and ova are more reproductive possibilities at this time.

An excellent, in-depth resource for cancer-related reproductive issues is Leslie R. Schover's *Sexuality and Fertility After Cancer.*

Chronic GVHD

If you have had an allogeneic transplant, there's an ongoing risk of chronic graft-versus-host disease (GVHD).

Unlike acute graft-versus-host disease, which appears soon after the transplant, chronic graft-versus-host disease appears three or more months afterward. It can be less serious than acute GVHD or it can be very serious, even fatal. Usually, the skin is affected first—it may itch or exhibit scaliness or a rash—although any organ can be affected, such as glands in the eyes or mouth. Often, the blood's liver enzyme values become elevated, signaling the beginning of chronic GVHD. You may have a painful or tender upper abdomen. Your lungs may also be involved. Graft-versus-host disease can affect connective tissue, tighten tendons, and make movement painful. It also occurs in the intestines, with symptoms of excessive diarrhea or painful cramping with bowel movements.

Immunosuppressive drugs given to control chronic GVHD can impair the immune system, rendering the patient highly susceptible to recurrent bacterial infections. Often, patients have recurrent upper respiratory infections of the sinuses and throat. These infections should always be regarded as potentially dangerous in patients with chronic GVHD, in whom the risk of infection that spreads through the bloodstream (sepsis) is always a concern. As a rule, these patients receive long courses of prophylactic antibiotics, such as penicillin or erythromycin.

Many researchers have observed that patients with GVHD also experience a graft-versus-leukemia effect (discussed under "Mini-transplants"). This seems to reduce the risk of relapse. It's not the GVHD itself that reduces the risk of relapse—it is the graft-versus-leukemia effect. For this reason, immunosuppressive medications may be carefully chosen to allow some GVHD, but not enough to cause serious health problems, to develop. It is considered *chronic* GVHD if it occurs after the first 100 days. Chronic GVHD may eventually burn itself out, though sometimes not for several years.

Sally, a classroom teacher, has had chronic GVHD since her matched unrelated donor transplant. Her doctors have not allowed her in her classroom for the past three years, but she is an amazing woman who deals with the physical effects of GVHD matter-of-factly—as just one more of life's lessons:

> I still think GVHD is a long-term daily battle with symptoms and side effects. Living with GVHD is no job for sissies. Recovery after a transplant is hard work. GVHD can be draining on the emotions and spirit, as well as the physical body. The thrill, excitement, and expectations of the transplant are gone and you're left to deal with unpleasant symptoms and the hard work of slow recuperation.

> GVHD is not as glamorous a disease as the cancer you once fought. Friends that may have rallied to help you battle the cancer may begin to lose enthusiasm in your recovery as your chronic disease turns into months or years of recuperation. GVHD is difficult to explain and may give friends the idea that you have turned into a "professional patient" with an endless list of complaints and ailments. Even family members may tire of the "symptom of the day" mentality and build communication barriers or avoid discussion with you. GVHD can be as mean and unrelenting as the cancer, and depression and loneliness take their emotional toll.

> However, I have learned some secrets to regaining control of life and coping with GVHD. Visualize your recuperation as a battle, an actual daily fight to get your life back. Encourage your efforts to fight GVHD, as you would against any invasion into your life or your family's life. My battle has turned into a challenge to be overcome.

Since medications are an important weapon in the battle against GVHD, Sally found that using a checklist to monitor her med dosages helps:

> I found that frequent dosage changes were necessary due to infections and new symptoms. I created a checklist of all the medicines, listing each dosage and the time to take it. (Creating this on a computer is very helpful so that you can revise it easily.) I used a checklist because sometimes I truly couldn't remember whether I'd taken the next dosage or not. I learned that survival depends on maintaining the correct daily dosage level. The checklist is a great help in communicating with my doctor and understanding the daily medicines.

Complications of immunosuppressive medication

Immunosuppressive drugs given to control GVHD pose their own risks. The main one is increased risk of infection. If you are taking immunosuppressive drugs, be careful not to break the skin. Stay out of crowds. Thoroughly wash and cook all foods. Avoid live vaccines and those who have had recent inoculations with live vaccines. Check with your doctor about avoiding other risks, such as bacteria and fungi in gardening soil. Most transplant centers provide extensive information about such precautions.

Long-term use of immunosuppressive drugs, such as cyclosporine, may raise blood levels of lipids and cholesterol, increasing the risk of blocked arteries. Different immunosuppressive drugs can be substituted, cyclosporine levels can be adjusted, or cholesterol-lowering drugs can be prescribed as needed.

Complications of radiation

Total body irradiation can cause several late effects. Fingernails and toenails will dry and fall off as new nails grow beneath them. Another big problem is intense dryness of the eyes, mouth, and skin, which can cause other problems. Moreover, cataracts are almost certain to develop a few years after transplant and can happen from certain chemotherapy regimens too. While the surgery to correct cataracts is usually easy to deal with, it can't be done while the patient is on chemotherapy or is otherwise immunosuppressed.

This patient tells of her experience with skin problems and nail loss after radiation. She managed to find some humor in what was happening:

> While I was in the BMT unit, I developed rough red spots on my fingers and on my heels. The doctors blamed that on total body irradiation. As the rash healed, the skin on my fingers dried out. The doctor had to cut off the dried skin so that I could do such simple things as brush my teeth and dress myself without immense pain as the skin pulled. They protected my heels from painful rubbing against the sheets by having me wear fleece-lined heel booties.
>
> Once I was out of the unit and past the two weeks of intensive outpatient care, my fingernails began to rise. I couldn't figure out what was happening at first. Then I realized that new nails were growing underneath, and my original nails were falling off. Sometimes that happened at

most entertaining times. I was being introduced to a new acquaintance
who offered me his hand—I took his hand and shook it, but as I retracted
my hand, a nail dropped into his hand. I wish you could have seen the
look on his face!

Other possible late complications

Shingles, peripheral neuropathy, cataracts, reduced kidney and liver function, infertility, weakness, fatigue, and cognitive and emotional problems can
follow a transplant. See Chapter 16 for more information. For women, premature menopause usually develops after transplant and should be discussed with your doctor.

Becoming a donor

Only a small percent of patients needing allogeneic transplants are able to
find a donor because there are too few donors in the marrow registries.

Family and friends of those with leukemia should consider joining the
National Marrow Donor Program. A blood sample only—not marrow—is
used for testing.

Many who have donated marrow describe it as one of the most fulfilling
experiences of their life, second only to becoming a parent. Most say they
would do it again, eagerly, and without hesitation. The process of harvesting
marrow or stem cells is described earlier in this chapter.

A decision to become a marrow or stem cell donor is a serious commitment.
You must remain on call, be willing to undergo additional blood testing, and
be willing to donate as soon as you're called, regardless of other plans or
even minor illnesses. You could be saving a life. A donor should never back
out once treatment of the patient has begun, because often this treatment is
intended to destroy all of the patient's marrow. Without donor marrow the
patient will die.

After you have donated, you may be asked to donate again later for the same
patient in case of relapse. Often, the second donation simply requires an
apheresis of stem cells even if marrow cells were used the first time. Once
you have donated for a patient, you will not be considered eligible to donate
for a second patient for twelve months. If you donate marrow or stem cells
to an unrelated patient through the National Marrow Donor Program, you

and the patient may contact each other after one year, if both agree. You may join the NMDP by calling (800) MARROW-2.

Appendix A contains resources for donation information. For an in-depth description of transplantation from the patient's perspective, see Susan Stewart's *Autologous Stem Cell Transplants: A Handbook for Patients* and *Allogeneic Bone Marrow Transplants*, available from the Blood and Marrow Transplant Information Network at (847) 433-3313 or *http://www.bmtinfonet.org*. You can also call the National Cancer Institute at (800) 4-CANCER to ask for their publication on transplantation, *Bone Marrow Transplantation and Peripheral Blood Stem Cell Transplantation*.

CHAPTER 10

Clinical Trials and Beyond

Why should anyone choose an experimental therapy with unknown risks over standard leukemia treatments that have well-known risks? Aren't clinical trials of new treatments dangerous? Aren't these experimental treatments just for people who have no other choices left? And why are they called clinical trials?

Many of the treatments now in clinical trials are of lower toxicity than some traditional/standard chemotherapeutic agents. Many experimental treatments, such as monoclonal antibodies and biologic treatments, use cancer-fighting agents found naturally in the body, which are doubled or tripled in number outside the body and are then reinserted into the body. Others, such as idiotypic vaccines, use your own white blood cells, retrained to attack the leukemic cells. Other treatments utilize substances that force immature cancer cells to mature; others aim for and destroy the parts of the cancer cells' chromosomes that keep cancer cells from dying a natural death. These new and possibly better treatments are available to leukemia patients in carefully controlled settings called clinical trials.

This chapter contains crucial information about clinical trials. We first discuss the structure of clinical trials and how they're run, explaining the advantages and disadvantages of trials, safeguards, and patients' rights. We describe why it's often to your advantage to do your own searching in addition to relying on trials your doctor may recommend. We explain how to evaluate different trials, what to expect, and what to do when you're finally enrolled. The chapter ends with a look at where new clinical trials are heading in terms of treatment options for the future.

If you are considering a clinical trial, there is a large group from which to choose underway and recruiting leukemia patients. For example, at the time of this writing there are 131 clinical trials for AML, 108 for adult ALL, 107 for CML, and 91 for CLL. In addition, there are 82 trials for adult T-cell leukemia, 51 for hairy cell leukemia, and 48 for prolymphocytic leukemia.

Although the following advice is contained later in the chapter, it bears repeating here: do not sign a consent form until you have received and read a copy of the full protocol, are sure you fully understand what you will be facing, and have considered all other clinical trials for which you might be eligible.

This chapter focuses on finding and evaluating clinical trials for treatment, not on trials for prevention, detection, or support. For the sake of readability, we use the word "substance" throughout this chapter, with the understanding that either new substances or new methodologies can be the objects of testing.

Who should learn about clinical trials?

The National Cancer Institute recommends that if you have acute leukemia, or chronic or acute leukemia that has not responded to standard treatment or that has relapsed, examination of clinical trials may be very much in your interest. However, all leukemia survivors should become familiar with methods for finding trials, and with the general structure and function of trials. If you wait until you have reached the point where you need a trial before you learn these things, you may run out of time.

What are clinical trials?

Clinical trials are the means by which promising new treatments are evaluated to see if they offer more benefit than existing treatments. The US Food and Drug Administration (FDA) requires successful test results by means of a highly structured, controlled environment (clinical trial) before it will approve treatment for wider use by doctors and patients in less controlled settings. Sometimes, two or more standard therapies are compared.

When clinical trials show that a new treatment is better than older standard care, and these results are duplicated and verified by objective third parties, then the treatment that was used in the clinical trial becomes a new standard for care.

Clinical trials are tests run in a clinical setting on humans. The word "clinical" distinguishes these trials from tests done on leukemia blood samples or on animals. Clinical trials are not started on humans until a substance has shown promise when tested first on human blood samples, then on animals—usually laboratory-bred mice.

There are many kinds of clinical trials. The trials that usually interest most leukemia survivors are those that focus on treatment, but trials also improve cancer prevention, detection, and support. A clinical trial can test either a new substance or a new method for administering treatment. For every 5000 compounds tested in laboratories and in animals, only five will be tested in humans. The FDA will approve only one of five drugs tested on humans for actual treatment purposes, so clinical trials are crucial.

Usually, clinical trials will not admit cancer survivors unless they have already tried standard treatments without success. There are a few trials, however, that admit only those patients whose cancer has never been treated.

Clinical trials are designed and structured to withstand the minute and critical scientific scrutiny necessary to determine if a new treatment is effective. By the time a new substance is being used as part of a phase III trial (explained later in the chapter), the group of patients receiving the new substance is so closely matched for so many characteristics that any difference in their progress against cancer can be attributed, with a good deal of certainty, to the new treatment—and to *only* the new treatment.

Three study designs that aid in ensuring the results of treatment are attributable to the new agent—not to chance or confounding factors—are randomization, blinding, and double-blinding:

- **Randomized trials.** Participants are closely matched on various characteristics—disease stage, prior treatments, health, age, sex, and so on—and assigned randomly via computer to receive either the new treatment or existing standard treatment. This means that you might not receive the new substance at all. Randomization is used to demonstrate, as clearly as possible, that a group of patients very closely matched in all respects to a second group did either better or worse, and that *only* the treatment given explains the difference in outcome.

- **Blinded trials.** Patients are not only randomized, they are also unaware of which treatment they're being given. This is considered necessary to rule out the placebo effect, defined as the ability of the human body to respond differently to treatment in measurable, physical ways, based on complex psychological and motivational factors experienced by the patient. Some patients might respond better to a treatment, for example, if they know they're getting a new treatment as opposed to an older one. Passive, compliant patients might report responses that they think will please the doctor and staff. The placebo effect is the subject of some controversy; some researchers maintaining it is truly measurable, while others believe its supposed effects can be attributed to other phenomena, such as inaccurate measurements or patient subjectivity.

- **Double-blinded trials.** Neither the patients nor the medical staff is aware which substance is being given to whom. Double-blinding is used to eliminate the possibility that subtle factors—such as motivation and mood on the part of the doctor or nursing staff, which might be sensed by the patient—could account for differences seen in the progress of the group receiving the new treatment, compared to those receiving the old.

In these respects, clinical trials differ from less rigorous tests designed and administered by doctors and researchers working independently on new substances. Independent researchers often lack complete records and consistent evidence that can be duplicated and verified by impartial observers. Often, their patients are not subjected to the necessary long-term evaluation—five years or more—that determines whether the new treatment truly made a sustained difference in leukemia regression.

In general, if trials are run by a university, an NCI-designated regional cancer center, or a pharmaceutical company adhering to NCI and FDA guidelines, the chances are very good that safeguards for the patient are part of the design. The NCI and FDA require that a committee of responsible and knowledgeable researchers known as an institutional review board (IRB), which is ultimately responsible for overseeing the trial, reviews and approves use of the substance in question. Therapies offered by independent researchers in their own for-profit clinics—especially those that involve ingesting or injecting an untested substances—should be avoided or, at the very least, approached with extreme caution.

Why participate in clinical trials?

Aside from the altruistic aspect of participating in a trial in order to benefit others—an aspect that may or may not motivate you—clinical trials offer you a good chance to receive more effective treatment, and perhaps a cure, years before it's available to the general public.

One patient's wife talks about the hope that participating in clinical trials have given to her and her husband:

> We have seen just two clinical trials recently for CML and AML that bring exciting hopes to the horizon. If one would choose to be ill, this is the age to do it in. I believe there is going to be a tremendous jump in knowledge regarding this terrible disease in these next few years.
>
> We are certainly taking one day at a time and praying that Cees remains in remission, hoping that this will be the end of his leukemia. However, we do realize that the possibility of relapse always hangs in the wings. This is why we will continue to be greatly involved in the pursuit of a cure, and will help the Leukemia and Lymphoma Society in any way we can. We have a great reason for doing so, right?

Rituxan, the recently approved monoclonal antibody treatment for NHL, is an example of a treatment that has been available for several years to those with leukemia who were willing to enroll in clinical trials testing this substance. Here's a story from a patient who is participating in a clinical trial using Rituxan:

> I'm just home today from six nights in Mt Sinai Hospital where I had my first cycle in the Fludara/Rituxan trial. The protocol has been slightly changed with a lower, slower dose of Rituxan the first day, and further doses the third and fifth days of this first cycle along with a 30-minute infusion of Fludara each of the five days. One also takes Allopurinol for fifteen days to protect the kidneys from toxins from dying cells. Cycles are every 28 days, and for the second through sixth (and last), Rituxan is given only on day one. Fludara is given all five days.
>
> My only bad reaction so far was a chill with bad shakes during the first Rituxan infusion. The infusion was stopped for a while and I was given another blanket. Then it was started again at a still slower rate and I had no further reactions. I hardly noticed Fludara at all; I certainly wouldn't have needed hospitalization if I'd been getting only that. I may be able to do cycles two through six as an outpatient.

All my counts have dropped some (both good and bad). My hemoglo-
bin fell enough that I was given two units of packed red cells last night, so
I'm feeling pretty good today. I'm being very careful about infections, and
have been preaching hand washing to my family.

Guinea pig?

In the US, the long and not altogether honorable history of the clinical trial
process has resulted in laws, procedures, and methods that safeguard the
patient. For example, each clinical trial has a lengthy protocol, which will be
given to you if you ask for it. The protocol describes what will be done,
when, and what action will be taken if certain undesirable effects occur. You
should always ask for, and thoroughly read, a copy of the full protocol.

Informing and obtaining consent from the prospective patient are time-
consuming and repetitive processes done to ensure that all risks and benefits are made clear. Unfortunately, there still remain cases of patients being
pressured to sign clinical trial consent forms without full information or at
the last minute, without time to consider other options.

Always ask that the consent forms and the full protocol be sent to you well
in advance of your scheduled visits.

Only institutions funded by the federal government or governed by pertinent local laws are required to abide by consent guidelines. If you're being
treated in a for-profit hospital that receives no government support, it's possible for you to be treated in a study without your knowledge or consent,
thinking that you're getting standard treatment. Ask your doctor if you're
receiving state-of-the-art treatment as defined by the National Cancer Institute (NCI) or if you're being treated in a study. In addition, phone your state
health department to determine if your state has its own laws regarding consent issues.

This patient caregiver is concerned about the level of information she and
her husband, the patient, are being given about a clinical trial:

My husband is a three-year survivor of AML (M2). He was in remis-
sion for almost two years as a result of high-dose chemotherapy. He
relapsed last October, and was scheduled for two more rounds of chemo, the

first of which put him in remission. In January he received an autologous BMT instead of using our 19-year-old daughter as a mismatched donor.

He is in a double-blind study involving a drug called linomide. The standard literature given to patients for informed consent is written at about a sixth-grade reading (and cognitive) level—not enough information for me. I told the doctors we wouldn't sign for informed consent unless we have a copy of the real protocol so that we know what we are really facing in this trial.

I know that the drug is made in Germany, is an immunostimulant that (they hope) boosts the number and strength of natural killer cells, and that it is not listed in the current Physicians Desk Reference (PDR). Supposedly, they have had good luck with this drug in producing long remissions for leukemia patients who do not have available donors, and the current trial is aimed at perfecting the dosage to be given.

Even though the test is double blind, we've been hoping that he is in the arm of the trial that gets linomide. The doctors, study director, and I think there's a pretty good chance that George is actually getting the drug because side effects that he has had match the side effects for it.

Placebos

For cancer clinical trials, true placebos are almost never used. A true placebo is a drug or treatment that has been made to look exactly like the active substance or the effective procedure, but it has no active ingredients. In clinical trials of antihistamines, for instance, the placebo used most often is a sugar pill.

For randomized cancer treatment trials—usually phase III trials, of which more will be said in an upcoming section—the new treatment is compared to existing, accepted treatment, not to a placebo. Exceptions to this ethical policy are new treatments for which no corresponding previous treatment exists, such as trials of the earliest efforts to purge bone marrow of cancerous cells prior to bone marrow transplantation. In that instance, standard care was represented by reinfusion of unpurged marrow, and the test treatment involved reinfusion of marrow purged using an experimental technique.

How clinical trials are run

Clinical trials are organized into three stages: phases I, II, and III. Each phase addresses different, increasingly complex, issues concerning the success of the new treatment. Some drugs are tested in trials that are a combination of two phases, such as phase I/II or phase II/III. Usually this is done if some knowledge of the new treatment's effect on humans is already known, so that its development and testing can be expedited.

There may be clinical trials in which you can participate locally on an outpatient basis, but many require travel and in-patient stays.

Here's the story of a peripheral blood stem cell transplant patient who came through the procedure well, and how his wife, Lynn, feels about it as he enters a new phase of a clinical trial:

> Cees came home on day +17 from his autologous PBSCT. He was infused on November 30 and has done tremendously well. He came home one week earlier than the doctor had anticipated that he would. It is wonderful that there is still hope, and some great treatment possibilities out there.

> For the record, Cees's counts on the day of his discharge were WBC 8.0, HCT 39.0, platelets 84,000, and ANC 6200. His doctors just were amazed at how well, at 62 years old, he had come through his fifth and hardest chemo (this one a high dose with busulfan and etoposide) despite severe mucositis of the mouth, throat, and digestive tract. He is now eating soft foods and only takes a morphine tablet under the tongue at night for pain. He says his taste buds are beginning to become more active, and realizes that it will take time for everything to heal.

> He goes back soon to meet with his doctors to decide with them when to start his Interleuken-2 injections. They'll be used to help boost his immune system and ensure that, should there be any lurking cancer cells around, his immune system will recognize them and destroy them. He'll continue these injections for a total of twelve weeks.

> It is a study that the Fred Hutchinson Cancer Research Center and the Virginia Mason Center are doing together. This is the next step in treating cancers by first doing the chemo, and then bringing in the biotechnology.

Phase I clinical trials

The primary purpose of a phase I clinical trial is to measure the safety and toxicity of different doses of a new substance in the human body. Some phase I studies may also assess leukemia response, the amount of drug that accumulates in the body, and the substance's general behavior in the body.

Phase I trials are preceded by animal studies that measure toxicity, so an estimated safe human dose is already known. Rigorous controls are enforced to help ensure that no patient suffers adverse effects. For example, blood or urine values of certain body substances may be measured several times a day to ensure that the liver and kidneys are not compromised. Doses that are found to be unacceptably toxic are lowered.

Phase I trials usually involve just a few patients, perhaps 10 to 30. Often these patients have a variety of different leukemias so the activity of a new substance against different leukemias can be studied. Sometimes one group of patients will receive only a low dose of the drug and a different group will receive higher doses. But in later studies, the same patients who initially received a low dose may be given a higher dose, if toxicity is not too great.

The advantages of a phase I trial are:

- You may receive a treatment that may be better than anything else currently approved by the FDA years before it becomes available to the general public.

- If this drug is already in use for other illnesses, its toxic effects might be already recognized.

- A candidate substance for cancer treatment is not approved for phase I trials unless the substance has shown activity against cancer in cultured blood cell lines and in animal studies. In addition, the substance shows reasonably acceptable toxicity. Of every 5000 substances tested in animals, only 5 enter phase I trials.

- Doses found to cause unacceptable toxicity are appropriately lowered.

The disadvantages of a phase I trial are:

- Because phase I trials are chiefly concerned with discovering dose-limiting toxicity, they are brief compared to phase II and III trials. You may receive too low dosages of the test substance to destroy effectively all of your cancerous cells.

- Phase I trials usually test one substance alone, yet experience has shown that, at least for the chemotherapeutic agents commonly used today, combined drug regimens are more effective against most cancers than single-drug regimens.

- The substance, although it may be an approved drug for other illnesses or even for other cancers, most likely has never before been used in humans for your illness. Although it has been tested in cultured cell lines and in animals implanted with leukemia, it may not be effective against your kind of leukemia, or it may be no better than existing treatments.

- The substance, although it may be an approved drug for other illnesses or even for other cancers, may be administered to you at a much higher, more toxic dose.

- The dosage will be varied among those enrolled, thus its effects on your leukemia may not be directly comparable to the effects on the leukemia of others enrolled in the trial, and patients do talk among themselves.

- The use of patients with different leukemia types makes it difficult for you to compare your progress to that of other patients.

- Toxicity may cause substantial discomfort, illness, or permanent damage, in spite of the safeguards designed to prevent damage.

- Often, phase I trials are run by one principal investigator at one institution. You may have to travel to participate in a phase I trial. (Phase I trials for pediatric leukemias, however, are sometimes offered at multiple locations.)

Unfortunately, for every 100 drugs tested in phase I trials, only 70 will prove promising or safe enough to carry forward into phase II trials.

Phase II clinical trials

Phase II trials measure the activity of new treatments against cancer. Some phase II trials also attempt to measure how best to deliver the drug to the leukemia—orally, by infusion, and so on—and how often the dose should be given.

Phase II trials involve many more patients than phase I trials—perhaps 20 to 100—so that the substance will receive a more thorough test, and the statistics collected will be more meaningful.

Sometimes, but not always, phase II clinical trials are divided into arms. One arm gets one version of the experimental treatment and a second arm gets another—perhaps the same experimental agent combined with an established, FDA-approved cancer-killing drug, or perhaps the agent delivered by another route, or on a different dose schedule.

Owing to the results of phase I testing, a clearer idea exists about what cancers will benefit most from this treatment when it is used in a phase II trial. The kinds of cancers considered eligible for phase II trials, therefore, are usually more narrowly defined than those eligible for phase I trials.

Phase II trials take more time than phase I trials because, unlike phase I trials, more of the new agent is administered in an attempt to cause leukemia regression.

The advantages of a phase II trial are:

- Candidate substances for leukemia treatment are not approved for phase II trials unless phase I trials have indicated that the substance has some activity against such cancer in humans.

- You'll receive a treatment that may be better than anything else currently approved by the FDA several years before it becomes available to the general public.

- Only doses that result in acceptable levels of toxicity, determined during phase I testing, are utilized.

- Randomizing and blinding usually are not used in phase II trials. Therefore, you are assured of receiving the experimental treatment.

The disadvantages of a phase II trial are:

- The substance, although it may be an approved drug for other illnesses or even for other cancers, may not prove to be better than existing treatments for your illness.

- Although its toxicity was determined in the phase I trial of this substance, the substance is still an evolving treatment with the potential for unexpected side effects.

- More of your time will be needed for a phase II trial than for a phase I trial if the dosage is spread over a greater period.

- You may have to travel to participate in a phase II trial.

Unfortunately, more than half of the drugs used in phase II trials will be found ineffective against cancer or too problematic for use. Of the original 100 drugs that entered phase I trials, and of which only 70 survived to pass to phase II, no more than 33 will survive phase II testing.

Phase III clinical trials

Phase III clinical trials test a new substance's efficacy compared to existing standard treatments by using patients who are closely matched on several characteristics, such as stage of disease.

Phase III trials are usually much larger than phase II trials, and are sometimes multicenter trials—that is, trials run simultaneously at many sites. Often they run for months or years, with long periods of follow-up.

Phase III trials are randomized and sometimes, but not always, blinded or double-blinded.

The advantages of a phase III trial are:

- A substance that has survived the scrutiny of phases I and II is very likely to be better than current treatments—either more efficacious, or equally effective but less toxic.

- You'll receive a treatment that may be better than anything else currently approved by the FDA a year or two before it becomes available to the general public.

- If, during the trial, a new treatment shows itself to be vastly superior to existing treatment, those receiving the existing treatment are switched to the arm of the study utilizing the new substance.

- If a new treatment shows itself to be clearly, or dangerously, inferior to existing treatment, those receiving the new treatment are switched to the standard treatment regimen.

The disadvantages of a phase III trial are:

- Randomizing and blinding may not appeal to those who are determined to receive only the new treatment, not the contrasting current treatment.

- The new substance may prove to be just as effective as, but no better than, the existing treatment.

Unfortunately, Of the 33 drugs that survived phase II testing, only about 25 will be found effective in phase III trials.

Selecting the best phase

As you can imagine, phase II trials might appeal to patients who find phase I trials too risky and phase III trials too controlled. It would be a mistake, though, to assume, based only on the structure of the system, that phase II trials are the only good choice. A phase I trial of a drug with a long history of use for, say, an autoimmune illness such as rheumatoid arthritis, might be a very safe choice for a leukemia survivor if animal studies have shown the agent is active against leukemia. A phase III trial using a new monoclonal antibody that just varies an ancillary feature of treatment, such as one antibiotic against another to control infection, might be as good a choice as a phase II trial of a less well-known, less promising substance. The patient is generally selected for a phase of a trial based upon diagnosis and stage, prior therapy, etc.

Where to go for clinical trials

Clinical trials are found most often at the NCI-designated Comprehensive Cancer Centers, Clinical Cancer Centers, and at other university medical hospitals that receive federal funding and cooperate with the NCI on clinical trials. Many regional groupings of oncology centers have been established for clinical trials, so you may hear your doctor mention SWOG (South West Oncology Group), ECOG (Eastern Cooperative Oncology Group), or others like those. Your community oncologist may participate through association with the NCI's community clinical oncology programs.

A clinical trial's location will be a factor in your decision of whether to join a trial. Because geographical proximity is often important to families, many trials are now offered in multiple centers. The following patient, who has strong feelings against using chemotherapy and radiation therapy unless it is needed, decided on a particular clinical trial because of its proximity and use of a biological substance for treatment:

> I have been through a period of remission and then relapsed about eight months ago. I was introduced to the possibility of the Maximine clinical trial about a month ago. I have not been following any allopathic routes with the treatment of AML because I am anxious to use only

natural ways of treatment; I am very much against using heavy doses of chemotherapy and radiation. I realize there will come a time when that is what will be needed, but up until now I have been successful using a more holistic approach.

On my last visit to the oncologist, we discussed treatment options I would be comfortable using if my blood test results were not moving in the right direction. My doctor suggested participating in a Maximine trial. There are clinical trials of it nearby, so I won't have too far to travel. The University of Florida at Jacksonville has one; my doctor suggested that I try getting into it. It appears to be the most natural route for me, if I have to take therapy, but I pray I do not. However, using Maxamine and Inter-leuken-2 produces a more natural fight against this disease—the hista-mines attach themselves to the phagocytes to save the natural killer (NK) and T cells so they have a chance to do their job. But I'm still checking into it and hoping my counts go in the right direction so I won't need any treatment just now.

Finding trials for leukemia

As an adult with leukemia, you would be wise to take an active role in find-ing the best care for your disease. Adults with cancer are seldom asked to join a trial unless they are being treated in a regional cancer center. The approach is different from that used for children with cancer, whose families are commonly approached regarding enrollment in clinical trials, and 75 percent of whom do eventually enroll in clinical trials. The NCI estimates that less than 5 percent of those adults who are eligible for clinical trials enroll and that minorities are very much underrepresented in the clinical trial process.

You can use several methods to find clinical trials:

- You can ask your oncologist which trials, current or planned, would suit your medical circumstances. This method has its advantages and disad-vantages, one advantage being that you need do very little other than have a passive acceptance based on trust. The disadvantages are described in the section "Why research trials on your own?"

- You can call the National Cancer Institute at (800) 4-CANCER and ask about trials for your type of leukemia, being sure to specify whether you're willing to travel—otherwise they'll send you local trials only—and asking for the full protocol document, not the summary. Be warned that if you call often with this request, which is not an unreasonable thing to do because new trials are added every month, eventually they may decline to send you any more listings. This has been the experience of some cancer survivors who've used this service, which is provided by various regional cancer care centers under the auspices of the NCI.

- You can research US and international clinical trials on your own at the NCI's web site, *http://cancertrials.nci.nih.gov*. This service alone may be worth the cost of a personal computer and the time spent learning to use it. Once available only to those who subscribed to the NCI's Information Associates program for $100 per year, now the NCI provides this tool free-of-charge on the Internet. We strongly suggest that you examine all trials available for leukemia, particularly those for your kind of leukemia.

- You may also track new cancer treatment trials using CenterWatch (*http://www.centerwatch.com*). CenterWatch has many good features, such as an email news notification service, but at the time of this writing the titles and descriptions of clinical trials posted at this web site are so general, you must do much more research. For example, it doesn't specify what agent is being tested or where the trial is really held. Just the city is shown, which is inadequate if you're searching for trials at a top-notch cancer center in a large urban area. The listings are by state, forcing you to read the same over-generalized titles again and again for each state if you're willing to travel and want to be familiar with all the trials available.

A survivor who is actively looking for answers to the question "Where do I go from here?" asks the Internet support community to give her help in the following letter:

Dear Friends,

Confusion reigns once again. The blood work from Friday shows that I am in hematological remission: all counts are normal or low normal. Palpation indicates no enlarged nodes or body parts. Ready to celebrate you think?

The latest biopsy report shows 50 percent involvement of cancer cells in the marrow. My cell counts are doubling at more than 50 percent. After the recent round of chemotherapy, the implication is that leukemic cell population was likely higher in the marrow before the chemo, and has dropped down to only 50 percent involvement. What to do?

The combination chemotherapy clinical trial I'm in now, fludarabine/ cytoxan, can cause immunosuppression, hemolytic anemia, and discourages growth of stem cells. I've had lots of chemo and don't want to become refractory this early in my life. You'll notice I'm still fighting, but I'm getting worried!

If I want a bone marrow transplant, Dana-Farber Cancer Institute's eligibility criterion is marrow biopsy showing 10 percent or less leukemia cell involvement. I believe the Hutch (Fred Hutchinson Cancer Research Center in Seattle) protocol calls for 30 percent or less. Suddenly, getting to either may be impossible for me. Frankly, I'm desperate for help. Does anyone have any clinical trial options to suggest that I haven't investigated? I can't wait for in vivo or animal trials. At this point, I need a blooming miracle!

In fact, she found a high-dose cytoxan trial, went through it with success, and had her bone marrow transplant three months later. This patient survived because she was willing to use any help she could find, and she appreciated the value of using clinical trials.

Why research trials on your own?

Some people who depend on only their oncologists for comprehensive and up-to-date information about clinical trials have been disappointed. In many cases, oncologists in clinical practice—and that means most oncologists— are aware only of the high-priority trials that receive emphasis in publications such as *Oncology Times* or those that are offered nearby. Some still do not use a computer to search the NCI's database for all applicable trials. Perhaps they haven't the time to do so—remember that most oncologists "in the trenches" must track information on every cancer known, whereas you have the opportunity to focus intensely on your own cancer, subtype, and stage.

If you have a hematological oncologist who is associated with a university medical school or cancer research center, you can usually expect very good to excellent treatment. Often, however, when consideration of clinical trials is appropriate, doctors are biased toward their own research or toward trials run by colleagues at their own institution. The ideal oncologist is one some-where in the middle: educated about all trials and aware of what's a good fit for you, but not biased toward his or her personal research or interested in work limited to his or her department.

Life isn't often ideal, so it's a good idea to learn to search for clinical trials on your own, and to repeat your search every month because new trials are constantly opening. Once you have found a trial for which you believe you qualify, you should bring it to your doctor's attention. What if you find several trials that seem to admit patients with your profile? How can you tell which trial would be best for you? Clearly, this is one of the most important questions that will arise during your experience with leukemia.

At this point, you need to acquire the necessary skills for searching Medline and Cancerlit, and for reading the studies that result from your searches. Medline searches are available using the National Library of Medicine's (NLM) new resource Entrez PubMed at *http://www.ncbi.nlm.nih.gov/entrez/query.fcgi* or the NLM's Internet Grateful Med, *http://igm.nlm.nih.gov*, which searches myriad databases. Cancerlit searches are available by pointing your browser to *http://cnetdb.nci.nih.gov/cancerlit.shtml*. Each clinical trial may have results published regarding the previous use of the substances in animals or in humans. These studies should be found, evaluated, and compared by you and your doctor to single out the substance most likely to benefit you. Tech-niques for searching Medline are discussed in Chapter 19, *Researching Your Leukemia*.

If your oncologist is unwilling to help you, is negative, or is at best non-committal about your proactive attitude toward searching for trials, consider finding a new doctor, because you'll need your oncologist's recommendation to get admitted to a trial.

Getting admitted to a trial

Once you have found one or more clinical trials for which you think you're eligible, you must ask your oncologist to consult with and refer you to the treatment center running the trial for an admission evaluation. If your doc-tor is unwilling to do so, seek a second opinion. You might try phoning the principal investigator listed in the trial description. Often they'll speak directly with patients about what's involved, but a few may insist on speak-ing first with your doctor.

You and your medical records will be scrutinized closely by your doctor, the doctors at the institution offering the trial, and, likely, your insurance company, to see if you're truly a candidate. Various physical parameters, such as the condition of your heart and liver, may be factors. The kind of leukemia you have, how aggressive it is, as well as the rate of progression must be considered.

One of the chief considerations in evaluating patients for most clinical trials is how much and what kind of previous treatment they've had. Some trials want only those patients who have been heavily pretreated; others require patients who have not had any treatment resembling that proposed for the trial. Still others seek patients who have had no treatment at all.

You should read all of the entry criteria listed for the clinical trial and become very familiar with the results of your previous tests so that you'll have a good idea whether you're eligible before you approach your doctor for a referral. (This is another reason it is important to keep copies of your own records.) Questions that overwhelm many other leukemia patients—such as how long the trial will run, where it is located, and what the side effects are—will not be a problem for you, because the description of the study will have answered many of these questions for you.

In order to be accepted, there may need to be a great deal of rapid communication between you, your medical care providers, your insurance company (which will almost certainly insist on pre-approval,) and others on the hospital team. The oncology nurse in charge of administering the trial at the center you've targeted, the social worker, the housing assistant (if you must travel for this care), and the principal investigator, a doctor running the trial, will all want to communicate at one point or another. You may need to make one or more trips to the cancer center for an evaluation. You may be pleasantly surprised by how kindly you're treated—for instance, some doctors phone personally. On the other hand, you may be dismayed by lost records, lack of communication, and red tape. If this has happened before, hand carry copies of records and x-rays to your meeting. Other patients experience heartache and anger when, after meeting all the criteria, a reviewing doctor, employed by their insurance company, denies payment for the treatment after finding some discrepancy. This topic is discussed more thoroughly in the section "Payment."

The evaluation process is the time to ask for your own copy of the full protocol. The protocol is the document that describes what will be done, when, and what action will be taken if certain undesirable effects occur. Remember not to sign the consent form until you have received and read, with real understanding, a copy of the full protocol, and have considered all other clinical trials for which you might be eligible.

Many principal investigators are willing to speak directly with prospective patients about the details of the trial and the patient's medical history. The names and phone numbers of the principal investigator and participating doctors can be found at the end of the document that describes the clinical trial.

You can expect to feel conflicting emotions at this time: the excitement of finding a treatment that may be a cure, and the fear that the treatment might have unknown or undesirable effects. You may have concerns about being away from home and nagging worries about financial considerations. All of this may be coupled with the thrill of empowerment on finding the best care. Some or all of these may suddenly erupt, overwhelming your emotions after months, or years, of coping relatively calmly with your illness.

No doubt, the very detailed information in the full protocol will answer many of your questions, and may raise many others. In addition, consider these less-than-obvious questions, which are adapted from Nancy Keene's book *Working with Your Doctor* (also published by O'Reilly & Associates):

- Who reviews this study, and how often?
- Who monitors patient safety?
- Why do the principal investigators believe that this treatment is better than standard treatment?
- What are all of the potential physical side effects of this treatment, both short- and long-term?
- Will participation in the study mean that I have to change oncologists?
- Must I be hospitalized to participate?
- What will be my costs, and what will my health insurance pay?
- Does the study follow patients for the long term?
- Who pays for any care I'll need if the treatment has unexpected negative effects?

Once you are accepted

Detailing exactly what to expect after you're enrolled in a clinical trial is not possible in this book because each trial is quite different. In general, most people find they feel well cared for in a trial setting. It might be wise, however, to expect the unexpected. Delays due to unsent paperwork that was never forwarded by those who promised to do so, especially insurance company pre-approvals for payment, are more likely than not. An excellent place to find out what to expect is Robert Finn's book, *Cancer Clinical Trials*.

Once treatment is underway, some people are surprised that the extensive and detailed protocol outlining the treatment is really just a guideline. The truth is that the protocol can be changed if you're suffering adverse effects. A change in protocol will not necessarily affect your chances of succeeding on the treatment. This is particularly true in a phase I trial that's measuring toxicity.

If at all possible, have a friend or relative with you during treatment to verify what medications are given, to provide emotional support, and to be an advocate if you need one. This is especially important if you have traveled some distance for care and do not have access to a local support system. If you are using morphine, to control side effects, for example, you may not be in full control of your thinking processes.

Remember that you have the right to withdraw from a clinical trial at any time, to read your medical records, and to ask that deviations from the protocol be made if you're experiencing very bad side effects.

Payment

Many people have difficulty getting their insurance companies to approve payment for care administered under the auspices of a clinical trial or for an investigational new drug. One might surmise that because cancer is a very expensive chronic disease, it would be to the financial benefit of insurance companies if better treatments were found. Nevertheless, individual companies are often unwilling to assume the costs of these studies.

The trend, however, is that more companies are paying for trials than in the past, or can be convinced to make exceptions for those who need treatment in trials. The federal government has set a good example by ruling that federally insured employees will be covered for their treatment within NCI-sponsored clinical trials, and the state of Rhode Island has passed a law requiring insurance companies to pay for cancer clinical trials. The state of Maryland has passed similar legislation that requires payment of fees for treatment given as part of a clinical trial for any illness, as long as the trial is approved by the National Institutes of Health. Medicare also has been mandated to pay for patients participating in clinical trials.

Some cancer survivors successfully convince insurance companies to approve payment by having their doctors supply evidence that previous tests of the new treatment showed some superiority over existing treatments, or writing "letters of necessity" demonstrating that this experimental treatment is the only remaining good choice available. Others have luck when their employers intervene. Still others use the news media to generate publicity that is embarrassing for the insurance company. Some cancer facilities offering clinical trials make provisions for those who want to participate but cannot pay.

Compassionate-use programs may offer drugs at a reduced price. Pharmaceutical companies may give patients access to drugs for little or no cost. In some cases, the pharmaceutical company may make a drug available to a patient who does not qualify for a phase III clinical trial under the compassionate use policy. In many instances, laws restrict compassionate use.

Importation of foreign drugs for single-patient use, under the FDA's strict guidelines, will almost certainly be an expense you'll have to bear on your own. But do check with your health insurance company, as policies vary widely.

The National Cancer Institute in Bethesda, Maryland, offers free treatment for those who qualify for their trials. This is a top-notch scientific institution run by the federal government that has some of the best cancer researchers in the country. Those who have used their services sometimes say, though, that they were very aware that they were in a research setting as opposed to a setting oriented toward patient care and comfort. Call (800) 4-CANCER for further information.

Non-US citizens are also admitted to trials at the NCI at the discretion of the principal investigator. Criteria weighed in making this decision include whether a US citizen would be denied treatment if a non-US citizen were enrolled, and whether treating this particular individual's illness would benefit medical progress.

Future treatment directions

During the past few years there has been much talk about new ways of approaching cancer treatment. Concerns about the toxicity of treatment and the loss of good, necessary cells as a result of therapy have made scientists look beyond chemotherapy. Ideas and theories from many areas of expertise are beginning to coalesce, and this should serve to bring about dramatically new methods for cancer treatment. Scientists are looking at cancer causes and ways to work with genes. They are identifying substances that may prevent the proliferation of cancer cells and providing new ways to deal with various genetic problems that might otherwise encourage unrestrained cell growth. They have identified the biological substances that work to enable cells to mature.

Many different avenues have been explored, and much has been done recently to improve upon and create new therapies for treating leukemia. This research is likely to continue.

Over the past decade, cancer research has tried the following:

- Targeting ways to identify the human genome, thus leading to a clearer understanding of the necessary genetic changes that must occur to set the stage for the development of leukemia

- Targeting specific antibodies, expressed by cells that are known to be present in leukemia, by using cell morphology, cytogenetics, and immunophenotyping

- Identifying and testing potentially useful anticancer substances that appear to help control leukemic cell growth so that the patient has a manageable disease and reasonable quality of life—without a cure *per se*

- Designing drugs that support the patient and his quality of life, that may not destroy cancer cells, but that contribute significantly to his survival by eliminating the secondary effects and illnesses related to treatment

Research in biological anticancer substances

This section deals with substances naturally made by the body to fight foreign substances. There are large numbers of researchers and of patients who view these substances as potentially curative while having lower toxicity.

Rituxan was approved by the FDA for use with non-Hodgkin's lymphomas, but is now in trials for leukemias as well. Campath-IH has been in phase II clinical trials and has been presented to the FDA for approval. Rituxan and Campath are monoclonal antibodies that are in trials to discover how well they work and to find their ideal dosages. Although these two antibodies have been billed as being less toxic, patients have reported some adverse side effects resulting from therapy.

Interferon alfa, approved for use in treating CML, is another example of a successful biological anticancer substance. Interferon alfa requires continuous use and produces flu-like symptoms, which are uncomfortable for the patients using it. However, researchers in Houston have shown that simultaneous Interferon alpha (IFN-alfa) and Homoharringtonine (HHT) is an effective regimen in Philadelphia Chromosome (Ph) positive chronic myelogenous leukemia, particularly in elderly patients (age greater than 60 years), because the presence of HHT alleviates some of the INF-alfa symptoms that occur when it is not present.

Antibody therapy

One kind of biological therapy that shows great promise is monoclonal antibody therapy. Antibodies are substances secreted by the white blood cells that turn into plasma cells. They attach to foreign material and pathogens so that the invaders can be destroyed by the T cells and macrophages. Antibodies that have been engineered in the lab to attach to only one cell surface receptor—called monoclonal antibodies—have been used to tag cancer cells for detection, quantification, and therapeutic applications.

Several antibodies are currently under study as possible treatments against leukemia. These include:

- Bexxar, a radioactive iodine-131 antibody that works for cells expressing CD20.

- CD47, an antibody that encourages apoptosis, killing off leukemia cells.

- H-LL2 (epratuzumab), anti-CD22 humanized monoclonal antibody, is also known as LymphoCide. It has two radioiodized forms Yttrium 90 and iodine-131.

- LMB-2, which is being tested against T-cell leukemias.

- Rituxan and Campath-1H, two antibodies active against CLL.

- Zevalin, a 90Y-labeled anti-CD20 monoclonal antibody. It is the radioactive form of Rituxan.

Bexxar is a radioactive monoclonal antibody that works with cells marked with CD20 (a B-cell antibody). The antibodies are welded to radioactive iodine-131. They target a protein called CD20, which is on the surface of B-cell leukemia cells. The treatment is thought to work both by delivering lethal radioactivity to the cancer cells and also by flagging them for destruction by the immune system. This monoclonal antibody is still in clinical trials.

The antibody CD47 appears to be very promising in creating a new kind of cell apoptosis (programmed cell death). It is being studied by researchers using AML, CML, and CLL cells, in hopes that it will produce alternative therapies to encourage cell apoptosis using signal-regulatory proteins which tell cells when it's time to die.

H-LL2 is a humanized immunoglobulin (Ig)G2a-kappa anti-CD22 anti–B-cell monoclonal antibody with proven targeting and therapeutic efficacy in the management of non-Hodgkin's lymphoma (NHL). It is in clinical trials for CLL.

LMB-2 is a recombinant immunotoxin (anti-Tac[Fv]-PE38) that targets an interleuken-2 receptor CD25. LMB-2 is being evaluated in clinical trials as treatment for hematologicalal malignancies. Cell lines derived from patients with hematological malignancies react to immunotoxins, not only with inhibition of protein synthesis, but also with characteristic hallmarks of apoptosis. Immunotoxins may be valuable in the treatment of cancers that are resistant toward apoptosis because their targeted killing is often facilitated by, but not completely dependent on, programmed cell death. Therefore, LMB-2 is another hopeful possibility for treating leukemias.

The original testing of Campath used a mouse antibody, however, the present Campath–IH is a humanized antibody that binds to the antigen CD52, which is expressed almost exclusively on lymphocytes and is not expressed on hematopoietic stem cells or progenitor cells. CD52 is expressed on greater than 95 percent of B cells and T cells. Campath destroys the cancerous lymphocytes. For example, Campath-1H combats CLL by selectively depleting only leukemic lymphocytes expressing CD52. Hematopoietic stem cells are not affected at all. This selective depletion permits the body to retain needed hematopoietic stem cells that are the precursors to, and repopulate the blood with, healthy lymphocytes that preserve normal immune function.

Rituxan is a chimeric IgG 1 kappa monoclonal antibody. This antibody recognizes the CD20 antigen expressed on normal B cells and in most malignant B-cell lymphomas. This antigen, important in cell cycle initiation and differentiation, is expressed strongly in over 90 percent of B-cell lymphomas. This CD20 antigen is also expressed in 97 percent of the patients with CLL, but the fluorescent intensity is markedly less in CLL than it is in low-grade lymphoma. As presently given, Rituxan shows activity with approximately 20 percent of CLL patients. Rituxan is being used in CLL therapy in clinical trials as a sensitizer to augment the concentration of chemotherapy drugs. Combination therapy using Fludara and Cytoxan with Rituxan and/or Campath is the latest clinical trial recommended for those with CLL (at press time).

Zevalin, the radioactive form of Rituxan also known as ibritumomab tiuxetan (IDEC-Y2B8), is an anti-CD20 murine immunoglobulin G1 Kappa monoclonal antibody. The tracer is Yttrium 90 and it is used for refractory or relapsed NHL and is in clinical trials for CLL. The radioactive form may cause additional killing of nearby cells, so if you didn't express enough CD20, using Zevalin might enable the destruction of additional malignant cells.

Merl participated in a phase II Rituxan trial for untreated patients and at this time is pleased with the results. One anecdote is never sufficient reason to sign up for a trial: by definition a phase II clinical trial tries to answer the question of whether a new agent or combination of agents will be more or less effective than current standard treatment. However, Merl's story of a measurable response and the lack of side effects is potentially encouraging to others who are considering participating in the wide range of clinical trials:

> Three weeks ago I completed eight weeks of infusions of Rituxan as part of a clinical trial at M. D. Anderson Cancer Center (MDACC) using Rituxan for untreated patients. I experienced absolutely no side effects during the infusions or afterwards. We would drive over to Houston from central Texas, a ride of three hours in the early morning, then have the Rituxan infusion taking four or five hours, and return home the same evening.

One month after completing treatments, my white blood counts were
still in the 100,000 range. Yesterday my white count was down to 57,000
with all other counts in the normal ranges. So I am back to watch and
wait until my next appointment at MDACC in three months.

As I am apparently one of a very few patients who has received this;
there is no past experience to predict what results might be expected with
Rituxan or how long the Rituxan might be beneficial.

Antiangiogenesis

Most tumors trigger the growth of many new blood vessels to support the metabolic needs of the tumor. This growth of new blood vessels is called angiogenesis. Antiangiogenic agents interrupt the body's ability to grow new blood vessels, causing tumors to shrink. An attempt to starve tumors by reducing the blood supply, antiangiogenesis is also likely to reduce the blood supply to normal tissues. In more recent findings, researchers found that angiogenesis is not limited to solid tumors, but is also linked to leukemia and other "liquid tumors."

Recent studies of leukemia cases show that this cancer of the blood system does, unexpectedly, involve growth of new blood vessels in the bone marrow. In other types of cancer, it was well known that new blood vessels must grow into solid tumors if they are to expand. But it was assumed that blood cancers such as leukemia would not require that because leukemia involves unrestrained growth of malignant cells in the blood, but no solid tumor formation.

Studies in children with leukemia have shown evidence of abnormally elevated levels of angiogenic growth factor bFGF (a hormone that stimulates blood vessel growth) in their urine. Microscopic examination found tiny new blood vessels growing in the children's bone marrow.

Antiangiogenic agents offer possibilities for treating adult and childhood leukemia in the next several years. Angiostatin and Endostatin are two examples of drugs that are being developed. Thalidomide is a first-generation antiangiogenic drug currently in clinical trials. However, Thalidomide is unsafe if a patient wishes to become pregnant (based upon the drug's previous history of causing birth deformities). Carboxyamidotriazole and paclitaxel, two additional antiangiogenic agents, are being studied for use with AML, ALL, and CML.

Antisense therapy

DNA wants to exist in paired strands, except when a cell is dividing. Because cancer cells are known to have one or more faulty genes somewhere along the length of their DNA, some researchers are experimenting with delivering short pieces of DNA or RNA that will match the faulty genes and couple with single strands of the cancer cell's DNA. It is hoped these short pieces of DNA or RNA might interfere with a leukemia cell's division and replication in a variety of ways—for example, they may interfere with the ability of the oncogene to produce protein.

Antisense therapy relies on agents that will alter disease processes by blocking reproduction of harmful proteins by cancer cells. These agents seek out and stop the diseased cells' messenger RNA (sense strand). Without the antisense intervention, the RNA would carry out its programmed job to provide basic directions for the production of disease-causing proteins. If the message can be intercepted by use of the antisense agent, new cancer cells will not be formed. If the agents prove effective, they will play an important role in preventing the spread of leukemic cells.

Bcr-abl stands for the name given to an abnormal gene that is the result of a fusion of material from two chromosomes (22 and 9). This has everything to do with the Philadelphia chromosome in ALL and CML. The Philadelphia (PH) chromosome is an abnormal chromosome that results from an exchange of material (DNA) between the normal chromosomes 22 and 9. In chromosome 9, there is a gene called c-abl. A break occurs beside this gene, and it is translocated to a place in chromosome 22 called bcr (breakpoint cluster region). What happens then is the fusion of these two pieces of DNA that gives rise to a fusion gene (bcr-abl). This fusion gene is involved in the development of CML and possibly other leukemias (e.g., ALL). Hopefully, bcr-abl might prove useful as a target for specific antisense treatment agents, which would prevent increases of leukemic cells, sparing normal tissues from the damage caused by chemotherapy (which is not selective for leukemic tissue).

An antisense agent that could prevent growth of bcl-2/Bax cells could also be an effective treatment for leukemia. Elevated bcl-2/Bax is a consistent feature of apoptosis resistance in B-cell CLL and is known to be associated with resistance to present chemotherapy agents. High bcl-2 levels are associated with chemoresistance, as in the case of acute myeloid leukemias and other malignancies. Important here is the finding that bcl-2 is not at all present in hematopoietic stem cells. That means that these stem cells would not be killed by antisense treatment and would become healthy cells available to combat leukemic cells.

Gene therapy

Gene therapy includes several kinds of cancer treatment that all involve modifying genes to cause them to die or to correct damage so that they will function as a normal cell does. Gene therapy in the strict sense means reinserting genes into cancer cells that lack properly functioning copies of these genes or inserting a man-made suicide gene into the leukemic cell to make the cell more susceptible to the toxic effects of certain drugs.

White cells can also be modified to attack leukemic cells, using a weakened virus that is genetically changed to contain a piece of the leukemic cell's DNA. When the weakened virus is unleashed in the body, normal white blood cells recognize it as an "invader" and destroy it. Since the virus is also expressing part of the leukemic cells' DNA, the normal white cells become sensitized to this protein and attack it wherever they find it—either on the virus coat or on the leukemic cell.

Leukemic cells are collected using leukapheresis, a painless process much like that for donating platelets. The collected leukemia cells will be sent to a central laboratory where they will be infected with the virus and tested. In the central laboratory, the cells collected from the leukapheresis will be infected with a crippled (unable to reproduce) cold virus that will add genetic material (DNA) to the leukemic cells. These cells are then considered altered. Because of the added DNA, your altered leukemic cells will make a protein (CD154) on their surface that is intended to stimulate your immune system to attack your own leukemic cells. At a later date, the altered leukemic cells will be given to the patient by infusing them through a needle placed in a vein in the arm.

Currently in the NCI's database there are more than 30 clinical trials classified as gene therapy for many different cancers. Invariably, trials are made with solid tumors before they are made in hematological malignancies, so gene therapy for leukemia is proceeding very slowly. Some current clinical trials do use gene therapy for leukemia however.

Cell cycle inhibitors

In a normal cell, DNA is surveyed for damage after it is copied in the early steps of cell replication. Cells go through this cycle on a regular basis. A substance called protein kinase C interacts with other substances to ensure a rest phase during which damaged DNA is repaired before the next step of cell division begins. If damage cannot be repaired in a particular cell, it is marked for destruction by the P53 gene. P53 is a key player in overseeing the orderliness of our DNA and its replication. It is called the guardian of the genome. P53 keeps the DNA pure and error-free.

Researchers believe that cell cycle inhibitors might be effectively used against cancer cells. Substances in this category, which are in clinical trials to test their effects against leukemia, include:

- **Bryostatin.** A protein kinase inhibitor naturally derived from a marine bryozoan. It appears to change certain leukemic cells into hairy cells and increases their response to interferon alfa and cladribine. Hairy cell leukemia is responsive to both agents.

- **Flavopiridol.** A synthetic flavone that is a potent inhibitor of cyclin-dependent kinases. Cyclins are proteins that govern the progression of the cell from one stage of cell division to the next. Like UCN-01 below, flavopiridol produces cytotoxicity independent of the patient's treatment status, which makes it an ideal agent for early leukemia testing. It is in clinical trials as a treatment for leukemia.[1]

- **GW506U78.** A nucleoside analogue derivative of Ara-G that shows great promise with adult T-cell leukemia in the acute stage. It is also being studied for fludarabine refractory CLL.

- **Lactacystin.** An inhibitor to the ubiquitin-protease pathway that helps in antigen processing. It has been suggested that there is an essential role of the ubiquitin system in apoptotic cell death control in CLL lymphocytes. Lactacystin sensitizes chemo-resistant and radioresistant human chronic lymphocytic leukemia lymphocytes to undergo apoptosis.[2]

- **STI-571.** A Bcr-abl–specific tyrosine kinase inhibitor, active and showing exciting results against an enzyme found in CML and ALL patients who have the Philadelphia chromosome transposition. STI-571 inhibits the expression of bcr-abl kinase, a mutated protein kinase linked to the uncontrolled proliferation of white blood cells. Clinical trials are actively underway for this exciting drug.[3]

- UCN-01. A derivative of the potent protein kinase C inhibitor stauro-sporine. UCN-01 may augment the activity of chemotherapy in drug resistant patients. UCN-01 has a different action mechanism than many other protein kinases have. It has been shown to be highly toxic to CLL cells by stimulating apoptosis.[4]

Vaccine therapy

Viruses engineered to target only cancer cells are being considered as one way to damage leukemia cells and spare healthy tissue. The virus itself could attack and kill the leukemic cells, or it could insert its DNA or RNA into the cell—DNA or RNA that has been modified in the laboratory to contain a killer-sequence or to weaken the cell's defenses or ability to replicate.

Cancer results from changes in the genes that give rise to altered cells that have either prolonged survival or growth advantage. This causes either a tumor or leukemia. The genetic changes can result in abnormal expression of proteins or the expression of new proteins that are different from the proteins ordinarily expressed by normal cells.

The strategy of fighting cancer with a vaccine is one that's based upon recently gained knowledge about how the immune system works and what can help to turn on immune responses. A critical protein appears to be expressed by helper T cells very soon after immune response is initiated. It acts somewhat like a light switch that can help to activate other cells in the immune system, and it makes them better at being able to present proteins and antigens to other T cells. A genetic defect in this protein may indicate immune problems.

This information provides hope that these new proteins, or altered expressions of proteins, will provide targets for the immune system to identify and use to eradicate the leukemia. Vaccines made from leukemic cells that have been removed from the body and cultured in the laboratory can cause our bodies to become resensitized, resulting in renewed attacks against the leukemic cells by the immune system. In other words, cancer cells may remain in the body hidden from the body's own defenses, ultimately allowing leukemic cells to grow and spread; cells grown in the laboratory, made from the patient's own cells, are reintroduced into the patient; the body recognizes those cells as foreign and mounts a defense campaign to kill them off; at the same time, the body becomes sensitive to the leukemic cells that have been hiding within the body and kills them off as well. Phase I trials have shown promising results and phase II trials will start shortly.

Researchers at Memorial Sloan-Kettering Cancer Center report that the vaccination of patients with chronic myelogenous leukemia with bcr-abl oncogene breakpoint fusion peptides generates specific immune responses and is safe for patients in the chronic phase of CML.[5] Clinical trials are in progress. The *Wall Street Journal*, August 4, 2000, has an excellent article in its Health Journal (B1) section about how vaccines work.

Research in chemotherapy

Chemotherapy is not a new form of treatment for leukemia; however, there are many chemotherapy clinical trials for leukemia. A trial might test a new drug that is thought to be promising, fine-tune existing treatments, or improve the results or reduce the toxicity of known treatments.

Several examples of new drugs in research at this time follow. Whether clinical trials of new chemotherapy drugs will prove to be more successful than existing standard treatments or not is unknown at this time:

- The new purine analog, Compound 506U78 (arabinosyl guanosine, Ara-G) has been studied in a broad range of hematological cancers. This drug has major activity in T-cell acute lymphocytic leukemia and is also active in mycosis fungoides and other hematological malignancies.

- A clinical trial of Compound 506U78 in fludarabine-refractory CLL patients has been initiated. A second study is investigating the potential of fludarabine and Compound 506 in combination based on *in vitro* studies suggesting useful synergism.

- 12-O-tetradecanoylphorbol-13-acetate (TPA) is being tested in treating patients who have leukemia that has not responded to previous treatment.

- The drug 6-hydroxymethylacylfulvene is being evaluated in patients with AML, ALL, or blastic phase CML.

Other clinical trials do not test new drugs, but test a standard chemotherapy regimen against a variation (in dosage, schedule, delivery method, combination of drugs, etc.) that may prove more effective or less toxic in treating leukemia. Active chemotherapy trials that are designed to test drug regimens include:

- Evaluating the maximum tolerated dose of combination bryostatin 1 and cisplatin chemotherapy in patients with advanced, incurable malignancies.

- Estimating the maximum tolerated dose of carboplatin plus topotecan given as a five-day continuous infusion in patients with recurrent acute lymphocytic or myeloid leukemia or accelerated or blastic phase chronic myelogenous leukemia.

- Evaluating the safety, maximum tolerated dose, adverse effects, and toxicities of cordycepin, given following a fixed dose of the adenosine deaminase inhibitor pentostatin, in patients with refractory TdT positive leukemia.

- Estimating the lowest dose of deoxycytidine (dC) that can be given as a host protective agent in conjunction with high dose cytarabine (HD Ara-C) in patients with refractory acute myelogenous leukemia or other hematological malignancies.

- Determining the maximum tolerated dose and dose limiting toxicity of dolastatin 10 in patients with chronic myelogenous leukemia in blast phase, refractory or relapsed acute leukemia, or myelodysplastic syndromes.

CHAPTER 11

Communicating with Your Medical Team

Once a treatment decision is made and it is determined that you are ready for treatment, you enter into a vital, long-term relationship with your doctor. It is important to communicate efficiently and clearly so that you are completely confident in your understanding of the information and directions you receive, and that you make your needs and concerns known and understood. Sometimes you will communicate with members of the doctor's staff more often than you will speak with the doctor.

Trust and communication are the foundation of the relationship between doctor and patient. The patient must feel that the doctor takes her concerns seriously, and that needs for information are being met fully. The doctor relies on the patient to communicate information about problems encountered, reactions to medications, adverse side effects, and other experiences in areas of concern.

With present medical practices, every patient must be a self-advocate. Ask questions, read IV bag labels, and be sure you're getting what you expect to receive. It helps a great deal if you have a family member go to the hospital or treatment center with you to ensure that you duly receive the expected medicines, treatments, and even proper meals.

This chapter begins with suggestions for establishing a relationship with your doctor—including letting him know your preferences, finding out who to call in what situation, and preparing for emergencies. It next discusses communicating with your doctor to achieve successful interactions. The chapter then describes medical case managers, the importance of a second opinion, and where to go for the most helpful, up-to-the-minute treatments. It ends with a closer look at the needs for communication and advocacy in hospital settings.

Establishing a relationship with your doctor

After you have chosen your oncologist, you should establish the kind of relationship you prefer. If you choose to let the doctor make the decisions and don't want too much information, share this with your doctor. If you need lots of information, but are concerned about taking too much of the doctor's time, tell your doctor that. If you know how to research your own illness, make that clear as well. Most importantly, if you want to be an active part of the team that makes decisions about your treatment, let your doctor know that up front. Only you can define what matters to you in your relationship with your doctor.

Responsibilities in communication

Both the doctor and the patient have a responsibility to communicate effectively with each other.

Be concerned if your doctor withholds information, or presents it in a cold, tactless manner. You would not expect the doctor to speak in a raised voice, talk down to the patient or family member, or hold medical discussions with you in hallways or waiting rooms. Similarly, you would be frustrated if your doctor peppered information with medical jargon that you could not comprehend or pressured you to make important treatment decisions without adequate knowledge, information, or time to think about it. Some patients have shared horror stories about how doctors belittle them or state that the questions being asked are dumb.

The doctor has reason for concern if the patient withholds information. It is your responsibility to inform your doctor about medical problems, stressful situations that could affect treatment, or the fact that medications are not being taken as directed. There is also no excuse for patients speaking in a raised tone of voice, taking an inordinate amount of the doctor's time, or pretending to understand something that is unclear. Your doctor deserves the same respect she shows to you. Be sure to ask your questions, record the answers, and ask follow-up questions as needed. Be direct about what you have to say—a long, roundabout story is wasteful of your limited time with the doctor.

Acknowledging that doctors are human

Doctors and oncology staff are human. A smile, a thank you, or an "I appreciate what you are doing for me," or some statement indicating that you can mentally put yourself in the other person's place, can sometimes transform an encounter from tense to pleasant.

Since staff members are human, they have good and bad days, light and heavy days. They usually try to do their best for each patient. So make allowances if someone is less efficient than usual or if you find yourself waiting longer than usual. There may have been an emergency or a terrified new patient whose concerns the doctor needed to allay. You can forgive that delay when you feel that the doctor would spend as much time with you in a similar situation.

Helping the doctor know you

Try to make your doctor aware of you as an individual. Consider that:

- Your lifestyle, profession, and interests need to be taken into consideration when a treatment program is prepared for you. Make sure you talk about your occupation and the amount of physical and mental stress you experience in your job.

- Inform the doctor of any members of your family who also have or had cancer and what type of cancer is or was involved.

- Let the staff and your oncologist know how much you understand about your disease so meetings can be held at your comfort level.

- The doctor should also be made aware of family, financial, or other current difficulties.

- Be very clear about your goals for quality of life during and after treatment, and whether you are thinking of having children in the future.

If you prefer that some information you share not go beyond your doctor's ears, ask that it not be written down in the records, so that there is no possibility that it can get into the hands of an insurance carrier or anyone else.

Who to call for what situation

In between office visits, patients may need additional information about side effects, supplemental medications to control nausea and pain, or what to do for any other medical problems. Patients and family members need to know the doctor's preferred procedures for such problems. Ask for advance clarification during an office visit so that you are prepared when the need arises. For example:

- Find out if you should leave voice mail messages for the doctor, speak with one of the oncology nurses—and if so which one, or if there is another way you should communicate with your doctor.

- It is wise to find out the doctor's policy about being paged on weekends and holidays.

- Tell your doctor and staff if it is okay to call you at work. Be sure to let them know whether they may leave detailed messages on your answering machine without violating your privacy.

- Clarify which problems to bring to the oncologist and which ones to bring to your family doctor or internist. Some oncologists request that all concerns come directly to them, while others want you to take colds, flu, respiratory infections, and similar problems to your family doctor. Be aware that while you are undergoing chemotherapy the rules may change, and everything may need to go through the oncologist. Many family doctors don't feel comfortable treating patients in active chemotherapy because they can't be aware of all the possible drug choices they shouldn't be prescribing during treatment.

The following leukemia patient handled the "What do I do if..." questions by speaking with her oncology nurse. She recounts that the exchange of information was helpful to both:

> One day, shortly after I began receiving chemotherapy, the treatment room was empty and the nurse had time to talk. "Tell me," I asked, "what do I do in case of emergency? Does he want me to call and talk with him, or am I supposed to talk to one of the nurses? I've been worrying about that."

> She smiled and said, "I wish everyone would think to ask that question. It sure would make things smoother around here. Call and ask for me or his other nurse. We can get his ear faster than any other staff members. Tell us exactly what is happening or what you need. One of us will be back to you as rapidly as we can. Don't hesitate to leave a voice mail message in our mutual mailbox. One of us checks it every fifteen minutes."

I smiled and said, "That's great, I feel much better knowing that! What do I do after the office closes?"

"That's when you call the exchange number. One of the doctors is on call every evening and on weekends, so some doctor in this office will be back to you very quickly. Just call the exchange number, and give your name and phone number. Don't even bother mentioning the problem; the doctor will talk with you and you can tell him then."

Having that information made my life much easier. I told other family members (and patients) what the procedures were, and although I've had to call the exchange number only three or four times in five years of treatment, the system has always worked like a charm. I find that if it isn't my own doctor who is on call, it's one of the other three doctors, whom I have met, and with whom I feel comfortable. I like the system and it works well for my family members and for me.

Preparing for emergencies

Find out what to do in an emergency. In some circumstances, if you are running a fever, the doctor may want you in the hospital immediately. Patients and caregivers need to know who to call to arrange that and who to contact if any other emergency occurs. Just having that information in advance is reassuring.

Another important issue to ask the doctor about is ambulance service. If the patient becomes very ill and needs emergency assistance, caregivers need to know what to say to the emergency medical technicians (EMTs) who come with the ambulance service.

You need to know which hospital you should ask to be taken to, and make the doctor aware you are in the emergency room. If you are well enough to have a family member drive you, do that—so that you are in better control of the situation. Sometimes the rules for ambulance calls require that the patient be taken to the nearest hospital, and that's not always one at which your doctor has visiting or usage privileges.

It's much more reassuring in an emergency situation to have your own doctor, or one from the practice that you know, instead of one with whom you have no relationship.

Documents and letters to have on file

If the patient doesn't already have a living will and a medical power of attorney, these need to be drawn up, to be prepared for all contingencies. Without these documents, there is no way to change normal procedures in grave emergencies—and medical practices may be carried out that are not what the patient wants. Check to find out how your living will should be written and where it should be filed. It makes sense to have one on file at the hospital to which your doctor is affiliated, and another copy in your doctor's records, so that no time will be wasted in an emergency.

One patient describes making plans for a living will and medical power of attorney at her daughter's urging:

> My daughter is an EMT who works with the Volunteer Ambulance Corps in our city. She drives the ambulance and does emergency first aid or follows doctors' orders given over the phone. She says that she is amazed that so few people know what hospital they need or have even planned for an emergency. Many don't know that emergency CPR and breathing apparatus must be used if an ambulance is called. This means that every attempt will be made to keep the patient alive. There is no "do not resuscitate" order in an ambulance.

If your children live out of town and aren't known to your medical team, but you want them to be able to talk with your doctors, do put on file in the doctor's office a letter stating that intent. In it, simply state that you wish your children (named in the letter) to have complete access to all your medical records, and to be able to ask questions of medical personnel and your insurance carrier concerning your health. Be sure your name, address, and phone number are on it. Sign it. Make copies for yourself and for each child, and have it on file in each medical office you visit.

Talking with your doctor

In general, the more directly you communicate, the better the chance of getting good care. It is hard for the patient to know when the doctor is being told enough. Or you may be overwhelmed by the emotional aspects that accompany cancer and the complexities of treatment options. The following sections contain suggestions for concise, yet complete, communication.

Between office visits

Document what has happened between office visits and jot your questions down in a small notebook that you can easily carry to the office with you. Between visits, don't hesitate to call your doctor's office with anything unusual that arises. At the next office visit, remind the doctor of those calls so he can be sure they are documented and be sure you understand the directions you were given to solve those problems.

Preparing for a visit

Before you go to an appointment to see the doctor, reread your accumulated notes. Then sit down with your caregiver and compile a list of problems you have encountered and concerns that need attention. It helps if you prioritize items. What seems unimportant to the patient may be very much a concern for the doctor.

Make another copy of your list to give to the doctor. This makes the doctor aware of your concerns so she may answer questions that have arisen between visits. This also lets you both know the agenda, and it keeps you from leaving the office with feelings of frustration because you forgot to ask a major question that you needed answered.

In today's medical world of managed care and limited doctor visits, it is very hard to get enough time from your oncologist to have all possible questions answered. One way to get the information you need is to research your disease outside of your visits and then distill the information into one or two questions to ask the doctor or oncology nurse. Don't walk into your doctor's office on a scheduled office visit with an inch-thick pile of papers. That is not a good way to keep the communication lines open. The doctor will feel put upon, other patients will have to wait, and you will be frustrated on being left with unanswered questions.

If you have many questions or have found lots of information on the Internet that you simply must discuss with the doctor, make a special appointment just for this purpose. It isn't fair to expect an extra twenty minutes of the doctor's time when you were scheduled for only a half hour office visit. Provide an advance copy of any articles you want to talk about so that the doctor isn't caught by surprise. That way you make the best possible use of time and opportunity.

Asking questions

It's fine to have questions. In fact, it's downright important that you have questions—and get answers.

Ask questions that the doctor can answer. A question such as, "How many patients with this type of leukemia have you treated," is more precise and easier to answer than, "Have you done this procedure a lot?"

Understand that sometimes you will ask a question that the doctor can't answer. A question such as, "What do you think of the new clinical trial for agent X that I found on the Internet" might be a topic so new that the doctor doesn't have any information. A question such as, "How will I react to chemotherapy?" have no definitive answer; there is general information that the doctor can share, but each person is different. Bear this in mind especially if you have an adverse reaction during chemotherapy. Some adverse reactions can be very unpredictable and it is impossible for any doctor to predict every possible reaction.

The following suggestions can facilitate communication with your doctor:

- Help out and remind the doctor about allergies, previous medicine changes, and other things that you believe may have slipped out of mind. Doctors see many patients in the course of a day and, with the best will in the world, they can't remember all the details of each individual patient's chart. Sometimes they may forget something basic that you shared previously.

- Ask your doctor to translate medical terms, so that you understand what you are told. Restate what you think the doctor said to be sure it is clear to you. By restating and confirming what you heard, any confusion may be eliminated. Doing this makes you feel more like an active member of your medical team and returns some feeling of control that you feared lost.

- Don't allow the doctor to distract you. If you are interrupted, be sure to get back to the question you still need answered. If you are interrupted often, simply comment that you need to get on with this thought before you move to another topic.

- Take a friend or caregiver with you to office visits, especially those during which you may be discussing new options or receiving new information. You may remember only part of what is said, and the caregiver may well recall the rest, so that between you, you have the essence of the conversation. Your friend or caregiver may note issues that neither you nor your doctor considered. Make it clear that you want the medical staff to communicate as fully with your caregiver as they would with you.

- If your doctor is comfortable with it, record the meeting, and then review the tape later with the person who was with you. If your doctor demurs, explain that you can't always remember the entire conversation, and that this way you can be sure you are complying with his instructions.

- Always ask for copies of bloodwork, pathology reports, and other medical records. Keep your own set of copies and understand what they contain. Make sure that your caregiver or family member knows where these are kept in case of an emergency.

Resolving problems

When communication problems arise, it is best to be open with the doctor and explain your feelings so the two of you can work to resolve such issues. It could be that the doctor is unaware that there is a problem. Some of the very best doctors have difficulty communicating with their patients. To make sure you are not part of the problem, ask the doctor and staff members how you can help improve communication.

If you have a complaint, voice it in a calm, objective way, and suggest possible solutions. Explain that you understand the pressure that medical personnel, as well as patients, are under, but that this current problem is causing you considerable distress. This leaves the staff with the impression that they are dealing with a reasonable individual who understands compromise and makes allowances for human error. It also allows you to become more direct later on if things haven't improved as they should. Going on the offensive whenever you have a complaint will not help communication. Keep written documentation of complaints in that same small notebook, so that you know how problems are being addressed.

If it's hard for you to share a problem with the oncologist face-to-face, you may prefer to put your concerns into writing and send the letter by mail. Explain the communication problem to a sympathetic nurse, social worker, or patient advocate, so that they may help you resolve the problem. Ask other cancer patients you know how they have solved similar difficulties. (However, don't confuse the particulars of your case with those of others. Each patient is unique and what applies to one may not necessarily apply to another, even if both patients have the same disease and the same treatment regimens.) Your family doctor might be willing to intercede and give you suggestions on ways to communicate with the specialist. If you are hospitalized, contact the hospital ombudsperson or a hospital official and ask for help.

If all else fails and you still can't communicate comfortably, it's time to consider finding another oncologist. This is a long-term relationship and it should fulfill your needs. Don't feel guilty or hesitant about it, just ask your family doctor, a fellow patient, or another doctor for a referral to someone else. Meet with the new doctor to make sure you are reasonably compatible in the way you think and operate. While changing doctors can be traumatic, civility makes it easier for both sides.

It is helpful to inform your new doctor that you are changing from your previous oncologist due to communication problems. Avoid being overly "descriptive" in voicing your complaints though; just focus on the kinds of communication you feel you need. A torrent of accusations aimed at your previous doctor will only make the new doctor wonder what he is letting himself in for, and put him on the defensive.

Medical case managers

Some types of managed care companies flag patients who have become "expensive" to the insurance company or who have been diagnosed with a catastrophic illness and assign those patients a nurse as a medical case manager. Medical case managers function as patient advocates and try to help patients conserve their lifetime insurance dollars. These nurses, for the most part, do not work for insurance companies, so their loyalty should be to patients. Medical case managers are available to advise about treatment options and to help keep track of the bills that may be accumulating, and can be very helpful in supplying patients with clarifying information. If you are assigned a medical case manager and are fortunate enough to get the right person in this role, the relationship can be extremely helpful to you and to family members.

One of these dedicated professionals shared one of her patient's stories:

> Six months ago I had a patient who underwent a bloodless stem cell transplant. Her religious beliefs precluded her from having a mixed blood transplant. Since it was an autologous transplant, and she was using her own blood, she was willing to let her blood cells be apheresed, knowing that her own purged blood would be returned to her. She was given IV iron, and lots and lots of epoetin, and had the transplant when her hemoglobin count was between twelve and fifteen. She was very closely watched and never required blood transfusions or platelets.
>
> The treatment was successful and she's still doing well. I was glad that I was able to help her arrive at the decision to have the transplant, because it has made such a difference in her life.

Second opinions

Sometimes in diagnosing and treating leukemias, the doctor, patient, or both feel that it would be helpful to have the advice of someone who specializes in the patient's kind of cancer.

If you have any concerns about the options presented and decisions made for your care, get a second opinion. While you may have to justify this to your insurance company, you should not have to apologize to your own doctor for wanting one. Most reputable oncologists are perfectly willing to recommend that their patients get a second opinion at a crossroad in the diagnostic or treatment paths.

It is important to get the second opinion from someone who is not in your own doctor's office; sometimes doctors who work in close proximity have very similar ways of thinking about a given situation. If you are in an HMO, the company may object to getting an opinion from another medical practice, but do not give in on the need for a different venue. This is the time to locate the best possible medical expert.

You can't be part of the cancer community for long before learning about the best hospitals and cancer centers for treating your kind of cancer. The word is passed from patient to patient, via Internet support groups and newsgroups, and among patients attending local support groups. Many times the referrals are to physicians at one or more of the group of comprehensive cancer centers established by the National Cancer Institute (NCI), part of the United States National Institutes of Health (NIH). The Cancer Information Service (CIS) at (800) 4–CANCER will provide you with the names of excellent doctors to use for second opinions. Unless your doctor is unhappy about your going for the second opinion, he will also be an excellent referral resource.

Merle Stock sought a second opinion on his treatment options for CLL after not being comfortable with the treatment recommendation from his oncologist. He tells other patients in his situation to educate themselves before making a treatment decision:

> Nine months ago my white blood cell count had climbed to 100,000, with no other symptoms. My oncologist wanted to begin immediate treatment with Fludara. I was not really comfortable with that option (the only one addressed) and I elected to do some additional research first.

> After much research and many telephone contacts I was able to make an appointment with Dr. Michael Keating at the M. D. Anderson Cancer Center in Houston for a second opinion. I was most pleasantly surprised with how accessible Dr. Keating was.

> My oncologist did not appear to have any interest in my obtaining a second opinion. It rather seemed that she felt it threatened her position as my doctor.

> I would strongly encourage everyone to follow the oft-repeated advice, "Educate yourself, learn all that you possible can before making treatment decisions." If you are not 100 percent comfortable with your oncologist or the treatment proposed, seek a second opinion. See one of the top CLL experts if at all possible.

Communicating with the hospital staff

There are several circumstances that might result in your being admitted to the hospital, such as treatment for infections that arise during chemotherapy, delivery of drugs that require offsetting with other protective drugs, or to receive the care required in connection with bone marrow transplantation.

It is important for patients to advocate for themselves during hospitalization. This statement is not a slur against hospitals or nursing care. With cost-cutting practices, many hospitals are understaffed and nurses are overloaded with patients. That's an open invitation to mistakes, and recent studies show that medical errors cause an alarming number of deaths in American hospitals.

Almost nobody wants to be hospitalized. The goal is to make the stay short and successful. Ultimately it's your life, and, in spite of perhaps temporarily diminished capacities, you're still very much in charge.

Here are three key points to remember:

- **Read your medical chart.** You may have to ask for access to your chart. Ask questions if anything is unclear. Ask for definitions of terms the staff may use, such as NPO (*noli para os*, nothing by mouth). If you're not well enough to do this, have a friend or relative do so.

- **Verify all drugs given to you.** Ask about oral medications before swallowing, and read the contents of the IV bags on your pole. If you're not well enough to do this, have a friend or relative do so.

- **Tell the nursing staff right away if something seems wrong.** Don't let seemingly simple things, like feeling constipated, become major problems.

The following patient has been hospitalized several times, the most recent while participating in a clinical trial using the monoclonal antibody Rituxan. Her approach to hospitalization is pragmatic and her advice is priceless:

> I had a port put into my chest the day before the infusions began. The worst aspect of that was sitting around all day waiting for an operating room to become available. I also hated missing all three meals that day and having to put my glasses, all unprotected, into a big plastic bag with my winter coat and abandoning them, then not having these things delivered to me until just before noon the next day. Since I'm very nearsighted, I can read without glasses, but I can't distinguish faces.
>
> A few bits of advice based on my latest hospital experience:
>
> 1. If you're having even the simplest surgery, be sure to take along a good strong case for your glasses so you won't stew about them for hours as I did. Also, I suppose, have proper containers for anything else that comes loose from your body such as false teeth, hearing aids, artificial limbs, etc.

2. *If you'll have a port in your chest, don't plan to wear anything that pulls over your head.*

3. *When any hospital personnel (from the lowliest nurse's aid to the most prestigious doctor) leaves your room saying (s)he will be "right back," immediately translate these words in your head to "anywhere from fifteen minutes to an hour and a half, or possibly never at all." Therefore, if this person has left part of your body exposed and it is cold, cover it right up. If (s)he has left the light on and you want it dark, turn out the light. Go back to sleep, for that matter. If the person returns in five minutes, don't be embarrassed, but rejoice that a miracle has occurred.*

4. *Go with the flow and don't sweat the small stuff. If someone wakens you at 3 a.m. and again at 5 a.m. to take blood (with some difficulty, out of your arm, because these particular tests can't be done on blood from the port) and then leaves with the words "Have a good night's sleep," just laugh cheerfully. It's the only way to survive.*

Actually, the staff was quite good otherwise, and this has been my best hospital experience of the three I've had in the last five years. I was in no pain and felt relatively well, so I must assume that most of the other patients were in greater need of prompt attention than I was.

Good interaction techniques and a positive attitude make an unbeatable combination. The following patient used humor to make a difficult hospital stay much easier for herself and others:

Once I moved into my room, I knew it would be my home for at least a few weeks. I decorated the walls and door with cartoons and quips that I had brought with me. Then, using my laptop and a printer, I printed out and posted on my window the joke of the day.

Within two days, the entire staff was making it a point to come in to check on me and to comment on my décor and the joke of the day, read some of the quips and cartoons, and generally let me know that they appreciated my efforts. I certainly received excellent care, and the entire staff knew me.

My health situation wasn't good, and every one of them knew it, but the humor bridged the gap and it let them know I was not going to take this lying down. Clearly it worked, because I am here to tell the tale.

Before discharge, have the staff answer all of your questions about aftercare. Make sure you understand:

- Whether you're really going to be able to handle being at home. If you're not reasonably mobile or pain-free, ask for additional time in the hospital.

- The medications you may be taking.

- Whether the hospital pharmacy can fill your prescriptions before you leave. If not, get the doctor to phone your pharmacy or get a family member to fill prescriptions beforehand.

- What side effects or aftereffects you should watch for that might signal a problem.

- What follow-up appointments should be scheduled and when, plus any diet restrictions.

- Your bill. Always ask for an itemized bill and take time to read it, no matter how complex it appears. You don't want to pay for a birthing room if you are a male cancer patient, and such accidents definitely happen with computer codes being typed in so rapidly today.

CHAPTER 12

Side Effects of Treatment

Too often we recall people who have had terrible experiences while receiving cancer treatment. Yet remarkable progress has been made in alleviating this suffering. The development of medications to relieve nausea and depression, and the development of low-scatter and high-voltage radiation equipment that reduces damage to healthy tissue is especially impressive.

This chapter describes both common and serious side effects of leukemia treatment, and what can be done about them. This chapter may serve as a reference for you as treatment unfolds. Knowing which effects of treatment are temporary, which are harmless, and what to do about those that are not is a useful beginning to dealing with treatment.

Because so many different chemotherapy regimens are used to treat the leukemias, it's not possible to list all side effects of treatment. Nor is it possible in most cases to state unequivocally which side effects are serious and which are not, as a side effect may be associated with more than one condition, and because patients' responses to treatments vary.

Several excellent books focus on treatment from the patient's perspective, including dealing with side effects. If you'd like much more detail about dealing with side effects such as nausea, hair loss, IV lines, appetite changes, or fatigue, look in Appendix A, *Resources*, for a list of titles.

General observations

Always err on the side of caution and call your doctor if you're having unexpected or unusual side effects. Please be encouraged that, although we list many side effects here, you may have very little reaction or no discernible reaction at all to treatment.

Although this text has been reviewed by medical doctors, the author of this book is not a medical doctor and is not familiar with the individual characteristics that make you and your illness unique. The information this chapter provides should never be substituted for your doctor's knowledge.

Report immediately to your doctor any adverse reactions that arise during or after treatment, and direct all questions to your doctor, regardless of other sources of information available to you.

Many cancer survivors expect that treatment will make them feel bad, but they're not sure exactly what to expect. Some are delighted to find that they experience very few side effects of treatment, or none at all.

Side effects experienced by any one patient vary greatly from those experienced by another. Your health before treatment, the type and stage of your disease, the type of treatments you have, and a host of other individual characteristics will impact the side effects you experience. It isn't possible to predict what you will encounter.

Here's a patient who is dealing with a combination of side effects resulting from an allogeneic bone marrow transplant:

> I have had an unremarkable year, which has been a wonderful blessing. I have a very busy life, considering I'm still on disability leave from teaching fourth graders. My health can be described as "medium rare." Most of the time I'm medium, but a lot of things in my routine are rare.
>
> My leukemia is in a very good remission, but I continue to have rejection episodes from the bone marrow transplant and lots of infections. I still take 25-plus medicines per day and I am pestered by daily symptoms and side effects of the drugs. On any given day I may have headaches, muscle fatigue, cataracts, vomiting, or a really bad case of the snots. (What a vocabulary!)
>
> However, most days I am able to get up and accomplish my routine without too much hassle. In November and December, I've been much stronger. My transplant oncologists can't give me timetables for reducing the antirejection drugs, because it's such a new science and every person responds differently.

Why do side effects arise?

Side effects of treatment can arise for several reasons.

First, the treatments commonly used today for leukemia affect not only cancerous cells, but many healthy cells as well. Radiotherapy and many chemotherapy regimens target cells that divide rapidly, as many cancer cells do. This targeting of fast-growing cells means that many healthy cells that divide rapidly—cells in the mouth, intestinal tract, hair, fingernails, and others—will be affected, too. After treatment, these cells die all at once, instead of passing through the life cycle just a few at a time. This rapid turnover of cells causes some of the most common side effects of cancer treatment, such as mouth sores and hair loss. Other side effects come about owing to the body's attempt to heal itself.

Many side effects of treatment are normal and pose no danger to you. Adriamycin, for example, will turn urine red. Mitoxantrone will turn urine blue. These phenomena do not indicate that something is amiss. Fatigue is another common side effect of treatment that does not necessarily herald a problem.

Your oncology team should provide you with information about what side effects to look for and how to deal with them. If your doctor doesn't offer this information, ask for it. If something you're uncomfortable with occurs, even if it isn't on the list, get in touch with your doctor.

It's wise to keep in mind that even commonly used drugs are known to have numerous side effects. Aspirin, for instance, is known to cause any of the following in certain people: vomiting, diarrhea, confusion, drowsiness, severe stomach pain, unusual bruising, bloody or black stools, dizziness, hearing loss, ringing in the ears, difficulty swallowing or breathing, hoarseness, or swelling of hands, face, lips, eyes, throat, or tongue. Like most other drugs, chemotherapeutic agents also are known to cause a large number of both common and rare reactions.

Before we begin discussing individual side effects, it's important to note one generality: worsening side effects may be the result of synergy, increasing in number or degree as the dose or number of drugs increase. Not surprisingly, newer, more aggressive regimens that use high doses of chemotherapy and/or total body irradiation cause more side effects than older, standard dosages. Keep in mind as you read further that a drug or combination of drugs may cause more or worse side effects if given in very high doses. For instance, the standard dose of cytosine arabinoside (Ara-C) causes suppression of bone marrow; high doses may cause damage to nerves, liver, or stomach and intestines. High-dose treatment, such as that used for the acute leukemias, or in preparation for a marrow transplant, may cause stronger side effects.

A word about prednisone

Prednisone, the most commonly prescribed glucocorticoid for controlling the growth of white blood cells, can be responsible for many side effects if given in high doses, and especially if long-term use is in order following allogeneic bone marrow transplantation. Side effects include a suppressed immune response, appetite increases, rapid mood changes, insomnia, stomach pain, gastric ulcer, pancreatitis, diabetes, depression, weight gain (especially in the trunk and face), changes in blood chemistry, menstrual irregularities, impotence, facial redness, thinning of skin, stretch marks, acne, bruising, changes in bodily hair, cataracts, glaucoma, protrusion of the eyeballs, weakening of muscles, osteoporosis, avascular necrosis of bone, high blood pressure, seizures, and, rarely, psychosis.

Fortunately, there is an excellent book available about prednisone and its side effects. *Coping with Prednisone*, written by patient Eugenia Zukerman and her sister, Julie Ingelfinger, who is a medical doctor, can answer just about all questions you might have about using this drug.

If you are taking prednisone for about fourteen days in a row as part of CHOP or a similar chemotherapy regimen, you may notice elevated mood or euphoria while taking this drug, followed by moodiness, depression, fatigue, and pain if the dosage is ended abruptly. Ask your doctor if you can taper the last two or three days of your dosage. Some physicians recommend a taper after as little as fourteen days' use. Other doctors feel that fourteen days is not long enough to disturb the interaction of the adrenal, pituitary, and hypothalamus, but many patients report these side effects when their prednisone dose is finished.

A friend talks about a patient who has been taking prednisone for a long time:

> When I first met Jane she was a petite, sprite of a woman, full of energy and ambition. Then she went on prednisone treatment. The first

thing I noticed was how moody she became—full of conversation and
non-stop talking one minute, and sullen and angry a few minutes later.
That was totally out of character for her.

As treatment went on she began to expand physically. She said the
prednisone made her hungry, so she would eat constantly, and she gained
lots of weight. Then her normally slim face began to fill out until it was as
round as the moon. I learned later these were characteristics of long-term
prednisone use.

Side effects of treatment

The most common (nausea, hair loss, fatigue) and most serious side effects
of treatment are listed alphabetically in this chapter. Included within the various sections are tips from leukemia survivors for dealing with side effects.

Abdominal pain

Abdominal pain may occur following treatment regimens utilizing vincristine or prednisone, but it also may signal a serious condition known as typhlitis, an inflammation of the cecum, which is the first part of the large intestine near the appendix.

Typhlitis is emerging as a side effect of newer, aggressive chemotherapeutic
regimens used against lymphomas and leukemias. Phone your doctor immediately if you experience these in combination: nausea, vomiting, swollen
abdomen, diarrhea, fever, and soreness in the lower right side.

Typhlitis results from unusual bacteria thriving in vulnerable parts of your
intestine when your white blood cell counts are abnormally low. Your doctor can confirm this diagnosis with an ultrasound. Typhlitis also is known as
neutropenic enterocolitis, necrotizing enterocolitis, or ileocecal syndrome.
It's more likely to follow aggressive, high-dose treatments, and can be fatal in
a high percentage of patients if not caught early.

See "Constipation," "Metabolic imbalances," and "Radiation enteritis," for
other causes of abdominal pain.

Appetite or taste changes

Chemotherapy and radiotherapy can affect your taste buds to such an extent
that you can't taste food, or it tastes metallic or disgusting.

Adequate nutrition in spite of food aversion is a very important part of your recovery. Eat what you like, but eat as much nutritional food as you can. Ask your doctor about vitamin supplements and liquid supplements such as Nutrical or Ensure.

Others note that, rather than craving particular foods, they are repelled by them, particularly by meat. Foods that once were favorites now have a repugnant or metallic taste and scent.

Bone pain

Steroid drugs such as the glucocorticoid prednisone or the colony stimulating factor G-CSF can cause aching bones and joints. Ice packs may relieve this pain; if not, ask your doctor if the dose can be lowered.

Bone pain associated with G-CSF is temporary. That associated with steroid treatment is usually transient, but may become permanent if it causes avascular necrosis of bone.

Severe back pain may be associated with degenerative changes to the spine following radiation therapy. The spine is not able to sustain as high a dose of radiation as some other organs can. Surgery to fuse spinal discs may alleviate this pain.

See also "Metabolic imbalances."

Breathing problems

Many treatments for leukemia, such as monoclonal antibodies, radiation, or certain chemotherapy drugs that affect the heart can cause difficulty breathing.

Rapid breathing (tachypnea) can be the body's effort to lower levels of excessive acid, called acidosis. Acidosis is a very early sign of certain conditions such as serious infection, kidney damage, or diabetic complications that should be treated immediately.

Rarely, circulatory or respiratory distress results from untreated, intractable constipation. Constipation in its most serious form, fecal impaction, can be fatal.

Call your doctor immediately if you have trouble breathing.

Cognitive changes

Many leukemia patients report that treatment makes them feel disoriented or forgetful. These symptoms should improve over time, although they may improve very slowly.

Steroid drugs such as the glucocorticoid prednisone and dexamethasone are particularly notorious for causing a wide array of aberrant mental processes, ranging from minor and rapid mood swings to severe mania or depression. These changes usually develop within the first two weeks of steroid use, but this is just a general guideline, as these changes may occur at any time, including during subsequent use following an uneventful first use.

Often the actions of these drugs or the cancer itself interfere with normal levels of minerals and metabolites. This is clearly the case with prednisone, which alters levels of cortisol and adrenaline. See "Metabolic imbalances."

Treatment consists of modifying drug dose, controlling symptoms with sedatives or neuroleptic drugs, or just waiting for the effects of the drug to wear off.

Call your doctor if these symptoms are very disturbing, or if you or a loved one feel that these side effects represent a danger to the patient or the family.

Many cancer patients complain about short-term memory loss. One patient discusses her experiences:

> Before chemotherapy, people came to me when they had word questions because I was so skilled at that. I could come up with synonyms and the best word usage in a situation.
>
> Since chemo, however, basic words elude me and I find it very annoying. I was speaking to a group of healthcare workers and wanted to remember the word "formulary," as in the pharmacy list of drugs covered by one's insurance company. It simply wouldn't surface, and I spoke for five minutes about formularies without once using the word that would have made it all clear to everyone. Talk about frustrating!

Recent research studies bear out the concerns expressed by cancer survivors. There is a loss of memory associated with chemotherapy. Tim A. Ahles, a psychologist, presented the results in March, 2000 at a meeting of the American Cancer Society. His findings indicate that ordinary doses of chemotherapy sometimes appear to permanently dull survivors' intellectual powers, leaving them with poor memories, muddy thinking, and inability to do math in their heads. Those having chemotherapy fared worse than those who were treated with radiation.

Constipation

Constipation can be a very serious problem during leukemia treatment, because inactivity, other illnesses, and certain drugs, such as painkillers, vincristine, vinblastine, antidepressants, or antihistamines, may slow or paralyze the intestine or mask the urge to move one's bowels.

Constipation in its most serious form, a total blockage of the intestine, called fecal impaction, can present as circulatory or respiratory distress, and can be fatal. Call your doctor immediately if you feel constipated for more than three days, or if you have difficulty breathing or symptoms of heart failure.

If your doctor agrees, experiment with small amounts of different foods until you have a sense for what will maintain a balance between constipation and diarrhea. Increased fluid intake, regular exercise, increased dietary fiber, warm or hot drinks, privacy and quiet time in the bathroom, easy access to a toilet or bedside commode, and stool softeners may ease constipation. Do not make dietary changes or greatly increase your fluid intake without first verifying these choices with your doctor.

Dehydration

Dehydration is a very serious side effect of vomiting or diarrhea, as cancer patients must have adequate fluid to remove toxins and proteins released by dying cells from the body. Moreover, the quantities of electrolytes and minerals, such as phosphorus, calcium, potassium, magnesium, and sodium, already are disrupted in the leukemia patient, both by disease and by treatment. Dehydration exacerbates this imbalance.

If you suspect you are dehydrated, call your doctor immediately.

The most reliable symptom of dehydration is thirst. Other signs include the inability to urinate about once an hour, the production of very little urine, or the production of urine that is both dark and low in volume. Other symptoms, such as faintness, dry lips, thick saliva, or loss of appetite too closely resemble the side effects of chemotherapy to be reliable indicators of dehydration.

Take in as much fluid as possible, but do not drink products containing electrolytes (such as the products marketed to sports enthusiasts) unless your doctor says that your kidneys are in good condition and that these drinks will do you no harm.

See "Metabolic imbalances" for hypercalcemia.

Diarrhea

Diarrhea is frequently caused by radiotherapy to the abdomen, as dying cells are shed from the intestine, and by chemotherapeutic drugs that disturb the balance of electrolytes, such as potassium and sodium.

Phone your doctor immediately if you experience diarrhea and a fever more than 1.5 degrees higher than your normal temperature, general malaise, severe chills, night sweats, burning or pain while urinating, headache, neck stiffness, coughing, or trouble breathing.

Your doctor can recommend anti-diarrheal drugs, such as Immodium or Lomotil, which you will have to balance carefully with stool-softening drugs to control constipation. Experiment with small amounts of different foods until you have a sense for what will maintain a balance between constipation and diarrhea.

Dry mouth, difficulty swallowing

Normal saliva contains an antibiotic. If saliva is not present, dry mouth can lead to serious dental problems that result in whole-body (systemic) infection and tooth loss.

Gentle but scrupulous dental care is a must. Avoid spicy, sour, or acidic foods. Examine your mouth daily for fuzzy white patches that might indicate a fungal infection. Ask your doctor for drugs to increase saliva flow, or for a homemade mouth rinse that can be used several times a day.

Problems with swallowing that develop after radiotherapy can be corrected with surgical devices that stretch the esophagus.

Extravasation

Sometimes, chemotherapy that is administered by IV can leak out of the vein into surrounding skin, an adverse event called extravasation. The reaction of the body to a high concentration of chemotherapy in the skin can be serious and painful. The vein may be unusable for chemotherapy thereafter; the skin may die, slough off, and fail to regrow. A response resembling an allergic response, known as recall sensitivity, may happen later—sometimes even years later—if the same drug is used again, even if the drug is injected elsewhere.

Symptoms of extravasation include pain, redness, swelling, or burning at the IV site during or after the administration of chemotherapy.

Notify the medical staff immediately if you have these symptoms during or just after IV treatment.

Eye problems

Cranial irradiation, PUVA treatments for graft-versus-host disease, or long-term, high-dose use of the corticosteroid drugs, such as prednisone, are known to cause cataracts, or the redness and soreness of the cornea known as keratitis in some leukemia survivors. While keratitis may resolve on its own, surgery is the only known cure for cataracts.

Fatigue and sleep disorders

Ninety-five percent of patients being treated for cancer report fatigue.

During treatment, you may be able to offset some of the effects of fatigue on well-being and performance by getting as much rest as possible, eating well, and exercising moderately. Nonetheless, you may do best to adjust your demands on yourself to these new circumstances: let the less critical things go and attend only to what matters most.

Symptoms of fatigue should improve after treatment ends; however, many cancer survivors report fatigue years after treatment. Sometimes the fatigue is accompanied by feelings of inertia, so just getting out of bed in the morning can become a major chore. Everything seems to be too much effort, too hard, and the feeling is pervasive. Sometimes patients report that they are hard pressed to get themselves up to go to the bathroom. As healing occurs, so does a return of energy in most cases, so relax and believe this is only temporary.

Sleep disorders are also common, and in some cases persist years after treatment. Insomnia, "night horrors," and corresponding daytime sleepiness plague many leukemia survivors.

Because fatigue can have so many causes—nutritional deficit, drug interactions, tumor activity, tumor death, inability to exercise, depression, changed sleep patterns—it is difficult to treat fatigue with other than trial-and-error methods. Ask your doctor for suggestions for dealing with this problem, and see Chapter 13, *Stress and the Immune System*, for additional ideas.

Fever, chills, sweats

Although fever is common following some chemotherapy treatments, such as G-CSF or certain antibiotics, fever should always be reported to your doctor, especially if other signs of illness accompany fever. Fever can be the first symptom of life-threatening infection when white blood cells have been destroyed by therapy.

Unattended fever in the absence of sufficient white blood cell numbers can be fatal and is a medical emergency requiring immediate attention.

Hair loss and growth

Radiotherapy and many chemotherapeutic agents cause hair loss (alopecia) although there is a wide range of individual responses to treatment in this regard. Some people lose just a little hair; others lose all hair, including body hair, eyebrows, and eyelashes. Others report losing gray hair earlier than hair that contains pigment. Those receiving radiation therapy may lose hair only on the spots irradiated.

New hair should regrow in the weeks or months after treatment. In some instances, it may not regrow, although this is more common after radiotherapy, busulfan therapy, or following the high-dose treatment associated with bone marrow transplantation.

Methods to spare the scalp from exposure to chemotherapeutic agents, such as ice-packing or tourniquets, are not recommended because leukemia cells may be sequestered in the skin or blood vessels of the scalp. Denying chemotherapy the opportunity to kill all leukemia cells may result in failed treatment or relapse.

Hair loss is a great trauma for most patients. One patient describes what it was like when her hair began to come out while she was in the hospital:

> Six weeks after the cytoxan therapy, when I thought I was going to luck out and keep my hair, I started collecting loads of hair on my brush. My white blood cell counts were low and I was put into the hospital for fever that morning. By that afternoon it was raining hair. It fell all over the bed, pillows, blankets, and it was really a nuisance. Did you ever eat from a tray that was rapidly being covered with falling hair? I didn't have the courage to pull it all out, but my first stop on the way home from the hospital was the beauty shop, where I had my head shaved.
>
> My eyelashes, brows, pubic hair, leg and underarm hair followed in the next two weeks. I sunburned my head a couple of times, but other than being cold occasionally at night, it's been kind of nice being able to shower and be dressed and ready to go in less than twenty minutes. The best thing that happened was a friend giving me a T-shirt that said, "I'm too sexy for my hair, that's why it isn't there."

Conversely, interferon and cyclosporine may cause excessive growth of hair (hirsutism). Some women taking interferon-alfa-2B report growing long eyelashes for the first time in their lives.

Heart damage

Radiation therapy to the chest and certain drugs used for leukemia, such as doxorubicin (Adriamycin), are known to be cardiotoxic. Although it is more common for damage from the anthracycline drugs to emerge slowly months or years after treatment ends, immediate and rapidly serious or fatal damage is also possible.

Call your doctor immediately if you experience any symptoms that resemble a heart attack, such as chest tightness or pain, difficulty breathing, or numbness in the left arm or shoulder.

Hypercalcemia

See "Metabolic imbalances."

Infection

Infection can result when neutropenia, a lowering of white blood cell counts, occurs after treatment. The danger period for most patients is five to ten days after treatment. In general, chemotherapy is more likely to cause neutropenia than radiotherapy, but whole-body irradiation can also suppress blood counts.

Preventive measures include hand washing, avoiding scratches and cuts by handling skin gently, such as using an electric razor and patting skin dry, rather than rubbing, thoroughly cooking food, reducing human contact, and avoiding gardening and handling kitty litter.

If you have a fever more than 1.5 degrees higher than your normal temperature, general malaise, severe chills, night sweats, burning or pain while urinating, headache, neck stiffness, coughing, or trouble breathing, phone your doctor without delay.

If an infection develops, your doctor will examine you, and you may be admitted to the hospital, placed in an isolation room, and given a combination of immunoglobulin therapy, antibiotics, antiviral agents, or antifungal agents.

Kidney damage

Temporary or permanent damage to the kidneys may occur with certain drugs, such as ifosfamide, CCNU, methotrexate, or cisplatin. Notify your doctor immediately if you have symptoms of kidney failure, such as unusually high or low levels of urination, swollen limbs, yellowing skin, decreased sweat, or heart or circulatory symptoms.

Liver or gallbladder dysfunction

Mild liver or gallbladder problems sometimes develop when you are fed only by IV line (TPN, total parenteral nutrition), and the problems go away when you resume eating normally.

Lung damage

Cyclophosphamide and bleomycin may cause pulmonary fibrosis; methotrexate may cause pneumonitis. Notify your doctor if you have any symptoms of lung impairment such as chest pain or difficulty breathing.

Metabolic imbalances

The drugs used to treat leukemia may disrupt natural levels of electrolytes, minerals, insulin, or antidiuretic hormone. Hypercalcemia, an excess of calcium in the body, is associated with certain leukemias. Disorders known as diabetes insipidus and syndrome of inappropriate antidiuretic hormone (SIADH) may also develop, or symptoms of delirium or adrenal disease may emerge.

Symptoms of kidney failure due to excessive amounts of calcium, phosphate, and potassium release are noteworthy and can be offset with oral or IV hydration, alkalinization of the urine prior to chemotherapy, careful monitoring of electrolytes, use of diuretics, and low initial doses of chemotherapeutic agents.

If you or your loved ones notice any unusual symptoms, especially excessive thirst, unusually high or low levels of urination, swollen limbs, yellowing skin, decreased sweat, abdominal pain, bone pain, seizures, heart or circulatory symptoms, severe mood changes, dementia, delirium, cognitive changes or psychotic behavior, call the doctor.

Mouth or rectal pain (mucositis)

Most people remember stories about vomiting when they think of chemotherapy, but treatments for leukemia and other cancers may affect the entire gastrointestinal tract, from mouth to anus.

If you experience severe mouth sores, rectal pain that feels like hemorrhoids, or painful or bloody bowel movements, don't suffer in silence. Painkillers and perhaps IV feeding for about a week will help immensely. Some oncologists may prescribe a rinse called Magic Mouthwash that contains a painkiller, an antibiotic, and an antifungal. Your doctor can provide a very helpful cream for hemorrhoids. One patient recalls what brought relief for a hemorrhoid:

> Between the radiation and the chemotherapy, I developed an enormous hemorrhoid. It was painful and gave no quarter. The radiation and high-dose chemotherapy had taken bowel control from me and the hemorrhoid just made a horrendous situation worse. Thank heavens for the magic cream my doctor gave me. Wearing gloves, after I had used the peri bottle extensively to cleanse myself, I'd slather that magic cream over the anal area and feel the first peace I'd felt since I entered the BMT unit.

*My doctor wrote orders for me to have a daily bath in an oatmeal
solution, and that helped shrink the hemorrhoid as well. That bath often
turned out to be the highlight of my day.*

Muscle cramps

Many survivors report muscle cramping, especially in the legs and at night,
during and after chemotherapy. Often the chemotherapy regimen in use contained vincristine or doxorubicin.

Various remedies exist, such as quinine, calcium, potassium, or magnesium.
As calcium, potassium, or magnesium can damage the kidneys, none should
be used until you have discussed this issue with your doctor.

Some leukemia survivors report that heat treatment, or alternating heat and
cold treatment, temporarily reduces pain. Others report that vibrators, massage, or acupuncture help. Bananas and fruits high in potassium often help
ease the situation.

Nausea and vomiting

Nausea and vomiting are the result of some of, but not all, the drugs and
radiation treatments used for leukemia treatment. It's important to control
nausea and vomiting, not just to reduce suffering, but to allow your body to
absorb nutrients to heal. You need to keep well hydrated for flushing chemotherapy drugs from the body, to support your kidney function, and to allow
the uninterrupted sleep during which the immune system can be rebuilt.
You should not suffer nobly through nausea and vomiting as a mark of
strength: you may harm yourself if you do.

Fortunately, excellent drugs are available today to control nausea and vomiting. Zofran (ondansetron) and Kytril (granisetron) are two such anti-emetics, and anti-anxiety drugs such as Xanax, a drug similar to Valium, may
work for brief episodes of nausea. Some steroids, such as Decadron, also
work for reasons that are unclear. Older drugs, such as Compazine, are also
still in use, sometimes in combination with newer drugs.

Phone your doctor immediately if nausea and vomiting are combined with
any of the symptoms described under "Infection."

Take your antinausea medications on time, even if you feel well. They work by priming your body before nausea sets in. Moreover, if you wait to take them until you feel bad, you may lose them as you vomit.

Keep your doctor informed about the success of these drugs, because they can be recombined and substituted by others until you find a good solution.

Some oncologists start by prescribing older, less expensive nausea drugs because their use is more acceptable to insurance companies—even though many patients report that drugs such as Zofran are more effective than other drugs. If your pharmaceutical insurance option is liberal, tell your doctor so that he will feel free to prescribe his best choice first.

Sometimes just the aroma of food can bring on nausea. If so, you might try eating foods that have been chilled. If you are unable to keep food down in spite of nausea medication, feeding by IV line for a period of time gives your stomach a chance to recover.

Anticipatory nausea is also normal for many cancer patients. If you had treatment in the past that made you ill, during subsequent visits your central nervous system may react with nausea to visual cues or odors in the doctor's office. You're not crazy; many people report this reaction, even years after treatment. Chapter 13 describes this subconscious and unbidden learning process more fully.

Neutropenia

See "Infection."

Numbness, tingling

See "Seizures, paralysis, numbness, tingling."

Pain

Pain can be caused by several of the drugs used for leukemia or by radiation therapy.

The vinca alkaloid vincristine is clearly associated with the development of peripheral neuropathy, which may include temporary or permanent pain in hands and feet. Vincristine's negative effects are made worse when G-CSF is also used.

Severe back pain may be associated with degenerative changes to the spine following radiation therapy. Surgery to fuse spinal discs may alleviate this pain.

Painful radiation fibrosis, a reaction of the immune system after exposure to radiation, can develop in any tissue that has been irradiated.

Many other examples could be listed, as pain is a symptom of many aberrant physical processes. The best treatment depends on a correct diagnosis. Consult your doctor or a pain management specialist to find the best treatment for your pain.

Pancytopenia

Pancytopenia is a lowering of all blood cell counts. It's treated with transfusions of red cells and platelets, or irradiated whole blood. See "Infection" for additional information.

Sometimes pancytopenia can affect your life in unexpected ways, as this patient describes:

> I'm cancer-free three years after my BMT. Now, for the first time I can go for the surgery that is needed to take care of an ovarian cyst and a gall bladder full of gallstones. For everyone else this is a serious concern. For me, it's time to celebrate the return of my platelets to normal levels so they can do the surgery without worrying that I will bleed to death. Leukemia sure changes your world view.

Paralysis

See "Seizures, paralysis, numbness, tingling."

Peripheral neuropathy

See "Seizures, paralysis, numbness, tingling" and "Pain."

Pneumonia

Pneumonia is a very likely side effect if you have had chemotherapy, radiation therapy, or bone marrow transplant. In all those cases, it is likely that you have a suppressed immune system making you susceptible to any airborne disease.

Fungal pneumonias are associated with leukemia after high-dose chemotherapy and the compromised immune system that may result. *Pneumocystic carinii* pneumonia causes problems only when there are defects in cell-mediated immunity, which is a characteristic of hematologic malignancies. Most patients have fever, dyspnea, and a dry non-productive cough that may evolve over several weeks or acutely over several days. Antibiotic treatment is given, and sometimes corticosteroids are prescribed as well. *Aspergillis fumigatus*, another fungal pneumonia, is very dangerous indeed, and needs immediate treatment or it can be fatal.

Pneumococcal pneumonia, a bacterial form of pneumonia, and streptococcal pneumonia are also possible side effects of chemotherapy and a compromised immune system. These forms respond well to antibiotic treatment. It is imperative not to neglect a dry, hacking cough, and to call the doctor immediately so that the symptoms do not get worse. More leukemia patients die of pneumonia post-treatment than of any other disease, including the leukemia.

This patient describes what she does when she suspects a problem might turn into pneumonia:

> *I've learned to call my oncologist every time I feel a respiratory illness starting, because when I don't and I try to "tough it out" without drugs, I invariably end up with pneumonia. For most people, it's just walking pneumonia, but for me with a compromised immune system, it's into the hospital for a few days of IV antibiotics and lack of sleep.*
>
> *Wouldn't it be wonderful if hospitals were places to rest and sleep as well as recover? And wouldn't it be even more wonderful if my immune system would start healing itself so pneumonia wasn't always hanging over my head?*

Radiation enteritis

Radiotherapy can cause abdominal or rectal pain, diarrhea, bloody stools, or mucus in stools when the abdomen is targeted. It may be a short-term effect that fades in four to eight weeks after treatment ends, or, in 5 to 15 percent of patients, it may become a long-term chronic problem.

Interference with the absorption of nutrients is the chief concern. Enteritis is treated by controlling diarrhea with Kaopectate, Lomotil, Paregoric,

Cholestyramine, Donnatal, Immodium, or narcotics. Steroid foam may be prescribed if the rectum is quite sore.

Radiation pneumonitis

When the lungs are in the path of radiation targeting leukemia, pneumonitis may develop. This is why lungs are partially shielded during total body irradiation. The symptoms of pneumonitis resemble pneumonia, and it must be distinguished from pneumonia. Pneumonitis is treated with steroids.

Seizures, paralysis, numbness, tingling

Side effects related to the central nervous system are sometimes seen after certain chemotherapeutic agents are used for leukemia.

Seizures may follow use of drugs such as methotrexate, cytosine arabinoside (Ara-C), cisplatin, or ifosfamide. Only about 3 percent of patients receiving these agents experience seizures, and it is more likely to occur in patients who have had cranial irradiation, but it is also possible that seizures will occur in a patient whose metabolic balance has been affected by leukemia or its treatment. Seizures can be controlled with antiseizure medication and are usually transient.

If you are receiving methotrexate or Ara-C administered under the scalp or into the spine, you may be at risk for ascending myelopathy (numbness in the legs and back), and the loss of bowel and bladder control. They usually develop rapidly, and may progress to paralysis. Seizures also may follow. Usually the symptoms abate on their own, but there are instances of permanent damage and even death. Some doctors administer these drugs only at intervals of 48 to 72 hours in order to reduce the chance of this side effect.

The vinca alkaloid vincristine is clearly associated with the development of peripheral neuropathy, which may include numbness, tingling, or pain in hands and feet, and, more rarely, twitches or palsies. Vincristine's negative effects are made worse when G-CSF is also used. Peripheral neuropathy usually is temporary, but may become permanent.

Some leukemia survivors who receive radiation report odd head, neck, or arm symptoms when they tilt their head or twist their neck. Called Lhermitte sign, some report this as dizziness, while others report it as an odd sensation that spans the gap between noise and movement. This is most likely caused by demyelination, a temporary form of radiation damage to the material that insulates our nerves. As electric wires are insulated by rubber, our neurons are insulated by myelin, which serves to protect our neurons from crossover electric current and loss of signal. Lhermitte sign is an indication that two nerves are crossing over in a demyelinated area and are confusing their signals. This symptom should abate in several months.

See also "Metabolic imbalances."

Shingles

See "Viral infections, shingles."

Skin problems

A wide variety of skin problems—pain, itching, burning, discoloration, scaling, wrinkling, dryness, rash, redness—are associated with just about all of the treatments for leukemia; many chemotherapies and radiation therapy can cause these problems.

Ask your doctor for help before tackling this on your own, because dermatology problems can be complex and hard to diagnose. Common remedies, such as lotions that contain alcohol, may make the problem worse, especially if itching is your chief complaint.

The change in skin color that may accompany treatment is often a tanned effect. This is not a true suntan that will protect you from the sun's rays. In fact, your skin will be overly sensitive to sunlight, and prone to wrinkling, freckling, or premature aging, and should be protected accordingly.

If you notice any unusual lesions in the treated areas, such as moles, tell your doctor. Several leukemias are associated with added likelihood of developing skin cancers such as basal cell, or melanomas.

Sore, red, stiff veins

If administered into the arms, vincristine (Oncovin) may cause pain and swelling of veins, even if no leakage occurs.

If you notice lengths of rigid, painful, swollen, or red veins in the days or weeks following receipt of vincristine, tell your doctor, because these symptoms are the same as those associated with blood clots.

Ice packs or warm (not hot) compresses may relieve the pain associated with veins that have reacted to chemotherapy.

To spare your veins from additional damage, your doctor may recommend that you have a venous access device such as a peripherally inserted central catheter (PICC) line or central catheter (port) installed.

Urinary bladder pain, hemorrhagic cystitis

Drugs such as cyclophosphamide (Cytoxan), ifosfamide, CCNU, and platinum-containing drugs, such as cisplatin, can damage the bladder. Simultaneous administration of a drug called Mesna (mercaptoethane sulfonate), along with hydration by mouth and IV, are critical to protect the bladder from this painful and sometimes chronic condition. Sometimes this combination is administered during a brief hospital stay to allow close monitoring to guard against bladder or kidney damage.

Radiation therapy that cannot avoid the bladder also may cause temporary or permanent changes to bladder function. The bladder may become less elastic, and the urge to urinate may become more frequent.

Viral infections, shingles

Viral infections are a major concern with leukemia treatments, and of them, shingles is the most painful and troublesome. All who had chicken pox as a child, and cancer survivors who receive marrow from a donor who had chicken pox, harbor within their nerve cells a herpesvirus called varicella Zoster, the virus that causes chicken pox and shingles, two manifestations of the same illness. There are many human herpesviruses; varicella Zoster is just one. It should not be confused with the genital herpesvirus that is transmitted sexually.

Patients who have had bone marrow transplants and those whose immune systems are compromised are very susceptible to shingles. When the immune system becomes suppressed or dysfunctional, varicella Zoster may re-emerge from nerve endings, causing quite terrible pain and blisters, called herpes Zoster or shingles.

The virus can affect any or all nerve endings within the entire body, but it is most likely to appear along the side of the face, neck, arm, or side of the body. Although 10 to 20 percent of those with shingles may never get blisters, they will still experience itching or pain, or both. The blisters tend to appear in lines, following the paths of nerves. Shingles that affect the eyes can cause temporary or permanent blindness.

If you suspect that you have shingles, contact your doctor at once. Treatment with acyclovir or Valtrex is very helpful at the onset, and so are prescription creams that help deal with the rash and painful, itching feeling. For severe shingles episodes, it is not unusual to require codeine or even morphine briefly. Neurontin (gabapentin) is a new drug that shows great success for the pain of shingles.

Shingles normally heal within four to six weeks, but some patients experience lingering pain for years afterward. If this happens, a procedure called a nerve block or glycerine block can be performed by a neurosurgeon. It should alleviate pain for several months and can be repeated if needed.

Weight gain or loss

One of the myths about cancer treatment is that it always causes weight loss. For any cancer treated with steroids, however, the reverse may be true.

The corticosteroid drugs used against leukemia, such as prednisone, may increase appetite and cause weight gain. When treatment has ended, the weight may drop away on its own, or changes in diet and exercise patterns may be necessary to lose weight. Attempting to lose weight while being treated is not recommended. Maintaining excellent nutritional intake to help your body slough off damaged tissue and rebuild new tissue is difficult enough during treatment without limiting the intake of calories.

It's quite common to develop chubby cheeks, known as moon face, if you're taking prednisone for leukemia. This accumulation of fat in the cheeks will abate after prednisone therapy ends.

If you are losing weight during treatment in spite of, or in the absence of, steroid therapy, notify your doctor, and see the suggestions included in the sections "Appetite and taste changes" and "Nausea and vomiting."

CHAPTER 13

Stress and the Immune System

Few things are more stressful than dealing with cancer. No matter how positive and optimistic leukemia survivors attempt to be, stress will likely still be there. Some people believe that their leukemia was caused by stress, or that it will be made worse by stress, or that perhaps they have a cancer-prone personality. The effects of stress and personality on the inception and growth of cancer are unclear and are still being studied. Animal models indicate that a wide range of tumor responses to physical and emotional stress are possible, depending in some instances on species, gender, stressor, season, previous exposure to stress, and biological state.

Regardless of the effect of stress on cancer, there are good reasons to reduce stress. Your sense of well-being will improve, and you can lessen or prevent the chance of secondary illnesses.

Many research studies have attempted to discover links between cancer, stress, depression, personality, and coping skills. The connections are complex:

- First, there is no consistent evidence that stress causes or worsens cancer. Studies done using animals and humans do not consistently show a positive association between stress and cancer, not even when underlying disease already exists. In fact, in some animals, some forms of stress cause tumors to shrink. More details are provided in the section "Stress and cancer."

- Second, the few studies that hint at a link between personality and cancer are not conclusive for various reasons, such as the design of the study. Details are discussed in the section "Is there a cancer personality?"

- Third, most of the studies have been done on men, and new evidence is beginning to emerge that implies that women react to stress, not in the "fight or flight" manner men do, but in a more social manner, called "tend and befriend." Women seek the support of others rather than become aggressive. This needs to be studied further.

Many research studies have attempted to discover links between cancer, stress, depression, personality, and coping skills. This chapter describes the known associations—or the lack of them—between stress, the immune system, illness, and cancer. A definition of stress is offered, then physical and emotional responses to stress are described, followed by a discussion of the evidence, or the lack of it, regarding stress and cancer. The chapter concludes with ways you can minimize stress or make stress a useful experience. An excellent resource for information about stress is *http://www.stress. org*, which puts out a monthly newsletter called *Health and Stress*.

What is stress?

Experts in various fields of medicine and psychology recognize many different circumstances and events as stressful. Depending on the circumstances or point of view, stress could be viewed as a threatening object or the event itself, the physical reaction within our bodies to the threat, or the state of mind that precedes our taking some action in response to threat.

To the psychiatrist studying brain chemistry, our awakening in the morning and the corresponding rise or fall in levels of several hormones may be considered a stressful event for the constantly adapting brain. For the psychologist, overcrowding of humans in urban areas can be considered a stressful event. An orthopedic surgeon considers the impact sustained by cartilage within the knee when one runs on concrete as stress.

The psychoneuroimmunologist, however, views the interaction of the immune system with the central nervous system as an *adaptation* to stress. This interpretation, which can accommodate both physical and emotional stress, will be the chief focus of this chapter.

For the sake of readability, we won't differentiate between responses and reactions, nor between anxiety and worry. We will assume that the stress of a cancer diagnosis causes distress, although some authorities maintain that not all stressors cause distress.

Most cancer patients and their families know, without consulting theoretical underpinnings, that a cancer diagnosis and treatments cause stress. Kim

Murphy, a leukemia survivor, recounts the stresses he has experienced in going through the assorted treatments:

> Regarding the side effects of CML and its therapies, for me the most significant side effect of this whole experience is the effect the diagnosis has had on the entire atmosphere surrounding my family and its future. It has changed everything. I was just starting my prime earning years, we had just moved into a new house and new neighborhood, my daughter had just started a new school, my wife had just started a new job. I was diagnosed on the day of our move!

> The diagnosis has affected the way we view our new house—for months I hated it, partly I think, because of its association with the day of diagnosis.

> It has affected my relationship with my mother, who comes to stay with us during holidays—she finds it impossible to resist comments regarding her perception of our financial status, including particularly the new house, now that we have the expenses of CML to deal with.

> It has affected my relationship with my daughter, who one day asked if the day I was going to die was coming soon (my daughter has been wonderful, by the way. She's 8).

> It has affected my relationship with my wife, with whom I am closer to now than I have been in some time.

> The physical effects of the interferon are negligible compared to those other intangible ones.

> I had a bone marrow transplant at the Fred Hutchinson Cancer Research Center in April '98. My twelve-month marrow was "clean" by PCR and cytogenetics. My eighteen-month marrow was "clean" according to both tests at the Hutch, but an excellent local laboratory found one single cell showing a "probable" 9:22 translocation. I informed the Hutch of this and they are going to get back with me.

> This just illustrates, again, what a roller-coaster effect the diagnosis, and now the follow-up lab tests, have on the patient and his family. I just want it all to go away! I want to be normal again! I feel great and have had a remarkably good course post-transplant. But just one test result can make me feel like maybe it was all for naught.

Responses to stress

Our bodies and minds respond to stress in many ways. These adaptations may change with the type and intensity of the stressor, the amount of time we have been exposed to it, previous experiences trying to adapt to similar stressful events, the person experiencing stress, and his or her physical and emotional state at the time.

Although many emotional responses to stress are possible, such as anger and withdrawal, the responses most often reported by cancer survivors are fear, anxiety, and depression. The National Cancer Institute reports that during and after diagnosis and treatment, almost half of all cancer patients report anxiety, and about a quarter report significant anxiety. Twenty percent experience transient or long-term depression, and 15 percent are diagnosed with post-traumatic stress disorder. Estimates by other researchers are sometimes much higher.

Fear is sometimes useful

Several bodily changes occur as a reaction to a fearful event. During fear, hormones that prepare us to adapt to stress are released in a chain reaction, first from the brain, which in turn triggers the release of antistress hormones from the adrenal glands. Our heart rate increases, blood is redirected to body parts associated with fight or flight, and extra sugar is made available in the bloodstream via the liver.

Fear can be a useful, goal-oriented reaction to a stressor. Each of these physical changes is aimed either at our fleeing from danger or conquering it bodily.

Fascinating research into brain structure and function has shown that the amygdala, part of the "old brain" conserved in most creatures from reptiles up through the primates, including humans, is the brain organ responsible for finding safety quickly when fear arises. Direct connections between the amygdala and our sensory organs bypass the higher brain centers of decision-making, allowing us to react very quickly to threats, sometimes without our being aware that we have perceived them. For instance, if you hike in the woods, have you ever stopped abruptly after sensing just a muted change of color or pattern, and upon closer inspection realize that subtle difference is a snake? This brain connection is probably responsible for the immediate, calm, highly effective, goal-oriented behavior that some people exhibit in unbelievably horrifying situations.

Although fear doesn't feel good, it can be a useful, goal-oriented reaction to a stressor. It galvanizes us and prepares us for action. The extreme and immediate physical reaction to fear, however, does little or nothing to prepare us to deal intellectually with a fearful situation that requires extensive analysis, planning, and decision-making, such as absorbing the technical medical information about our cancer diagnosis. On the contrary, research has shown that both very low and very high levels of the antistress hormones from the adrenal gland interfere with learning new tasks. Short of our ability to jump up and flee the doctor's office or our sudden acquisition of strength with which to throttle the bearer of bad news, we have been poorly prepared by evolution for dealing with the stress of cancer.

As a result, an out-of-phase mismatch of events is what many of us experience when being told of the cancer diagnosis—we may remember forever, and with great acuity, the perceptual cues that were present, instead of the key points that the doctor attempted to relay.

Anxiety is unhealthy

Most adults have experienced the difference between fear and anxiety. Fear is an acute, strong, visceral response to stress. Anxiety is a nagging, chronic, or generalized fear response. Although some would choose the chronic physical distress of anxiety over the pronounced physical distress of fear, anxiety may be the more physically harmful of the two experiences. Unresolved fear may convert to anxiety as we begin to grow accustomed to a threat.

When we're anxious, the same physical changes that accompany fear occur at lower levels, with deleterious effects on our body. Sustained increased heart output and constriction of blood vessels to rechannel blood to certain organs can contribute to the development of high blood pressure and cardiovascular disease. Altered sugar metabolism can worsen diabetes. The tendency for digestive activity to increase in times of stress can exacerbate underlying gastrointestinal disease.

Worry and anxiety involve recycling the same fear, repeatedly examining the outcomes and evaluating interventions. We sometimes use this activity to justify worry, assuming that repeated scrutiny will result in knowing what to do if worse comes to worst, but this continual rehearsal of negative events in search of solutions may not benefit us should danger actually arise. The two thought processes, worry and planning, occur in different parts of the brain. In magnetic resonance imaging, those who worry show activity in the emotional part of the brain, whereas those who plan show activity in the opposite hemisphere, the so-called logical half of the brain. This may mean that, from the standpoint of providing a good solution in the face of danger, worry is not the best strategy. Worry does not determine the best solution and enable us to move on to the next problem; it prevents us from detecting and dealing with new problems in a timely and effective way.

Physical symptoms of anxiety may include: shortness of breath, sigh breathing, dry mouth, inability to swallow, trembling, weakness, incessant crying, circular or obsessive thoughts, inability to concentrate, paralytic or manic movements, insomnia, headache, recurrent nightmares, or extreme fatigue.

What feels like anxiety is not always caused by worry. Sometimes it can have physical causes. In some cases, symptoms that are indistinguishable from anxiety can be caused by the leukemia itself.

These anticancer medications can also cause anxiety:

- Corticosteroids, such as prednisone

- Bronchodilators and certain other drugs used for asthma

- The newer antidepressant drugs to control nausea and pain, such as Prozac

- Cessation of the use of the quick-acting antianxiety drugs, such as Valium or Ativan

Certain physical changes that accompany incipient medical conditions are heralded by feelings of anxiety:

- Pneumonia

- Heart attack

- Electrolyte imbalance

- Angina

But the chief cause of anxiety among cancer survivors is worry and sustained, unresolved fear. Fear of pain, abandonment, dependency, financial ruin, professional ruin, relapse, or death. For parents, there is overwhelming fear for their young children, if the disease makes it impossible to care for them.

When we worry for a long time about one problem, new electrical circuitry is laid in our brains. Sometimes conditions resembling or related to our problem will trigger anxiety symptoms or symptoms of physical distress. Many cancer survivors report anticipatory nausea just smelling the rubbing alcohol used to clean the skin over a vein before chemotherapy is administered or blood is drawn. Studies have shown that this response can cause blood counts to drop—even if there will be no chemotherapy or blood draw at that time.

Obviously this reaction, called a conditioned response, can have a direct impact on the immune system, as has been demonstrated many times in animals. For example, when rats in one experiment were fed a combination of immune suppressant and saccharine dissolved in water, their white blood cell counts dropped afterward, as expected. When the experiment was repeated using only saccharine in water, white blood cell counts still dropped. This demonstrates that the association of event and outcome does not require knowing, for example, what chemotherapy is intended to do. Physiological cause and effect can occur in the absence of the cognitive processes as we know them today.

This does not imply, of course, that you can skip chemotherapy because just thinking about it may have some of the same effects. There's no evidence that a conditioned drop in blood counts coincides with an attack by the immune system on leukemia cells.

Depression

Research has shown that those who are depressed often have suboptimal immune system function.

Most cases of depression that coincide with cancer are called situational depressive episodes, directly related to the stress of adjusting to cancer. These depressive episodes differ from organic disturbances such as manic depression or unipolar depression, unless the person has had episodes of these diseases in the past, well before the leukemia diagnosis.

Depression may be diagnosed if one or more of the following symptoms persist for more than two weeks:

- Despair
- Excessive sleepiness
- Insomnia

- Appetite disturbance

- Irritability

- Inability to function

- Loss of interest in sex and other pleasurable activities

- Thoughts of suicide

Cancer-related problems that seem to have no solution can cause depression. When problem-solving efforts repeatedly don't work or are punished, we cease trying. Experts call this learned helplessness, but we know it as despair, and it is linked to depression. Subsequently, when new problems arise that we could indeed solve, or when new methods of dealing with old problems emerge, those exhibiting learned helplessness fail to act. A therapist trained to deal with depression can help overcome learned helplessness and despair.

In addition to the psychological factors surrounding cancer that can cause depression, see the following. Please note that these are possible side effects that do not necessarily occur in every person:

- Chemical treatments for cancer that are neurotoxic or toxic to the thyroid, such as prednisone, interferon-alfa, or interleukin-2, can cause chemically induced depression.

- Hemorrhagic stroke, which may result from untreated symptoms of some leukemias, can cause depression after blood products that cannot be cleared settle in the brain.

- High doses of cranial irradiation for BMT therapy, even if they are not accompanied by steroid therapy, may cause depression. Depression is but one of a constellation of symptoms that may result from cranial irradiation.

The following patient tries to describe what it was like for him in the days after his acute leukemia diagnosis. He didn't realize that he was deeply depressed until his alert oncologist caught on to what was happening:

> The day I was diagnosed was like any other day, but I left work early to be at the oncologist's office by 4:30. My wife had arranged to meet me there and we planned to go out for a meal and to talk about what he had to say. I don't know what we expected, but it wasn't, "You have acute myelogenous leukemia and you need immediate treatment, followed by a bone marrow transplant."

For days afterward I was in denial. I couldn't make decisions about work issues because the treatment question was hanging over my head. I couldn't decide about treatment options, because I couldn't believe that I had AML. It got so bad that I couldn't make any decisions. I could barely get myself out of bed in the morning, and I'd drag myself into work feeling like nothing at all. The doctor's office called to ask when I wanted to come in for chemotherapy and I just told them I'd call back because I couldn't decide. My wife began pushing me to start chemotherapy, but even she couldn't tell how depressed I was.

I had no idea how bad things had become until my oncologist called to ask what was holding me up. I think he expected me to say I was on a project at work, but when he asked, I simply couldn't answer. Fortunately he put two and two together and told me to come in immediately. My wife literally got me up and into the car and dragged me to his office. He started chemotherapy, made me an appointment with a psychiatrist, and gave me samples and a prescription for Prozac. I honestly couldn't have done any of those things myself at that point.

The effect of stress on the immune system

The stress hormones released by the adrenals during episodes of fear and anxiety also affect white blood cells, the infection-fighting army within our blood. Initially, the surge of brain and adrenal hormones that accompanies stress causes an increase in circulating white blood cells. When cortisol remains high, however, white blood cell numbers drop. As stress, anxiety, or depression continue unabated over weeks or months, output of the adrenal hormone cortisol is consistently high and white blood cell numbers remain reduced.

Stress and cancer

If prolonged stress and resulting anxiety affect the number of white blood cells in our body, does this mean that cancer can be caused by or made worse by stress? The answer, based on animal and human research, is unclear.

Animal studies support what many recognize intuitively: if stress had an unequivocal link to the development of cancer, just about every one of us would develop cancer. If stressful life events within the last three years were responsible for the emergence of cancer, then everyone who survived imprisonment in Auschwitz and other Nazi annihilation camps ought to have been diagnosed with cancer soon after being freed by the Allies. Continuing with the same analogy, all people who are diagnosed with cancer should either develop a second cancer triggered by the stress of the first diagnosis or should never be able to recover from the first cancer. Likewise, all loved ones of those diagnosed with cancer should then develop a cancer from dealing with the stress of their loved ones' suffering.

In fact, animal studies show a very wide range of tumor response to stress, depending on the type of stressor used, the ability of the animal to modify or escape the stressor, the species tested, gender, the animal's previous experience with this stress, whether the tumor was chemically induced or transplanted, whether the tumor is primary or a metastasis, and so on. In some cases, stress causes animal tumors to shrink.

Human studies have been somewhat less direct in measuring stress and tumor response, because few humans would tolerate having tumors chemically induced or transplanted, or being deliberately subjected to stress. The best study design would follow cancer-free people for years, recording stressful events and subsequent cancer diagnoses.

Most human studies so far have relied on retrospective self-reports of stress levels prior to the cancer diagnosis. This method of collecting information is often criticized as dubious. For instance, a person who has just been diagnosed with cancer and who has agreed to fill out a questionnaire on life factors may report that other recent stressful life events were not very stressful. Compared to this newest problem, cancer, these events may in retrospect seem not to be very stressful. Yet at the time the previous stressful events occurred, they may have been perceived and reacted to as very stressful events.

In short, while stress has been undeniably linked, over and over, to increased rates of some illness, such as upper respiratory infection and certain auto-immune disease, there is no clear causative link between stress and cancer. Several excellent texts on the topic of stress, the immune system, and cancer are listed in Appendix A, *Resources*.

Is there a cancer personality?

If stress causes both emotional and physical changes, but does not consistently have a part in the development of cancer, what other factors might be responsible? Can the ways a person adapts to stress affect his or her health? Do habitual ways of adapting hint at a "cancer personality"? The evidence, based on animal and human research, is conflicting.

Obviously, animal studies on this topic are difficult to perform because we can't know with certainty what animals are feeling, so most studies are done on humans. Often, the design of these studies is criticized.

For instance, melancholia, or what we would call depression today, received attention in the past as a personality trait possibly linked to cancer, but we know today that depression is less a personality trait or coping mechanism than an imbalance in brain chemistry with many different causes including genetics, situational adjustment, influenza, and stroke.

What can we do?

If fear is not very useful in dealing with cancer, and anxiety and depression pose risks for long-term health problems, what reactions and responses deal effectively with cancer-related stress? And if stress is not linked conclusively to the inception or growth of tumors, and may in some cases shrink tumors, why attempt to reduce stress associated with the cancer experience?

First, most people prefer feeling good to feeling bad. Stress reduction techniques can help you feel better.

Second, increased levels of stress are clearly tied to the worsening of certain illnesses, such as upper respiratory infections. If you've decided on a course of chemotherapy or radiation therapy, your immune system may be compromised for a few days or a week during each cycle. It's best to avoid infections and to minimize those that may arise during these troughs. Stress reduction techniques may help you keep secondary health problems to a minimum while undergoing anticancer therapy.

Third, high levels of stress for long periods of time can contribute to the development of high blood pressure, gastric disease, migraine headaches, certain autoimmune diseases, and other stress-related illnesses.

This patient has learned to deal with some of the stress of her illness and treatment, and writes to others in her support group:

> Instead of boring you with the details of the life of a couch potato, I'm going share some lessons I've learned. My timing doesn't always match God's timing. My priority all year was to return to teaching. Rejection and my suppressed immune system prevent me from being with walking germ squadrons—a.k.a., fourth graders. I've learned that what seems like empty, wasted time away from the lives of children, must be redirected to a productive life until I can return. So for now, I'm trying to be a good steward of my time.
>
> Big things aren't always important, and small things can be essential. Sometimes we're led by the "urgency of the generally insignificant." Are the people that you work with so valuable that you invest more than 40 hours a week with them instead of your family?
>
> We let a lot of stuff that seems urgent cram into every cranny of our lives. Sometimes paying the bills or attending every rehearsal isn't as vital as spending an hour to write a letter, read to the kids, or meditate on God's mercy.
>
> Pretend tea parties with little girls or real tea parties with girlfriends are the best medicine.
>
> Maintain an extremely healthy sense of humor. I watch funny movies, collect cartoons, and rent comedies. Share your funny stories with as many people as you can. Total strangers in the produce department are looking for a smile. You may fear their strange responses, but most often they will motivate your good mood. I have a list of silly things to do in an elevator and it's a real bang to see how many people you can challenge to smile.

In the next sections we discuss behavioral and medical ways to interrupt the worry cycle.

Stress reduction techniques

A chapter of this length cannot do justice to the history of theories of stress and stress reduction, and the ways of life that arose to accomplish this. Stress reduction has always been of interest to humans, albeit under different names, and has received close scrutiny in the 20th century, after the delineation of the chemical link between stress and hormones. Thus, various ways to reduce stress have been discovered or rediscovered.

The following sections comprise an alphabetic list of techniques that many have found useful for reducing stress. Not all of these will work for any one person; in fact, it's possible that none of these will work for you during particularly stressful times, such as during periodic checkups, or if you have a symptom that causes fear of relapse. Hopefully, however, the following ideas will help you discover your own ways to unwind.

Acupuncture

Acupuncture is a versatile way to reduce stress and pain, and is particularly good at relieving certain kinds of pain.

The ancient Chinese mapped the flow of energy in our bodies through pathways called meridians. These pathways are thought by Western medicine to be neuroelectric, although there continues to be discussion about the exact nature of these meridians. Eastern medicine believes that the misdirected flow of energy through these meridians accounts for most of the imbalances that occur within our bodies, and that these imbalances cause illness and can be detected in twelve pulses.

The central nervous system produces hormones for which receptors exist on the surfaces of white blood cells. Recent gains in knowledge regarding this interaction of the central nervous and immune systems may explain more fully some of acupuncture's mode of action.

An experienced acupuncturist spends at least an hour taking a comprehensive medical and emotional history; will use few needles, perhaps no more than six; may prefer Japanese to Chinese needles because they're thinner; and will be skilled at using the needles in a way that is not perceptible or barely perceptible.

The needles come in packets for single use only. You'll be able to see your practitioner opening these packets, which is reassuring if you have well-justified doubts about the reuse of needles. All body surfaces on which needles are used will be cleaned first with rubbing alcohol.

If you have asthma or hyper-reactive airway, tell the practitioner. Certain acupuncture treatments call for the burning of an herb called moxa, which may irritate your breathing. When moxa is used, only a sensation of warmth is felt on the skin.

Shoes should come off last and go on first. The easiest and most regrettable way to find a tiny, thin, lost acupuncture needle on the floor is with your bare foot.

It's becoming increasingly common for health insurance companies to pay for part or most of acupuncture treatment, although they generally pay less for psychological diagnoses, such as stress, than they do for medical diagnoses, such as migraine or endometriosis.

In some states, acupuncture practice must be supervised by a medical doctor. Verify the license and credentials of your practitioner with your state health department.

Biofeedback

Biofeedback is a way to relearn how to relax, usually monitored by a psychiatrist or psychologist.

During initial biofeedback sessions, sticky sensors are attached to various muscle groups on the part of your body that seems tense or is in pain, and a graph of muscle tension is displayed on a monitor. Relaxation tapes or the guiding voice of a therapist establish a calm atmosphere.

You can tell you've succeeded relaxing these muscle groups because the indicators on the screen change.

After a few sessions with the sensors and the screen, you no longer need them to indicate success, and you switch to doing relaxation exercises on your own. It is important to rehearse this stage of independence over and over with a therapist so that you can do the exercises independently in any setting.

As with acupuncture, it's becoming increasingly common for health insurance companies to pay for part or most of biofeedback treatment, although they generally pay less for psychological diagnoses, such as stress headache, than they do for medical diagnoses, such as migraine.

Counseling

Counseling sessions with a mediator or therapist who is experienced in cancer survivorship issues have proven very helpful to many people. Group counseling or support with other cancer survivors is a wonderful way to reduce stress. The group generates camaraderie, reduces feelings of isolation, offers practical as well as sympathetic support, and can become the source of many new friendships. See the section "Support groups" for more information.

Some people prefer to talk privately with a counselor while they attempt to deal with emotionally charged concerns. For those people, individual counseling is available.

A counselor might be a psychiatrist, a psychologist with a PhD or a master's degree, or a licensed social worker. Some insurance companies pay a larger percentage of the cost for sessions with a psychiatrist or psychologist, but often, social workers charge less to begin with.

Exercise

Moderate, regular exercise is a wonderful, well-documented way to reduce stress, as well as to improve overall health. Exercise also generates endorphins, the body's natural opiates, which reduce pain and ease depression.

Be careful, though, not to be too strenuous, for very strenuous exercise, such as training for a marathon, can lower white blood cell counts for about 24 hours. Do only what feels good, stopping before the point of exhaustion. Check first with your oncologist before starting a new exercise regimen, especially if you have had doxorubicin chemotherapy or radiation therapy in the chest area. Both of these treatments, if given in high doses, entail a risk of cardiac damage.

Mind-body exercise programs, such as yoga and tai chi, have shown to help manage stress. Mind-body exercise couples muscular activity with an internally directed focus. The participant enters a temporary self-contemplative mental state, resulting in a feeling of well-being and stress relief.

Family

Of all social support factors that appear to contribute to the positive outcome of an illness, including cancer, the support of family or very close friends appears to be highest. This effect has been shown most clearly in studies of white males recovering from heart conditions, though. The beneficial effect is less clear when other illnesses, females, and members of non-white ethnic groups are studied.

Most people are both blessed and cursed with family. Cancer survivors report family members who range from saintly, indispensable soulmates to those seemingly hatched by fate as an example of how not to behave. Nonetheless, at times, there's something uniquely comforting about being surrounded by those who resemble you, share your body language and your mother tongue, regardless of their inclination, or lack of inclination, to offer support. If nothing else, the less helpful ones can unintentionally provide wry entertainment.

Occasionally, people have family members who need more support than the cancer survivor does, or who are tooth-grindingly insensitive to what the patient is going through. And once in a while, stories surface about family members who actually blame the cancer survivor or family "rivals," such as a daughter-in-law, for the cancer.

Don't berate yourself if you find you frequently need a vacation from family members who put themselves first at all costs. Often these unhealthy imbalances in family dynamics were present all along, but remained subtle and bearable until the cancer experience exacerbated them.

Friends

Few other stress reducers are as good as sympathetic, listening friends.

When friends offer to help, don't be too noble to say yes. Keep in mind that often they don't know quite what to say when they learn of your cancer, especially at first, so they may prefer to act instead.

If they're good listeners, let them know if you do or do not feel like talking about cancer today—and that tomorrow might be different. Undoubtedly, there will be days when reducing stress means talking about cancer, and other days when one more word about cancer will make you want to run for cover. Try to sense or ask if *they* feel like listening, too.

Far too many cancer survivors report that friends, even very good friends, disappear when cancer appears. These friends are speechless, sad, frightened, or guilty that they're healthy—never mind that perhaps we're much more sad and frightened than they are.

Each of us has to decide on a way to handle this abandonment that meshes with our system of ethics. Many cancer survivors say that they just don't need additional sources of sadness and stress in their life, and they move on to find new friends, often in cancer support groups. Other cancer survivors try to keep their old friends by never talking about cancer. Bear in mind, though, that for those who are very fearful about cancer, just being around someone with cancer might be frightening.

If you have healthy friends who have remained a presence in spite of cancer—lawn-mowing, grocery-buying, baby-sitting friends; friends who have listened to you when you're scared; or friends who have just spent time with you if talking about cancer is not your style, you're very lucky. Show them that you're glad they're around. The harmony that results is a guaranteed stress-reducer.

Hobbies, volunteer work

As a form of healthy denial and, in some cases, a form of exercise, hobbies are an excellent stress reducer. Immersed in an activity you enjoy, you're likely to forget cancer, breathe and laugh more easily, and feel capable.

Hobbies are especially important for reducing the stress that may be linked to the lowered self-esteem of those who are temporarily or permanently unable to return to work.

Knowledge

Not surprisingly, a book such as this supports the belief that gaining knowledge about your cancer, and thus gaining some control over your cancer experience, is an excellent coping mechanism. Learning about your illness and your options has been proven to reduce anxiety and stress, and may be the crucial factor in your illness and its outcome. Not only can obtaining a correct diagnosis and learning about new, more effective treatments result in sound choices, but animal studies have shown that those who perceive that they have a means to escape stressful situations maintain better white blood cell counts than those who perceive otherwise. Bear in mind as well that, while our doctors often must master information about a broad variety of cancers, or are immersed deeply in their own research projects, you can have the luxury of going narrow and deep, learning a great deal about your own illness.

If your doctor seems unreceptive about things you've learned, seek a second opinion or consider changing doctors. *Working with Your Doctor*, by Nancy Keene, is an excellent book on this topic.

Worthy of mention is the observation that some doctors react badly to the idea that their patients find information on the Internet, because the information available on the Net ranges from abysmal to superb. If you use the Internet to research your illness (see Chapter 19, *Researching Your Leukemia*), avoid using the word "Internet" when discussing your findings with your oncologist. Instead, use terminology that credits the sources on which your findings are based: Medline, the PDQ database of the National Cancer Institute, Cancerlit, certain reputable medical journals, and so on.

Laughter

In his book *Anatomy of an Illness as Perceived by the Patient*, Norman Cousins says that we should take humor seriously. Cousins was diagnosed in 1964 with ankylosing spondylitis, a degenerative disease of the connective tissue that causes disability and pain. He undertook to improve or cure his condition by focusing on positive, happy thinking, and he believes he succeeded.

Funny friends, books, and movies are good ways to forget about cancer for a while, and can invoke some of the healthy bodily changes that come about when people laugh and relax. Two studies have found that mirthful laughter reduces blood levels of the hormones associated with stress.

Massage therapy

Back rubs and neck rubs given to you by loved ones will release endorphins that reduce pain and depression.

The lymphatic strokes practiced by massage therapists, on the other hand, are location-specific and utilize pressure. In a four-year research study, published in *Psychology Today* and *Massage Therapy Journal*, patients at the James Cancer Hospital (Ohio State University) were given massages as part of their treatment. Researchers found that the immune system was stimulated during the massage, blood pressures dropped, and circulation improved. In many cases, there was a dramatic drop in pain in as little as fifteen minutes.

In its April, 2000 issue, *Massage* magazine suggests that understanding the client's type and stage of cancer is essential information for the therapist wanting to help the cancer patient, so be sure you share that information with your masseur or masseuse. The concern has been that massage might exacerbate leukemia. In fact, no studies exist that conclude massage is contraindicated. Some oncologists suggest relaxation massage. Deep tissue techniques should be used with care.

Massage therapy is licensed by some states, and recognized by a national organization, the American Massage Therapy Association (AMTA). In some states, massage therapy can be performed only under the supervision of a doctor, nurse, physical therapist, or chiropractor. Your local phone book will list the nearest chapter of the AMTA for verifying your practitioner's credentials, or you can contact the national office at (847) 864-0123 or online at *http://www.amtamassage.org.*

Meditation

Meditation is a way to interrupt negative, cyclic thinking by focusing on one soothing word or peaceful scene. Those who practice meditation regularly are eventually able to lower their blood pressure and levels of stress hormones. These reductions persist beyond the end of the meditation session— sometimes well beyond.

Lowering of blood pressure is beneficial for those who have cardiac or vascular damage following doxorubicin or radiation therapies.

One study has shown that those who meditate have higher levels of melatonin in their urine, and another study has shown that higher levels of melatonin are found naturally in those with certain cancers. The significance of higher levels of naturally produced melatonin, or melatonin supplements, in leukemia survivors is not fully understood, but a few studies have shown that melatonin can increase the growth of myeloma cells in the test tube. (Myeloma is a cancer of the blood and bone marrow, related to leukemia.)

Owing to this unquantified risk, the FDA requires a warning on melatonin dietary supplements made or distributed in the US about possible health risks for those with white blood cell disorders.

It is likely that naturally elevated levels of melatonin associated with meditation do not have an undesirable effect on tumor growth, and that only the higher doses associated with dietary supplements do. It is also possible that all relaxation efforts, not just meditation, increase only urinary levels of melatonin, and that future studies will demonstrate this—or that blood levels, not urinary levels, are significant for an effect on cancer. Clearly, more research on melatonin's effects on leukemia is needed, but it's not likely that meditation will harm you.

Mini-vacations, healthy denial, and escapism

Denial is a healthy coping mechanism as long as it doesn't cause us to neglect the care we need for cancer. Some healthy ways to take a mini-vacation from cancer are:

- Drive to work along a prettier route.

- Schedule day trips away from daily stress.

- Buy your favorite author's latest hardcover edition instead of waiting for the paperback or library version.

- Grant yourself permission not to worry for one hour, one day, one week, and so on.

- Take a nap on your lunch hour.

- Buy a pair of wild golf pants or lipstick that "isn't your color" and wear it anyway.

- Spend all day Saturday in your bathrobe reading old *New Yorker* cartoons.

- Write a limerick and mail it anonymously to a friend.

- Odd though it may sound, you might enjoy celebrating the parts of your body that still work. Most of them still do work, of course, and rejoicing in this and using our bodies may have healing effects as yet unknown to medicine.

Music, song, and dance

Dr. Albert Schweitzer once said that he couldn't imagine life without music or cats. Schweitzer was an extremely productive, altruistic, humorous man who lived and worked in a difficult setting well into old age. He was a strong believer in the doctor within each of us, and thought himself but the facilitator of his patients' own healing processes.

Music can lower stress and enhance emotions. You can experiment with music to see which type suits your needs at different times. Some people find the relaxing or soul-thrilling effects of classical music best. Others find that loud pop or rock music numbs pain, and that its relatively simple, repetitive rhythms and singable melodies interrupt incessant worries. Still others enjoy ethnic music. Listening to a type of music you've never heard before, such as the Australian didgeridoo or Tibetan chord-singing, might distract you from the worries of cancer.

Singing can release cares from your soul, and may realign anxious breathing. Singing out loud in the car when you're alone, like screaming, can lower tension levels.

Classes in dance for people of all ages and both genders are available in many community centers. If you feel that you need greater control in your life, ballet's discipline, controlled breathing, and classic beauty may make you feel better. If, on the other hand, you feel there's too much control in your life, jazz or aerobics may allow you to set free some inhibitions. Flamenco might help you rediscover the sexuality that may have gone to sleep when you heard the word cancer. Yoga, tai chi, and Feldenkreis movement, all of which span the disciplines of exercise and dance, are fine ways to stretch and relax.

Nutrition

In general, the diet that is recommended for those without cancer—a diet high in vegetables, fruit, and grains—remains the best diet for those with cancer, although those who are losing weight and suffering from loss of appetite should consult their oncologists before substituting vegetables for meat.

A few nutritional factors seem to have some effect on mood:

- A diet high in animal protein has been linked to anxiety and panic attacks. Other studies have found that certain flavonoids, compounds found in plant but not animal tissue, are similar to Valium in their relaxing action. This might mean that it's not reducing meat intake, but increasing vegetable intake, that lowers anxious episodes in some people. If you're suffering from severe anxiety symptoms related to your cancer diagnosis, you might try modifying your diet to contain more vegetables and grains—but check first with your oncologist.

- Drinking milk at bedtime or eating turkey for dinner are known to help with relaxation. These foods are high in tryptophan, an amino acid that aids sleep. Tryptophan is used by the body to make serotonin, a neurotransmitter that affects mood and is the target of many of the newer antidepressants.

- Low blood levels of zinc correlate to treatment-resistant depression and to an increase in the undesirable immune system inflammatory response sometimes seen in depressive patients.

- Cachexia, the weight loss experienced by some cancer patients, has been linked to depression, which is thought to be triggered by nutritional deficits, or by the leukemia's commandeering of dietary substances otherwise needed for the manufacture of brain neurotransmitters.

Note that chemotherapy regimens that contain procarbazine may require that you avoid certain foods high in tyramines, including bananas and some cheeses. Always verify a change in diet first with your oncologist.

Pets

You may find that your pets, considered family members by some, are a unique solace to you through the cancer experience. Animals seem to have a knack for knowing when we need help, and they don't care if we smell funny or if our hair is missing. They don't become instantly bashful because of our diagnosis, and they aren't afraid they'll catch cancer from us. How many humans will sit by us for an hour in the bathroom while we're sick, as our dogs will? And who's funnier than the puppy who barks at the wig on the dresser?

Positive thinking and visualization

Positive thinking and visualization have been shown to increase immune system function. Oddly, one study has shown that when cancer survivors visualize an immune system attack on the leukemic cells using attack images that are incorrect according to what is known today about immune system function, immune system parameters still improve. This may reflect the "taking charge" phenomenon: the belief that you can escape stress tends to lessen the effect of stress on the immune system.

Visualization can be used to attempt to direct inner forces against the cancer or to relax by calling to mind pleasant experiences, places, or dreams. Initially, it might be useful to practice visualization in a quiet, relaxed atmosphere—but eventually you can do it anywhere.

Reading

As a form of escapism, reading is a good way to reduce stress.

As a means of learning more about your illness, reading may make you feel more stressed temporarily, but this may be offset by long stretches of peace of mind, after you're able to make better medical decisions based on what you've learned by reading.

Reading from and writing to the various cancer discussion groups on the Internet can provide a cathartic outlet. See the section "Support groups."

Relaxation training

This technique is similar to biofeedback, discussed earlier, and incorporates visualization techniques, described in the section "Positive thinking and visualization."

Sleep

Research shows that even one night of missed sleep lowers levels of natural killer (NK) white blood cells. Although NK counts recover quickly once sleep is restored, persistent lack of sleep is an opportunity for illness.

Animal research on the artificial shifting of the phases of lightness and darkness shows that the immune system is depressed by the shifting. Fishes that occupy parts of the ocean that receive low light in winter experience an additional breeding cycle if artificial light is increased, and simultaneously their white blood cell counts decrease.

Spirituality, religious beliefs

Your religious beliefs may provide comfort when little else is making sense. Some people find that their spiritual beliefs sustain them in spite of a seemingly arbitrary infliction of suffering, either because their religion provides answers for the question of human suffering or because of theological beliefs they have developed independently.

Other cancer survivors, however, experience a crisis of faith after their cancer diagnosis. They find it difficult, for instance, to reconcile the emergence of a seemingly undeserved, life-threatening illness with their belief in a kind, nonpunitive deity.

On a more human level, the support that fellow church or temple members furnish to those who need help is clearly an asset in stress reduction. Support might take the form of emotional support (cards, calls, hugs, visits), prayer, practical support (rides to and from the doctor or casseroles for supper), or financial support for someone who is underinsured.

The May, 1995 issue of the *Journal of the American Medical Association* contains an article showing a correlation between religious practice and prayer, and increased good health. At least one other study has shown that a person who is prayed for improves when ill, even if he or she is not aware that prayers are said.

Support groups

For some of us, support groups can be the difference, literally, between life and death. The opportunity to exchange information with those who have already weathered leukemia can provide you with everything from emotional support to the knowledge to question your treatment and seek medical help elsewhere. Support groups are an immeasurably useful way to do this, bringing together a variety of skills, sometimes including medical and legal knowledge.

Moreover, Dr. David Spiegel's work with breast cancer survivors shows longer survival among those who were part of support groups—a serendipitous finding from a study intending to highlight other aspects of survival.

Support groups are offered locally in many areas by organizations, such as the Leukemia Society of America, the Wellness Community, or local hospitals.

Support groups are also available on the Internet. See Chapter 14, *Getting Support*, for instructions about subscribing.

Touching and hugging

Being kissed, hugged, and patted by people who love you causes the release of endorphins within the central nervous system. Endorphins are natural opiates produced by our bodies, capable of reducing pain and depression, and producing feelings of well-being.

Hugging, kissing, snuggling, and giggling with a child who has cancer has been shown in several nursing studies to lower the child's pain and anxiety levels.

Hugging and kissing your partner can be enjoyable and healthy, even if you're feeling too tired at the moment to enjoy all of the sexual activities you enjoyed before diagnosis.

Water

In the 1930s, marine biologist Sir Alister Hardy noted that humans have features in common with water mammals, features not found in any other primates, such as a subcutaneous layer of body fat, hair that grows in one direction to reduce water resistance, a protective dive reflex within the respiratory system, a nose that blocks water during a dive, residual webbed toes, and fully webbed toes in 7 percent of humans. He argues that we humans may have spent a period of our evolution in water.

Anthropologists may settle this point eventually, but for our immediate use, it means that, for some of us, water is a wonderful way to relax. A good swim or a warm tub with salts and a good book can make you briefly more than just human.

Writing

If you have an urge to write, you'll be encouraged to know that those who write very honestly and emotionally about their frightening, negative experiences increase the function of their white blood cells. You can write for yourself in a journal, write letters to friends, write letters for your children to read when they're older, or write email to cancer discussion groups on the Internet. Journal-keeping is presently being recommended as a very successful stress reducer for survivors.

Stress medications

Stress associated with cancer responds well to antianxiety and antidepressant medication. Research has shown, though, that these medications are most effective when used in combination with counseling and behavior modification training.

There are many drugs to choose from to ease anxiety or depression or to aid sleep. The newer drugs available today have fewer side effects and are less likely to be addictive than drugs used just a few years ago.

Antianxiety medication

Antianxiety drugs (anxiolytics) fall broadly into two groups: the fast-acting drugs and the slower-acting drugs. The fast-acting benzodiazepine drugs, such as Valium, Ativan, or Xanaxm, are potentially addictive and can cause rebound anxiety when they're stopped. The newer anti-anxiety drugs, such as BuSpar (buspirone), cross the boundary between anti-anxiety and antidepressive drugs, are not addictive, and can be stopped abruptly with no ill effect. They take two to three weeks to work.

The mood change following use of the older anti-anxiety drugs in the Valium family is pronounced and rapid, similar to the effect of alcohol. It's unwise to drive or operate heavy machinery when using drugs in the benzodiazepine family.

The mood change following use of newer anti-anxiety drugs, such as BuSpar, is more subtle and gradual, and sleepiness, if present, is less pronounced than with the benzodiazepines.

The anti-anxiety drug Ativan, a benzodiazepine, is often used just prior to chemotherapy to control nausea.

Antidepressant medication

The availability of today's more effective, safer antidepressants is a blessing for those coping with cancer. Unlike the antidepressants of a few years ago, which caused sleepiness, weight gain, or other undesirable side effects, today's antidepressant medications are far safer and less disruptive to weight and sleep patterns.

Some of the newer antidepressants can cause restlessness and insomnia for the first two or three weeks they are used. You might discuss with your doctor the temporary use of a sleeping pill until your body has adjusted to the antidepressant.

Antidepressants are also good pain relievers, although their mechanism as such is not entirely clear.

Improvement in mood is gradual with most of the antidepressants used today, changing slowly over a few weeks or months. The fullest effect is gained if the drugs are used continuously for months. Always check with your doctor before stopping an antidepressant, lest gains in improved mood be lost.

The best source for information about antidepressant medications is a psychiatrist. This specialist is the one most likely to be familiar with all antidepressants and their side effects, and can rotate you through several, until you find the best one for you.

Sleep medications

Sleep medications range from the very mild, including over-the-counter antihistamines and Tylenol, to the stronger medications necessary for those using prednisone or coping with moderate to severe anxiety.

The anti-anxiety drugs in the benzodiazepine family, such as Ativan, are also used as sleep aids. The section "Anti-anxiety medications," contains cautions about these drugs.

One of the newest sleeping pills available is Ambien, a drug that aids those who have trouble falling asleep. It's cleared very rapidly from the body, so it's less useful for those having trouble staying asleep. When Ambien was first approved by the FDA, it was marketed as a nonaddictive sleeping pill, but postmarket experience has shown that, for at least some people, it may be addictive.

Drugs prescribed for severe pain, such as codeine and morphine, also induce sleep.

Some people use melatonin, a substance marketed as a food supplement, to aid sleep. Melatonin has been shown to increase the quantity of white blood cells. This is a risky phenomenon for a person with leukemia, a cancer of the white blood cells, because the white blood cells increased could be cancerous. Accordingly, the FDA requires a warning on melatonin dietary supplements made or distributed in the US about possible health risks for those with white blood cell disorders.

Always consult your oncologist before using any drug, whether it is a prescription, nonprescription, or a "natural remedy" marketed as a food supplement.

CHAPTER 14

Getting Support

Cancer can be a terrible burden in its physical aspects alone, but to face leukemia without support is far worse. Cancer can be an isolating experience for the patient, because for others, it calls to mind issues that many people dread, such as chronic pain and the surrender of physical independence. Many people, especially younger people, have never experienced any form of long-term illness in their families, much less the chronic and very serious aspects of cancer or cancer treatment. More than any other diagnosis, cancer brings home a sense of mortality in the patient, family, and friends.

This entire book is, of course, about getting you the support you need. Support can take many forms. Various organizations offer an almost staggering variety of services to leukemia survivors, most of them free. Appendix A, *Resources*, contains a full list of such services, including emotional, informational, medical, financial, travel, research, and legal services. Still other forms of institutional support are discussed in other chapters, such as Chapter 19, *Researching Your Leukemia*.

The goal of this chapter is to get you the help you need by priming you to anticipate difficulties in communication, to offer tips on articulating needs in a reasonable way, and help you re-evaluate your expectations of others. How can you ask for what you need, and how can you reconcile yourself to being disappointed or to seeking help elsewhere, if support is lacking? How do you keep the physical problem of facing leukemia from growing into additional emotional and social problems if you have a misunderstanding with someone who tries to help you? The support you ultimately receive is, in some measure, a result of how good you are at asking for help and expressing appreciation.

This chapter first details specific issues that may require the help of others: the emotional and practical support needed to deal with everyday issues, such as transportation, child care, housecleaning, medical care within the home, workplace issues, keeping a positive attitude, and so on. Next, we address a few general aspects of communication and support, such as some typical reactions that the "healthy unaware" have to serious illness. We then look in detail at the variety of sources from which you might seek support.

Specific needs

The word "support" means different things to different people, or different things on different days, depending on what you're dealing with at the moment.

First, there are tangible, instrumental ways others can support you, such as:

- Offering to locate and interpret medical information about your illness.
- Offering their points of view for your decision-making process.
- Organizing blood donor or marrow donor drives.
- Helping you move around at home after treatment.
- Offering to do some of your cooking, cleaning, laundry, or shopping.
- Driving you to and from treatment visits.
- Acting as an advocate for you when you're not well enough to express your needs or demand better care.
- Keeping track of medications you must take if you're too groggy to do so on your own.
- Monitoring your reactions to specific medications and your health in general.
- Organizing fundraisers.
- Calling insurance companies, medical offices, or employers to iron out misunderstandings.
- Being a surrogate parent to your children.
- Offering to stay overnight with you if you need nursing care.
- Offering to assume temporarily some or all of your workplace responsibilities.
- Understanding that fatigue is the most common long-term effect faced by cancer survivors, often lasting for years, and remaining constant in their efforts to help and understand as time unfolds.

Next, there are ways that others can provide emotional support:

- Empathizing, at least in principle, with the terror of facing a life-threatening illness.

- Attempting to understand how you feel, however alien it may seem to them.

- Just being around when you want company.

- Sending gifts and cards if you're house-bound or hospitalized.

- Attending to your children's emotional needs.

- Not assuming to know how you feel.

- Avoiding nosy or inappropriate questions, offering instead to listen when you're ready to talk.

- Saying, "I'm sorry this happened to you. Please let me know what I can do for you."

These issues are faced by almost all cancer survivors. There also are several issues leukemia survivors face, especially those with chronic disease, that other cancer survivors may not face:

- Lengthy but uncertain survival for chronic disease in the absence of an absolute cure.

- Inaccurate, frightening, and frustrating comparisons of leukemia to other cancers, especially to non-Hodgkin's lymphoma or to other cancers that metastasize to lymph nodes and bone.

- The financial devastation that may accompany the lengthy course of some leukemias. They may require repeated treatment or transplantation, entailing fatigue and side effects that impede your ability to work.

- Looking and seeming healthy while harboring a malignancy, and the misunderstandings about this that develop among the healthy unaware.

- The loss of support over time. Frequently, others get tired of hearing about illness from those who have low-grade disease.

Communicate these details

Those who have no experience with leukemia seldom can understand intuitively what you're facing. You should consider communicating very clearly about the following issues.

For slow-moving, chronic disease, others need to be told that:

- For some chronic leukemias, watchful waiting is the best way to handle the disease. You don't look ill, you may not feel ill, and you may only have higher than normal white counts.

- Your illness may recur after several years; that is, long remission does not currently equate to cure.

- The path is an uncertain one regarding recurrence of disease and the success of subsequent treatment.

- Your disease may progress to a more active or aggressive state.

For all subtypes of leukemia, the healthy unaware need to be told that:

- It's characteristic for leukemia to arise or lodge in bone marrow or lymph nodes, and that this is not necessarily a spreading of disease (metastasis) that signals no hope for treatment or cure.

- Repeated treatment, and the fatigue that may follow, may leave you unable to work for long periods of time. Following transplantation, for instance, you might be unable to work for half a year or more, yet the bill for transplantation still must be paid. Insurers often will cover only 80 percent or less of the cost, which can range from $150,000 on up, depending on the follow-up care required and the type of transplant performed.

- The path and long-term side effects of this illness may be lengthy, perhaps requiring their patience and understanding for many years.

- There are differences between the few subtypes of leukemia that generally enjoy a good chance of cure and the many subtypes of leukemia which vary considerably in behavior, treatment, and prospects for survival, and that are still considered non-curable at this time.

Typical reactions

In an ideal world, you would be surrounded by people who come forward as soon as you need help. They would know what you need before you need it, would give lovingly and unselfishly, and would never become exhausted. Money would flow without a second thought, and those who help you would expect nothing in return. In reality, it's not often that way.

Often, others are only partially aware of what you're going through. Nausea? Fatigue? While they may have had nausea or fatigue in the past, it's likely that it was quickly remedied. They may not realize what it's like to experience nausea for days each week, even before the chemotherapy treatment has begun. They don't truly understand what it's like to be tired all day, every day, as soon as they wake in the morning. Most people may have considered their own mortality, but seldom have they done so with the sense of immediacy that a cancer diagnosis entails.

At times, others would like to offer support, but don't know what to do or say. They may say the wrong thing. In some instances, others find it easier just to avoid discussing the issue of your illness. They hope—it is presumed—that if they dwell on other topics you (and they) will feel normal again. Carried to extremes, these people just avoid you whenever they can.

In very rare cases, the motives of others are not at all honorable, and they may say or do things that are despicable.

Frequently, there are good explanations for what you may perceive as the failure of others to provide adequate support. Other people, being mortal, have finite logistic, emotional, and financial resources. They still have their own responsibilities and needs to address.

If they are loved ones, they may have assumed some of your responsibilities as well. They might attempt to manage this on a reduced income if the leukemia survivor is unable to contribute financially. They may be concerned that the time they're missing from work to provide care will jeopardize the family's only remaining source of income. The thought of losing a loved one is probably highly threatening to them, perhaps causing anger, terror, sadness, and a host of other debilitating feelings. None of these issues justifies unkind behavior, of course, but hidden concerns might cause loved ones to seem distracted, inattentive, overly controlling, or insensitive.

Fortunately, it appears that many leukemia survivors receive most of the support they need when they need it, with just an occasional bump along the way—if they make their needs known.

How to communicate about needs

There's no one way to communicate successfully with others about your needs. Even among people who believe they know each other well, misunderstandings and hurt feelings arise because of daily variations in mood or circumstances of which they're unaware. Your own skills in dealing with leukemia come into play, too, when what was not upsetting yesterday may be upsetting today, and if you're sick, tired, and discouraged.

Despite these ups and downs, many leukemia survivors have learned by experience about communicating with others. The following sections contain details regarding how to discuss your illness, but some very general guidelines are:

- With your closest loved ones, be as honest as possible as gently as possible.

- With those to whom you're not very close, use your judgment about what, and how much to say in order to protect yourself and them from undesirable consequences, until you can assess the quality of their responses. You may choose, for example, to tell some family members, social acquaintances, and coworkers a few things about your treatment while avoiding lengthy, painful discussions or topics they're likely to misunderstand.

- For that group in the middle, comprised of good friends and perhaps some other family members, try to sense the boundary. Just as you have limits to what you can bear, few friends are able to absorb all of your pain all of the time. Asking, "Are you in the mood to listen to this today?" or "Do you have the time and energy to be my sounding board?" are two possible approaches. And the reverse is true: you need to be clear but tactful if you don't feel like discussing your circumstances, or if you aren't feeling sturdy enough to have visitors.

Exceptions to the rule

These general suggestions are probably no surprise to you. Nor will be the fact that there are exceptions to every rule.

The general guidelines of telling your closest loved ones the most, with greatest honesty, may not hold. For example, you may have a close relative who handles bad news better if you joke about it a little, but who will never be able to react appropriately to the rawer emotions. He or she may turn tail and run if you cry, for instance. Conversely, you may have a casual friend with a medical background who is a skilled listener, and who can at times provide you with more objective support than your family can. From such interaction, a very deep friendship may grow.

At times, you just can't predict how someone else will react. Trudy, a leukemia survivor, puzzled over her husband's reaction to her illness:

> It is funny how different things affect people. My husband finds it terribly hard to accept my illness. He never talks about it, smirks if I talk about the importance of hand washing, and things like that. He is kind, though, and does the heavy work now.

> The other day, I was reading the support list and I read about the death of one of us. He just happened to stand behind me and looked over my shoulder. I heard him sigh and say, "Only 40 years old." It seems finally to have come home to him. While it is hard on those of us with leukemia, it must be much harder for the people living with us.

Although most loved ones will support you, it's not unheard of for some family members and friends to disappear when they discover you have cancer. There's no one solution to this very painful problem. Often, leukemia survivors just move on to find new friends, but some justifiably neither forgive nor forget. Sometimes the absentee friend will reappear and apologize, perhaps not until years later.

Cultural and gender differences

Gender and cultural differences in communicating about illness can affect the outcome of asking for help, especially in the US, as its population is composed of so many cultural groups.

In short, there can be obstructive differences in the styles of different groups of humans as they confront illness. Keep in mind that any method of expression is simply a trait, not a fault or virtue—that is, each style is adaptive or maladaptive in different settings. For example, keeping a stiff upper lip and trying to be the strong, silent type might be maladaptive when you need to ask for help.

This patient had real cultural differences with the oncologist and it definitely affected the doctor-patient relationship. Life perceptions were in conflict in this relationship:

> I am still trying to forgive my oncologist. The hematologist, a young woman from India, gave me the news. She was unhappy that I was very upset at being diagnosed with cancer.

She told me "You Americans are too afraid of death. It is ridiculous that you are so concerned with dying. True, this cancer will likely kill you, but you have to get over this obsession with dying."

She went on and on for about three or four minutes chastising me for having a "poor reaction" to my diagnosis. You can imagine how that made me feel.

Sources of support

The rest of this chapter examines the people you might ask for support. The groups described work outward from the circle of intimacy, first discussing your strongest, most abiding relationships with family members and loved ones, then friends, support groups, coworkers, and social contacts. Please note that emotional issues specific to the end of treatment and the beginning of remission are discussed later in Chapter 16, *After Treatment*.

Cancer counselors point out that those people that patients must deal with tend to fall into three categories—nurturing, supportive, and toxic—whether they're family, friends, or acquaintances. In other words, your closest family members, upon whom you may hope to rely, might be negative and unsupportive, emotionally toxic to you. Those who are less close may actually be more nurturing than family members. In the discussions that follow, the term "loved ones" implies those who are nurturing, even if they are not related to you by blood or marriage.

A teacher with leukemia discusses the wonderful support she received from family and friends while undergoing a stem cell transplant in Boston:

> *My family was there for me all the way, and it made a huge differ-*
> *ence. My husband packed up and moved to Boston so he could be with me*
> *daily. I know it took its toll on him, because he hated the mask and gloves*
> *that he had to wear all those long hours in my room. I tried to encourage*
> *him to take long walks and just get out of the room so he could breathe,*
> *yet he was staunch in his support. His whole routine was upset, and he's a*
> *creature of habit, so I know what an upheaval it was for him. My daugh-*
> *ters came from the Midwest and the West Coast to spend what time they*
> *could and to donate platelets for me.*
>
> *My son and his wife handled laundry with a smile, driving 45 min-*
> *utes in Boston traffic to come spend time with me. Once I was out of*

isolation, my son and daughter-in-law cooked meals, using the strict neutropenic diet rules, and brought them into Boston to my hotel room so that I wouldn't have to eat frozen meals every night. I'll never forget and I'll always appreciate that kind of caring.

My brother and sister-in-law called daily, and came to stay with me. They came again when my husband had to go home to make sure our house was still standing. My sister-in-law deserves a halo. She was there during the worst post-radiation days and did things for me that I never expected to have to ask of another individual. Moreover, she did them matter-of-factly and with a smile.

I cannot begin to tell you how heartening it was to learn how many friends I had made in the school where I teach. My colleagues were just wonderful, arranging a card chain, so that daily, in the BMT unit, there were good wishes from individuals and whole grade levels of teachers. It was the most overwhelming and generous support I'd ever received.

Best of all was meeting my Internet buddies. People with whom I'd been corresponding for years were suddenly in my vicinity. They were very generous with their time, coming over and over again, and went out of their way to see that we had whatever we needed, even to the point that one friend, whom I did not meet, got me free Internet access through his own Internet provider. That was one very appreciated gift. Another friend took us home for dinner and then out to the museum to play before I went into the isolation unit. One special friend even made tapioca pudding for my husband, who had mentioned how much he loved it in a casual conversation.

I am firmly convinced that had it not been for all the support, concern, and dozens of prayer lists that I was on, the outcome of the treatment might not have been so successful.

Some people may be limited in access to support, but still combine sources of support into a system that works for them. Karin Laakso, although isolated much of the time with infections, finds companionship and support from several sources: an online support group, her daughters, and her cat:

I am immuno-compromised on three fronts: CLL, congenital immune deficiency, and no spleen. I find the frequent, prolonged infections a drag.

I am unable to work or even volunteer because I'm sick most of the time. Since I am divorced and live alone, the isolation is difficult.

That's where the online support list I belong to is great. I do have two wonderful, caring daughters in the area. But they are married and have busy careers.

I have one special cat, who is immuno-compromised three ways himself. We keep each other going and seem to have the proverbial "nine lives" together.

Loved ones

Some families work better as a team than others. It's rare for any team of people to respond perfectly when it comes to dealing with a crisis. Lapses in teamwork can happen often in the workplace, but can be hurtful within families.

Owing to the many variations in group behavior, it's not possible to cover in this section all family behaviors with which you might have to contend. Instead, we will discuss the most common problems and solutions.

For many people of all ages, a new crisis tends to elicit behaviors that worked well in the past, especially at first. These reflexive behaviors might be arguing, escapism, intellectualizing the problem, or taking control. For children in crisis, you might see a return to the dependent behaviors they had outgrown. The overall impression in a crisis may be that those around you revert to immature, maladaptive behaviors. Keep in mind that leukemia is a brand-new experience and learned coping behaviors can be hard habits to change, especially in a time of great stress.

It may be harder for your loved ones to help you if you don't communicate clearly about your circumstances. With loved ones, don't be shy or proud. Ask for all the help you need, even if it embarrasses you. Many family members express chagrin at the seeming reluctance of cancer patients to "trouble" them. In turn, they hesitate to invade the patient's privacy by prying or being dominant. Consequently, the already upsetting cancer experience can transform into an even larger menace than it is, because nobody will talk about it.

On the other hand, if your family is closely knit, sharing and verbalizing just about everything, the stresses associated with leukemia might *appear* to be taking a greater toll than one might see in a family with fewer emotional ties and more independent members. The telling point is the success of your family's long-term adaptation, not any temporary disequilibrium, emotional flotsam, or distancing you may experience.

What you need from loved ones may change as your experiences evolve from diagnosis through treatment. Different relatives and loved ones may prove good at handling different things. Unlike coworkers and casual acquaintances, close family members and loved ones probably won't surprise you too often with their reactions, because it's likely you already know their weaknesses and strengths. You may find yourself occasionally disappointed, but perhaps not surprised.

Communicating needs to adults

Ideally, communicating your needs to the loving adults in your life should be relatively easy. Honesty, gentleness, and especially gratitude work well. With a couple of exceptions, such as a relative who's mentally ill or otherwise frail, adults who are nearest and dearest should be trusted to handle every aspect, even the worst aspects, of your illness appropriately.

But cancer challenges a family's beliefs and myths about their family unit, and may alter the established dynamics of the family. If the father, mother, husband, or wife has always been a wise and strong provider, for example, the balance of power may shift temporarily during treatment for leukemia. If the partner without leukemia has developed an untoward reliance on the strong one, it may be a difficult transition to assume control for a while. The partner with leukemia may suffer lowered self-esteem when roles shift. It's important to keep in mind that often these shifts are temporary.

Many leukemia survivors note that their loved ones become ill, too, while trying to help them deal with treatment and emotional issues. Upper respiratory infections such as sore throats, persistent GI tract problems, such as diarrhea, emergence of autoimmune disorders, and worsening of certain other chronic illnesses, such as herpes or diabetes, often go hand in hand with the extreme emotional stress associated with a loved one's having cancer. At times, though, leukemia survivors report that a relative seems to want to be sicker than the person with cancer. This does indeed happen in some families, and if it happens in yours, chances are you've seen this kind of behavior before from that individual. The deciding factor in determining if the sickness is real is whether the ostensibly ill person continues to provide help to the best of his or her ability, or uses the illness as an excuse not to help—or even to punish you.

If you find that the adult loved ones in your life react to your needs in unhelpful ways, do ask why. It may be a simple thing to put right. They may be angry that you have cancer—of course you needn't apologize for having cancer. It is also possible that some older, unresolved issues are being forced to the fore by the stress of dealing with leukemia. They may feel, for instance, that they owe you little because in the past you were not supportive of them when they needed help. Communication, humility, and open-mindedness may work to break the impasse.

If attempts to communicate don't make much difference, it may be a disappointment to realize that the strength you thought existed in the relationship does not exist—or at least not for this set of circumstances. Perhaps you could rely on someone else temporarily for what you need. Sometimes loved ones just need some time to settle down and get used to the changes and increased responsibilities cancer brings.

Avoid asking a third family member to intervene if you have difficulty getting along with a loved one. Triangles such as this seldom succeed because they hint at two against one and talking behind each other's backs.

If reasonable attempts to get the help you need fail, you might discuss attending family counseling with the person who seems to be acting out of character.

If none of these attempts work, then find alternate support or a way to live without such people, temporarily or permanently; this is in your best interest. Because of the seriousness of leukemia, your concerns must be put first, at least for the time being. You may be surprised to find that, in spite of leukemia, your life is more serene and enjoyable in the absence of such difficult people. A decision to not deal with someone is also a way of dealing with them.

Sometimes family members just don't know how to deal with another's illness, and then the patient feels very much alone. The following patient finds solace in her support group that she can't find in her family, and expresses her thanks for the group:

Thanks for this group. I can talk to people here who are going through the same thing. My family will not acknowledge that anything is wrong. They won't even talk about it, no matter when I bring it up. My husband looks at me as if I am crazy, and my sister says, "I don't want to talk about it until I have to."

Sometimes I feel as if I am all alone and I get scared. Right now I'm in remission, but for how long? I just wanted to say I think this group is great.

Another member of the group answered the first patient with a suggestion from her own experience:

You need to convey to your husband and sister that you need to be able to talk with them about your illness. Bottling everything up inside is not fair to you. Of course we don't want to "live" in sympathy for ourselves, but we need to be able to talk about our problems and feelings.

While my husband, son, sister and close friends knew of my leukemia, my 80-year-old parents did not. When we finally had to "let the cat out of the bag," my wonderful husband did it for me. Then I came in to show my parents I still was the same person. I have never felt so relieved in my life as I did after we told them.

When I could finally say things like "I'm going to see the oncologist today" or "Yes, I know I look tired, but that's just part of this stuff," you wouldn't believe what a load was taken off my shoulders. The neat thing is, my parents can deal with it too.

Talk with a counselor or minister or whomever and see if you figure out how to get your family to open up. Do it for yourself and I promise it will help them too.

Communicating with children

Communicating needs to young children should have different goals than communicating with adults. While it's true that children sometimes provide instrumental support if no other family members are available, generally it isn't necessary or fair to expect a great deal of help from children. More often, they can be asked to help with small, safe chores in order to make them feel part of the solution, and to reinforce the honest relationship they've grown accustomed to.

Human children are inclined, by biology, to think the world revolves around them. Very young infants do not understand, for instance, that Mommy is a separate person who can leave them with Daddy and go grocery shopping, and they may become quite upset when they discover that Mommy is gone. This bonding trait is probably essential to survival for a species whose young have a long and vulnerable nurturing period, such as humans and some other mammals.

This egocentric thought process lingers well through childhood, though, and causes children to think that the bad things that happen are their fault. They may think that you developed cancer because they were very angry with you when you once punished them, for example. They may even have wished you were dead, and now it appears to be coming true. Depending on their religious upbringing, they may believe that God saw them misbehave and is punishing them.

For many reasons, your children see you differently than you see yourself. Lack of experience with emotions, fear of abandonment, or just plain being shorter than adults means their perspective is truly different. Often, small children can't distinguish a sad adult face from a grouchy one, for example, and because adults are all-powerful from their perspective, unconsciously they hedge their bets by tailoring their actions to forestall anger instead of sadness, which from their perspective is the worse of these two in terms of the consequences for the child.

This difference of perspective may also cause efforts to explain leukemia to backfire. If you try to compare leukemia to any illness they've had, it may create an extreme fear that becomes obvious when the next normal childhood illness strikes them. For these and other reasons, honesty with children about leukemia is essential.

Kathy, a social worker and leukemia survivor, describes to a friend the importance of telling her children about her husband's leukemia:

> You asked about how to deal with your children. I will put on my social worker's cap to reply to your question. It is important that you talk to them soon. Kids will pick up nonverbal cues that something is wrong and they will often imagine the worst. You might be thinking that they couldn't imagine anything worse than what is really happening. Children are very egocentric and their worst fear is usually that of abandonment. So, they need to be reassured that even though Daddy is sick, there will

always be someone available to take care of them. Tell them in very simple language that Daddy has a disease called leukemia (yes, use the word). If you avoid the word, you are giving them the message that this is something too horrible to even talk about.

Reassure them that the doctors are taking care of him and have medicines to give him. If you know of expected side effects, such as hair loss or vomiting, prepare them in advance. Basically, you want to be honest with them, but you want to keep it short and simple so as not to overwhelm them. You can tell them that you want them to come to you if they have any questions or worries. Although they need to feel that you are in control, it can be helpful to share some of your feelings, so they see that it is safe to talk about their own feelings.

At some point, you might want to mention that nothing they ever did or said caused their daddy to get sick. Children believe in magical thinking, so if they were ever angry at Daddy or wished that something bad would happen to him, they now believe they are responsible for his cancer. Also, reassure them that the cancer is not contagious.

Kathy describes how she has talked her daughter about having leukemia:

When I was diagnosed, my daughter was 9 years old. Her first question to me was, "Are you going to die?" I told her that I hoped that I wouldn't die for many, many years and that she would be all grown up by that time. But I did tell her that people can die from leukemia. If our children discover that we lied to them, they will have trouble trusting us again, and this will only create additional fears and insecurities for them. My daughter is now 15 and I still find it a challenge to know how much to tell her. But if I watch for cues, she usually lets me know how much she can handle.

Communicating needs to teenagers

This is a topic on which an entire book could be written. An adolescent trying to break away from the family and become independent is likely to experience quite ambivalent feelings if a parent is diagnosed with cancer. Just at the time in his life when he'd rather avoid talking to any adult, circumstances may force him to become intimate and empathic with a parent. He must be patient and caring toward one of the people most likely to make him angry by holding him to high standards, enforcing rules, denying him privileges, or restricting his freedom. Some find that teens turn surly or run amuck when faced with the physical, emotional, and financial hardships associated with cancer.

Nonetheless, some people find that their adolescent children are extraordinary in their ability to comprehend what's needed, and that they follow through with a maturity that's well beyond their years.

But—even more so than younger children—teens can appear to be knowledgeable and well-adjusted when in fact they are not. This group may have an intellectual maturity that is beyond their level of emotional maturity. A willingness to overlook unexplainable lapses, and an honesty that is geared to their level of understanding are wise attitudes. Frequent offers to chat candidly are a good tactic. These offers confirm their belief that they can approach you about difficult subjects.

If you have a teen who is developing behaviors that are a danger to herself or others, such as acting out rage, violating laws, or considering dropping out of school, find a counselor who specializes in the adaptation of children to serious illness. Attempts to handle these problems by yourself may risk compounding your health problems, may make you a psychologically abused parent, and may fail anyway. A teen may carry "cancer anger" formed during these especially rebellious years well into adulthood.

If you have a teen who is doing housework and assisting with medical care while continuing to carry academic responsibilities, thank him at least daily.

Good friends

We expect our good friends to stand by us while we're facing serious problems. Close friends can offer us help, such as emotional support, occasional running of errands, some cooking, household chores, baby-sitting, or an escapist night on the town. As with loved ones, we may occasionally be disappointed or surprised if they fail to live up to our opinions of them. On the other hand, many leukemia survivors have discovered that good friends earn their wings in heaven by way of loyalty and selflessness, and that some come to mean as much to us as our families do.

Because they usually have a lower emotional investment in the relationship than family members do, at times, good friends can be easier to deal with than your family. They can be more objective about some problems.

This objectivity is purchased with their relative distance. Good friends, in order to remain good friends, may need an occasional vacation from you and your problems. If you give them space to refresh themselves, they are able to return to you with more emotional vigor.

Most people will find that at least some friends or acquaintances will have responses that are disappointing. You can't control how other people react to cancer. Here is one patient's experience with a friend who disappointed her:

> I needed a ride to treatment on Friday and my mother was willing to stay at the house to be there when the children came home. She didn't have the car, so she couldn't take me to treatments. I asked a good friend if she could drive me to treatment at the doctor's office and come back for me a few hours later when treatment was done. At least I believed that she was a good friend.

> Her answer puzzled me, because she said she'd happily drop me off, but she wasn't going to come pick me up. I was really confused, but took her up on the one-way offer. While we were driving to the hospital office building, she told me that she didn't want me getting sick in her car and she had heard that patients after chemotherapy were always getting sick. She was quite clear that she wasn't going to try to deal with that. Needless to say, I haven't asked her to help since, and I will take a cab before I ever ask such a thing of her again.

Some people find support from a wide range of friends or other sources. Judy Archer tells of some of her grown son's sources of support, after a stem cell transplant:

> My son is on temporary retirement from the Air Force and lives in the Phoenix area. He feels good and has had a remarkably trouble-free year since the transplant.

> Jay has an attitude which we believe has made a world of difference in his recovery. He is happy to share with others who need encouragement. Jay has had some pretty amazing experiences and support from (among others): the 69th Squadron at Luke AFB, the Spencer NASCAR racing team, the Chaplain Antique Air Museum of Mesa, AZ, the F-22 team at Lockheed-Marietta, and the Garden Railway Club of Phoenix.

> Needless to say I love my bald-headed fly boy of many and diverse talents...and am happy to report he is doing wonderfully, 378 days post-transplant.

Support groups

It would be difficult to say too many good things about the effect of a support group on an leukemia survivor. In addition to the personal testimonials from people who feel they found sanity, love, and knowledge from the members of their support groups, research by Dr. David Spiegel has shown that emotional support can extend the lives of cancer survivors.

Support groups are the one place outside of your inner circle of loved ones where you can ask or say just about anything. In some cases, you can ask help of support group members that you would be afraid to ask of family for fear of overburdening or frightening them. Moreover, regarding candid speech, the setting is sometimes freer than the family setting because everyone present understands all too clearly what you're going through.

For some, support groups can be the difference, literally, between life and death. The opportunity to exchange information with those who have already weathered leukemia can provide you with the knowledge necessary to question your treatment and seek medical help elsewhere. Support groups are an immeasurably useful place in which to do this, because they bring together a variety of skills, including medical and legal knowledge.

Support groups are offered locally in many areas by groups such as the Leukemia Society of America, the Wellness Community, and local hospitals. Telephone support groups are overseen by several of the nonprofit organizations dedicated to curing leukemia. If you have a computer, support groups are also available on the Internet.

Local, telephone, and Internet support groups all have their advantages and disadvantages. Many people use several.

Local support groups

Local support groups are useful for those who are able to get about easily, have access to a car, and enjoy face-to-face discussion, even about topics that might be upsetting. If you're in a local support group, you're likely to have a stream of visitors if you're hospitalized, and friends to offer you instrumental support, such as help with groceries or baby-sitting. Often, members trade phone numbers and form deep friendships.

Local support groups may contain only a small number of people, perhaps ten or less, who all may have different kinds of cancer. They meet only at certain times of the week or month. Some people find small groups like this advantageous, because they provide a chance to become more intimately involved and more opportunity to speak. The size of the group can affect the quality of the information shared. For example, if no group member has traveled for care, you'll have to make your travel plans with less foreknowledge. Some members of local support groups report that they feel excluded when things take a turn for the worse, as if some group members want to shield themselves from the possibility that similar bad things may happen to them, too. This is sometimes less likely to happen if the group is moderated by a trained therapist.

Hazel, a witty, caring, and extremely bright senior citizen, shares her appreciation for her local support group:

> After surviving breast cancer for twelve years, I was diagnosed with leukemia. This completely and totally devastated me! For months I was unable to function normally. My family tried to be supportive, but in their own way it was as hard for them as for me. I needed help. I had heard about the weekly support groups for cancer patients at the Wellness Community. Participating in one has helped me to cope by providing me with encouragement and helping me to rebuild my sense of control. In addition, the load I am carrying feels so much lighter because others are sharing it with me.

> Though the group involves a variety of cancers, we find a commonality in our problems, experiences, and feelings. Over time, we have laughed together and cried together. We celebrate our successes and bolster one another when there are setbacks, but above all, we are there for each other. I have met many wonderfully courageous people—people I feel privileged to know, people I have learned to call friends.

Internet support

Internet support groups offer several hundred friends, available at all times of the day. You can communicate at 3 in the morning when you have insomnia, and you can communicate with other survivors even if you have trouble getting around for various reasons. The people you meet will be from all over the country, and in most cases, all over the world, and will represent a tremendous amount of experience. Furthermore, if you're a little shy about expressing emotion in front of other people, an Internet group is a good choice because you can write a message and read what you plan to say before you decide to send the message. If you need to cry, you can do so without feeling conflicted about crying in front of other people.

Many of the Internet support groups schedule in-person reunions and gatherings. Often, members form personal friendships and write private email, or trade phone numbers to form even closer friendships. Sometimes, members discover that they're living quite close by and become very good friends.

A list of leukemia-related Internet support groups follows. Because the Internet is a dynamic resource, this list may not be comprehensive. The number of subscribers given was approximate at the time of writing and may vary.

The Association of Cancer Online Resources (ACOR) has pointers to many of the hematologic cancer email discussion groups. ACOR offers a handy automatic subscription feature for these and other discussion mailing lists. You can find them on the web at *http://listserv.acor.org* and join or leave a list from their web site. Lists for long-term cancer survivors, about cancer pain, cancer fatigue, and cancer sexuality are also available. (If you don't have web access, you can send email to *listserv@listserv.acor.org* with the message: subscribe listname [put in the name of the list you wish to join] your first and last names.)

- HEM-ONC. Offering medical discussion and emotional support for all survivors of hematological malignancies, this is the grandmother of hematologic malignancy lists. It's even run by GrannyBarb, and several oncologists subscribe to this list. Hem-Onc has about 750 subscribers from 36 countries of the world. *http://listserv.acor.org/archives/hem-onc. html.*

- HEM-ONC-FR. A French language discussion group for all the hematologic malignancies. *http://listserv.acor.org/archives/hem-onc-fr.html.*

- ALL-L. Medical discussion for acute lymphocytic leukemia, this list was formed in early 1999 and has about 215 subscribers. *http://listserv.acor. org/archives/all-l.html.*

- AML. Discussion and support for those with acute myeloid leukemia. About 340 subscribers participate. *http://listserv.acor.org/archives/aml. html.*

- BMT-TALK. Medical discussion and emotional support for those who will be having or who have had bone marrow transplantation for any cancer. Several oncologists subscribe to this list. About 1,200 subscribers get the list daily. *http://listserv.acor.org/archives/bmt-talk.html.*

- CLL. Medical discussion and emotional support for chronic lymphocytic leukemia. This list has over 1,870 subscribers from 32 countries. *http://listserv.acor.org/archives/cll.html*.

- CLL-CN. Medical discussion of the problems of getting leukemia treatment in Canada. People on this list generally belong to the CLL list as well. The list was started November, 1999 and has more than 85 members. *http://listserv.acor.org/archives/cll-cn.html*.

- CML. Offering medical discussion and emotional support for chronic myelogenous leukemia. Several oncologists subscribe to this list. About 480 subscribers are involved. *http://listserv.acor.org/archives/cml.html*.

- CARINGKIDS. A discussion group just for children of cancer patients, but supervised by adults. It is available using email. To join, email to *listserv@maelstrom.stjohns.edu* with the message: subscribe caringkids [your first and last names].

- GVHD. A discussion for those with chronic graft-versus-host disease to support one another and share ways of handling chronic problems. The list has about 220 subscribers. *http://listserv.acor.org/archives/gvhd.html*.

- HAIRY-CELL. A discussion group for those with hairy cell leukemia. This is a new list as of November, 1999, with about 50 subscribers at present. *http://listserv.acor.org/archives/hairycell.html*.

- MPD-NET. Since CML is a myeloproliferative disorder, many of those with CML congregate on MPD-Net, where they keep company with a group of others with essential thrombocythemia, polycythemia vera, primary myelofibrosis (agnogenic myeloid metaplasia), and secondary myelofibrosis. The membership includes about 1,685 participants. *http://listserv.acor.org/archives/mpd-net.html*

- WARMNET. A general information and support group from the Anderson Network at MDACC. To join this group, make a visit to *http://www.mdacc.tmc.edu:80/~andnet* and sign on.

Subscribers to these Internet support lists can quickly find community. The following is a first post from John Woods, who lives in Australia, and had never before communicated with someone with his disease. He found out quickly that he wasn't the only Australian on the list:

> *I'm a recent subscriber and have been flat out trying to keep up with the flood of mail that comes in every day. My greetings and acknowledgment to you all. I stumbled across the list by pure chance. I am finding*

*daily inspiration in the mail. I am a 53-year-old male living in Northern
NSW, Australia. So far I've only noticed US and Canadian correspondents on the list. Am I the only Australian?*

*I was diagnosed with leukemia in December 1995 and have gone
through two courses of Chlorambucil, or Leukeran, and have just started
another course after some wildly fluctuating WBCs and protracted ill-
health through winter. I also use naturopathy, and while it clearly hasn't
cured me, it has certainly improved how I feel, both physically and
mentally.*

*I've never met nor spoken to another person with CLL, so finding the
list has been something of a "homecoming" for me. Sorry if my ramblings
lack continuity, but I'm feeling my way. I have a suspicion that were I to
give way to my emotions at finding myself in communication with fellow
sufferers, I might open the floodgates.*

John Le Noury describes how finding an online support group of others with
leukemia helped him:

*Learning I had leukemia was extremely devastating for me, as I had
just retired and was looking forward to many good years after a fully
involved 35-year career in education management.*

*Then I discovered this support web site. From the people on it, I know
I am not alone. My confidence has grown and my knowledge of this disease has been multiplied by 1000%. I again feel confident about the future
and am taking a very active role in managing it so that I shall enjoy the
years ahead rather than dwelling upon the adversity, which can be overcome.*

One of the problems of an Internet support group is that the loss of a friend
is very difficult when you cannot say good-bye in person, when you have no
photographs to remind you of them, and no grave to visit. Sometimes group
members simply will never hear again from another member, and they never
learn what really happened. Some group members deal with their grief by
creating memorial web pages dedicated to a lost friend, containing photos
and examples of wisdom learned about living with leukemia.

Internet support groups may include cultural differences that can cause mis-
taken communication. Some people cannot deal with the intensity of the

material and stories of pain or problems that may be posted. Many groups have heavy mail volumes about topics that may not pertain to your circumstances. Incorrect medical information does appear, but is usually corrected in the next posts by others who are more experienced. Social and communication skills span a wide range. The cost of a computer and access to the Internet must also be considered.

A recent survey has shown that the over-65 age group is among the most active and fastest growing groups on the Internet, seemingly not reluctant to acquire the new skills needed to use a computer. That fits in well with the statistics on who gets leukemia, and Internet use for leukemia survivors is climbing.

Telephone support

Telephone support is offered by certain nonprofit groups dedicated to curing cancer and supporting cancer survivors. They offer to act as a clearinghouse for one-on-one telephone contact between those who would like to speak with others in their situation. They are listed in Appendix A.

A woman who had just been told she had leukemia shared her reactions to a call from a matched patient-volunteer this way:

> I was reaching out to anyone and anything I could find that would give me some information about what this disease was and the treatments I would have to undergo. A friend suggested that I call the Leukemia Society, and they put me into a First Connection contact with a patient-volunteer with AML.
>
> It was such a relief to know that there was someone out there with this disease who was still alive. That was the biggest relief.
>
> Then, when she was able to talk about the various treatments and the various levels of the disease, I really felt so much better. The reassurance was the biggest thing, and the knowledge that I wasn't alone in dealing with this disease was another.

Coworkers

What you can ask of your coworkers depends on the structure and size of your workforce, the level of competitiveness, your professional experiences, and the degree to which your work relationships drift into friendships. The minimum we can ask of coworkers is patience and discretion, but frequently they give us much more. Often, the feelings your coworkers express and the support they offer are a tremendous reinforcement for your well-being. To know you are needed and missed can be uplifting.

In general, though, we must exercise some caution when asking favors of coworkers who are not also friends, because the request may seem out of bounds, or may backfire if we're deemed too sick to perform well after revealing a weakness or need. As with some friends, coworkers may want to know everything about your illness, nothing, or some intermediate subset of information that is hard to define and may change daily.

The good news, though, is that many leukemia survivors report that coworkers pitch in and offer assistance without being asked: blood donations, bone marrow donor drives, bake sales, shopping, baby-sitting, cheering visits, and so on may materialize without your having to ask. Many leukemia survivors report that coworkers donate unused sick days to them, or pinch-hit for them if they miss time or feel sick or tired.

If some coworkers are reluctant to recognize your illness owing to their own fears or lack of social skills, they might never refer to it, not even to wish you well.

You can feel free to say nothing to the potentially unsympathetic coworker if you choose, but there are disadvantages in not keeping your immediate supervisor informed about your health status. For example, if your supervisor is unaware of problems you're experiencing as a result of your illness or its treatment, you may have difficulty winning a favorable decision if a dispute about your performance arises.

Remember that cancer is considered a disability under the Americans with Disabilities Act (ADA). Therefore, negative reactions in the workplace that result in demonstrable emotional or professional harm to you, such as denial of a promotion or censure for using earned sick time, don't have to be endured without legal recourse.

Employee assistance programs (EAP)

Increasingly, employers find that it's to everyone's benefit if they offer formal assistance to employees who have special needs at difficult times. Employee assistance programs are designed to help the employee weather life changes and become happy and productive again. If your employer has an EAP, you should ask what it has to offer.

You should be aware, however, that if a health-related dispute over job performance goes to court, employers can subpoena any doctor's records, and so are given access to records that accumulate when you use an EAP. This includes material that most people assume is confidential, such as the notes a psychologist or social worker takes during a therapy session, even if they don't bear directly on your job performance.

If you're seeing a psychologist privately, your employer may not know this or who it is that you're seeing. Clearly, this makes serving a subpoena more difficult. But if you use an EAP, the wolf is guarding the chickens, so to speak. In spite of safeguards that supposedly shield irrelevant material from non-privileged eyes, your employer may become privy to information, for example, about a dependent child who began using drugs after your diagnosis. These confidential documents also may be admitted as evidence into the permanent and public legal record, should you have a workplace dispute that is settled in court.

Computerized self-help programs

Although not yet widely used, computerized self-help programs provided by one's employer or healthcare provider are another means of finding support. The Comprehensive Health Enhancement Support System (CHESS), developed at the University of Wisconsin, is one of the first and most comprehensive of such products. CHESS is planned to be made available to patients through their health care providers and employers. CHESS is a web-based source of patient support. Topic-specific content is available for AIDS, breast cancer, heart disease, asthma, Alzheimer's disease, and alcoholism. The addition of other specific topics is underway.

For more information on CHESS, contact its offices in Madison, Wisconsin at (608) 263-0492 or online at *http://chess.chsra.wisc.edu*.

Individual and family counseling

Many leukemia patients find the disease profoundly difficult to accept and deal with. For those patients, it is often helpful to get a referral to an individual or family counselor.

Kathy Lebedun, MSW, an Oncology Social Worker, made the following suggestions:

For many people, working with an individual therapist is the best way for them to meet their emotional needs. There are a growing number of psychologists, psychiatrists, and social workers who specialize in counseling patients and families dealing with cancer.

The patient's first experience with a mental health professional may occur during a hospitalization. Social workers and/or psychologists are usually an integral part of the cancer treatment team. Upon hospital discharge, they can refer the patient and the family to counseling agencies, such as Cancer Family Care, or to individual therapists for on-going services.

One-on-one counseling provides an opportunity to establish a confidential and trusting relationship with a skilled and caring professional. Many people find it helpful to explore their feelings with a non-judgmental counselor who can help them understand and accept that their feelings are a common reaction to the stress of cancer.

Often, it is difficult for family members to share their emotions with each other, and a therapist can help facilitate open communication. The counselor can aid the family in making practical decisions and in adjusting to the change in roles and responsibilities within the family. Whether one seeks individual counseling, family counseling, or both depends on the needs and desires of the people involved.

The emotional strain of living with a life-threatening illness can be overwhelming. However, the burden can be made easier with the appropriate help. For many people, counseling can make all the difference in the way they cope with their illness. In addition, psychiatrists can prescribe antidepressants and antianxiety medications, when indicated. Social workers familiar with community resources can link people with the appropriate assistance. Most insurance companies now recognize the importance of emotional health to a person's over-all well-being and provide at least partial coverage for professional counseling. You do not have to struggle on your own; individual and family counseling are available to you.

Organizations that focus on help

Your religious group, local chapters of the Elks, Rotary Club, Shriners, or other civic groups may be able to offer you help ranging from transportation for treatment, financial assistance, and pitch-in efforts for lawn care and cooking. Moreover, an enormous collection of nonprofit organizations exist to help you in various ways. Leukemia-specific groups—those for general needs, bone marrow transplantation, children's aid, young adults' aid, home care or temporary hospice care, and pain management—can be found in Appendix A. The Leukemia and Lymphoma Society (LLS) offers an especially helpful program called Patient Aid. They will reimburse up to $750 a year for your out-of-pocket expenses for the cost of prescription medicines and chemotherapy drugs and treatment, radiation and blood and marrow transfusion and testing, and travel for treatment or to local LLS support groups. Co-pays and deductibles for items covered by the Patient Aid Program are also reimbursable. You must register with your local LLS chapter, meet their eligibility requirements (not financial), and be approved in order to participate in this program. See Appendix A.

Challenging moments

Almost every cancer survivor has had a verbal exchange with a "healthy unaware" person that has left him angry, hurt, or speechless. It is sometimes helpful to know that a wide range of rude questions have been asked of other patients and survivors, and that a few people have found comebacks that were satisfying to them.

What you choose to do or say to such remarks depends on what consequences you're willing to endure. In most cases, the classic reply from Judith Martin (also known as Miss Manners), "Now, why would anyone ask such a rude question?" is right on the mark, but not always socially adroit. If someone asks you a rude or outlandish question, there's no rule that says you must be serious in return. Nor do you have to stretch, in your reply, to soothe and comfort the person who asks it, as if his or her discomfort with your illness were the most important issue.

In summary, your experience with leukemia may be your most vulnerable, powerless experience since early childhood. Getting the support you need is critical to adequate recovery, especially during and after relatively risky procedures, such as bone marrow transplantation.

We humans are imperfect. It's unfortunate but true that if we don't communicate clearly, if old resentments linger, or if altruism dries up, the formidable single problem of facing leukemia might evolve into six or seven additional problems.

While nobody knows better than you how to interact with your family, acquaintances, and coworkers, the past experiences of other leukemia survivors may help you spot problems before they arise, or to view old problems in a new way.

To tell or not to tell others about the diagnosis is a problem for those with leukemia diagnoses. Here's one thoughtful patient's way of looking at the question. Paul Hoffman describes his reasoning about sharing his diagnosis so he gets the support he needs, but doesn't get unwelcome reactions:

> *For many of us, this is a very difficult issue and each of us has to find our own way—much like the issues regarding treatment for CLL.*
>
> *In my case, I decided that I would tell my close friends and my siblings. In talking with my sisters, we decided that I would not tell my mother because I did not want to have to address her reaction as well as deal with my condition.*
>
> *I also decided not to tell any of my coworkers. I made that decision because:*
>
> - *I felt that I could continue to perform my tasks as I always had.*
> - *I did not want this to be the basis of any decisions about my status. In fact, subsequent to my diagnosis, our department reorganized and I found myself promoted. I firmly believed that I could handle the additional responsibilities that accompanied this change.*
>
> *I like coming to work and not having to deal with my health. Having people, however well meaning, come up to me and ask how I'm doing all the time would interfere with this. Believe me, I'm not trying to deny my state—I'm just not wanting to deal with this all the time.*

I have been able to receive six rounds of treatment with 2-CDA, three with fludarabine, and four doses of Rituxan, all with a minimum loss of time from work. Fortunately, I work at UCLA, where I also receive treatment. So I arrange for the earliest times available, generally at 8 a.m., and am back to work usually by 10 or 11. We have a generous flex time and nobody has even asked where I've been. I've also been fortunate that I could return to work directly after all of these treatments.

When the time came that I thought I might need a more invasive protocol, such as a BMT, I discussed my situation completely with my boss. I felt that it was my responsibility to ensure she had sufficient information for long-term planning in case such a treatment would be needed.

Additionally, I also finally told my mother. She has been supportive of me, so this has worked out as well.

As I'm not married, it is also a dilemma for me whether or when to tell people I'm dating. This situation has been more problematic. In at least one case, a woman, who initially was very supportive, just stopped talking to me. This really helps to determine what people are like, but still can be difficult to handle emotionally.

Each of us has to evaluate our own situation and determine who and when to tell to get the support we need from those who are important in our lives.

CHAPTER 15

Insurance and Finances

Recovering your health should be your primary focus after being diagnosed with and treated for leukemia. Unfortunately, the side effects of cancer frequently go beyond the physical, impacting your social, professional, and financial well-being. Families often feel the greatest impact. If you're an American with leukemia, you're apt to find it necessary to become an instant, though reluctant, expert on finances, insurance, and workplace issues.

You can ease the nonmedical aspects of your cancer experience in some ways. By becoming familiar with the somewhat harsh and impersonal business side of cancer, keeping careful records, and anticipating problems, you may be better able to handle hospital billing convolutions, insurance payment denials, employment pitfalls, and financial devastation.

This chapter discusses some of the more common problems you may encounter. It gives tips to avoid problems and steers you to up-to-date resources that may provide helpful solutions to these problems. We begin this chapter with a discussion of insurance, including being a savvy consumer of managed care plans and weighing your options for Medicare coverage. We then look at financial issues, such as various sources of disability income, employment issues, record-keeping, and defraying expenses when you travel for healthcare.

It is not the intent of this chapter to address in detail all issues concerning health insurance benefits, federal legislation such as ERISA, Medicare, and Medicaid coverage, unemployment insurance, and financial issues. Appendix A, *Resources*, lists many excellent books and other resources that explore each of these topics much more thoroughly. Some issues mentioned in this chapter, such as estate planning or declaring bankruptcy to protect your house and car, clearly require the aid of professionals, such as financial planners or tax attorneys.

Health insurance

Cancer patients in the US complain about health insurance issues more than any other single issue except the cancer itself. The delays and denials of managed care companies are the most common complaint, but concerns exist in many other areas. The rising cost of prescription drugs is another huge problem. The never-ending telephone calls and the recycling of paperwork are also lamentable. It is a deplorable situation if hospitals are calling when you are sick, to dun you for care on which your insurance company—if you are covered—is delaying payment.

Health insurance in the United States is a conglomeration of various plans that include a wide variety of options. With the advent of managed care, concerns about the financial stability of Medicare, and the creation of health maintenance organizations (HMOs), cancer survivors may find themselves feeling confused and trapped. Insurance companies see cancer survivors as a high-risk group and cancer treatments can be very expensive. Survivors feel resentful toward a system that has taken their money for years and now gives them trouble when they need to tap into its resources. Survivors face unnecessary obstacles to obtaining, maintaining, and collecting on medical insurance, along with finding and receiving medical care. In order to survive, you must be a very canny consumer who makes the system work for you. You need reliable sources of information about your rights and a good understanding of what is covered in the various healthcare packages available to you. Always use the open enrollment period, when it is available, to update your insurance coverage to get a package that meets your personal health insurance needs. You cannot be turned down during open enrollment. At other times, you may be asked to fill out a health questionnaire, and sometimes there is a requirement for a physical examination, as well before coverage will be provided. You do not want that. Try not to get yourself turned down for insurance because once you are turned down, that information stays on file and decreases your chances of ever getting decently priced coverage.

There are several types of health insurance, including managed care plans, Medicare, fee-for-service (indemnity) policies, and medical savings accounts. In addition, catastrophic insurance, long-term care insurance, and hospital indemnity policies can provide additional coverage.

Losing medical insurance coverage if you change or lose jobs is a problem. In addition to various state laws, two federal laws exist to help you retain coverage:

- **COBRA.** The Consolidated Omnibus Budget Reconciliation Act of 1985 provides for a continuation of your old employer's medical insurance coverage for a temporary amount of time—from 18 to 39 months, depending on your circumstances. You will have to pay the total cost of the premium, but at least you will have coverage. Always elect COBRA continuation coverage until you are certain that your new employer's policy will cover expenses associated with your care.

- **HIPAA.** The Health Insurance Portability and Accountability Act of 1996 is a federal law designed to prevent the permanent denial of medical coverage based upon pre-existing conditions. It covers companies with twenty employees or more and says that if you have had medical insurance coverage for more than twelve months, your new medical insurance company cannot refuse to pay for medical care for your previous health problems.

Some states have older, stricter laws that resemble HIPAA but provide better coverage. Call your state insurance commissioner for details.

Self-insured companies, usually businesses with large numbers of employees, are governed by the federal Employee Retirement Income Security Act of 1974 (ERISA).

Managed care plans

If you've spent any time around long-term cancer survivors, you know that most of them are very, very wary of managed care plans. HMOs are for-profit companies. They pay their administrative executives very well. In 1998, *Oncology Times* reported that the President of the Oxford HMO received $29 million in salary alone, along with stock options, and other benefits and perks.

Unfortunately, not all HMOs pay your benefits as generously as they imply that they will. Once you sign up for an HMO, you will go to the doctors who are employees of that plan or are under contract to the plan. The doctors in that plan may be paid a flat rate for each patient, or be limited in the number of tests a patient may receive. There is now a law prohibiting HMOs from keeping a primary care doctor from telling patients about expensive treatments. The HMO will usually not pay for treatment out of the plan.

In order to see any medical personnel, you must go through a "gatekeeper," the primary care physician, to get a referral and pre-approval. Some HMOs make it difficult for the primary care physician to make a referral, and they may limit the number of tests that can be ordered. The advantage is that the patient isn't bothered with paperwork of any kind. All that is necessary is to pay the required copayment with each doctor visit.

Somewhat less rigid are Preferred Physicians Organization (PPO) plans. Here, the doctors are part of a network, but the patient may choose to see any doctor without a referral, and go to any hospital in the system as desired. A variation of the PPO is the Point of Service Plan (POS), where the patient can see any doctor in the system just as in the PPO, but the POS plan will also pay for out-of-system doctors and hospitals on a preset percentage. For example, it may be 70 percent paid by the insurance carrier and 30 percent paid by the patient. The penalty is that the premiums are higher and out-of-pocket expenses increase as the plan becomes more flexible. Also, the patient must deal with the paperwork in order to see an out-of-network doctor or hospital.

If you are considering a managed care plan, try to choose one that will not restrict your access to the best oncology care. Get the list of doctors and hospitals in the network before you sign on, and make sure those you wish to use are in the plan so that there are no surprises later. Remember, however, that a given doctor's participation in any plan is subject to change.

Before you select any insurance coverage, investigate what you are getting. Some questions to ask about managed care plans:

- Do my physicians practice in this network?

- Are the specialists and treatment centers I may need some day in the network?

- Will everything have to go through a gatekeeper or will I have some flexibility? How often can I change my primary care physician? If there is some real dissatisfaction, is there an escape clause?

- Will the plan pay for me to see an out-of-network specialist if there is no doctor with that specialty in the network?

- What percentage of the fees I pay are used for patient benefits and what percent for administrative costs?

- What is specifically excluded from the plan? Is the BMT I may need some day explicitly excluded? (If so, walk away from this plan!)

- Is the plan accredited by the National Committee for Quality Assurance (NCQA)? (While such accreditation doesn't guarantee the patient anything, it does say that the plan has met basic requirements.)

- What provisions or limitations exist if I am traveling and need medical help?

Medicare

Medicare is funded through the Social Security system. It is provided by the Federal government for those over 65 and those on disability (SSD) after two straight years of SSD. If you are legally blind or on kidney dialysis, you also qualify. Medicare and its partner Medicaid, which covers low-income individuals, are public health insurance programs. Created by Congress, they have over time evolved into bureaucratic nightmares.

This book cannot explain all the facets of Medicare and Medicaid. Call your local Social Security office for that information, since it changes yearly, or get a copy of the annually published *Mercer Guide,* available at libraries and bookstores. Another excellent resource is the book *Medicare Made Easy,* published by the People's Medical Society, 452 Walnut Street, Allentown, PA 18102, (610)-770-1670.

If at all possible, cancer patients should elect Medicare Part B coverage for doctors' visits as well as Medicare+Choice supplemental coverage at Level C or above. Medicare+Choice plans fill the gaps in the original Medicare plan coverage and are also known as Medicare Part C. These policies range from levels A through J, with J being the highest. If you want prescription drug coverage, only levels H through J offer that.

Medicare+Choice plans include the original fee-for-service Medicare program, managed care plans, such as health maintenance organizations (HMOs), HMOs with point-of-service (POS) options, preferred provider organizations (PPOs), provider sponsored organizations (PSOs), private fee-for-service plans (PFFSPs) and medical savings accounts (MSAs). This is intended to give individuals the same opportunity for health coverage enjoyed by those who are not covered by Medicare.

At present, you are permitted to enroll in or withdraw from a plan on a monthly basis. If you've just become eligible for Medicare, your initial election period begins three months previous to your 65th birthday, or when you become entitled to Medicare, and ends the last day of the month preceding the month of entitlement. You will have only one initial elections period. Starting in 2002 and beyond, special periods are designated as the initial election period, annual coordinated election period, and the special election period. See a Social Security employee who can explain the new rules to you, because they are complex and your ability to change from one Medicare+Choice program to another is limited.

Be aware that Medicare doesn't pay the full amount of what your doctor charges. You may be billed for the difference, even though with the coverage you had through your employer, you only had a small copayment. Try to find doctors, therefore, who will accept Medicare's reimbursement as payment in full. Such doctors agree to "accept assignment."

The following leukemia survivor is in her early 40s and is now facing Medicare enrollment after two years of SSD payments. With her experience in working with hospitalized patients, she knows that Medicare does not cover all costs or situations:

> It was reassuring to hear that there are rarely personal expenses if one has Medicare and a good supplemental insurance. The Social Security Administration sent me the latest editions of their pamphlets and booklets. Now, I need to investigate my current health-care plan and learn what the benefits will be as a secondary payer. One of my questions is whether they will cover care that is denied by Medicare.
>
> As a medical social worker, I frequently had patients who were in the hospital on IV antibiotics. Once a patient was medically stable, Medicare determined that the patient could be discharged on IV antibiotics. However, Medicare doesn't cover IV antibiotics at home, so the patients were sent to Skilled Nursing Facilities to continue the medications. I certainly don't want to be faced with that scenario! So, I still have some research to do before taking the Medicare plunge.

It is wise for cancer survivors who are approaching 65 and eligible for Medicare, to meet with an advocacy or patient service organization usually found in your local hospital, to find out about costs, benefits, restrictions, and coverage. The last thing a cancer survivor requiring a bone marrow transplant needs is a policy that strictly forbids payment for them. Cancer survivors must carefully analyze the "deals" that Medicare managed care plans (HMOs) purport to offer. When you read the fine print, it's astounding what coverage, that you previously had before Medicare, is missing in your Medicare policy.

Be very wary of any Medicare managed care (HMO) offers that appear to offer you everything for practically nothing. You must read and understand the coverage, based upon your health needs, not on how low the premium will be. Will it cover chemotherapy drugs and other treatments that leukemia patients need? Will it cover the growth factors needed to bring up low counts after chemotherapy and monoclonal antibody treatments? Will it cover a bone marrow transplant? Most do not. If a bone marrow or stem cell transplant is possibly in your future, make sure it will be covered by the Medicare+Choice plan you buy.

Fee-for-service (indemnity) policies

Fee-for-service policies are the traditional policies that pay health care providers on a fee-for-service basis. Individuals under 65 should have a basic and a major medical policy. If one policy covers both basic and major medical, it is called a comprehensive policy. All of these policies have a deductible that the patient pays, and a lifetime cap (often one million dollars). After you have met your deductible, the policy pays 70 or 80 percent of the usual and customary charges for approved medical treatment and you pay the rest. Many also have a stop loss feature, so that after you have spent a certain amount, the policy pays the remainder of the bills for the rest of the calendar year. Most major medical policies cover prescription drugs, home health care, durable medical equipment (like a walker or wheelchair), limited mental health coverage, and some private duty nursing care. The key to this kind of coverage is that the higher you set your deductible, the lower your premiums will be.

Medical savings accounts

The promotion of MSAs could make catastrophic policies more common in the future. You finance regular medical expenses yourself, using a tax-free savings account you have dedicated to that purpose, and use the catastrophic policy to pay the bills for major illness. There is a catch to this and you must be aware of it. Often the money in the dedicated account must be fully spent or it is lost at the end of a predetermined period of time. This means that you must plan very carefully how much money you think you will need in that tax-free account. The problem is that this depends on people being well, and leaves the ones who need insurance coverage most, like cancer patients, in the regular insurance pool.

Catastrophic insurance

Catastrophic insurance policies are like major medical policies. They cover the cost of cancer treatments, for example and the costs of major illnesses. They are helpful to cancer survivors if your medical plan has a low lifetime cap, or a cap on a certain illness, such as cancer. A catastrophic policy makes a good supplement to your medical insurance plan. However, such a plan is often inadequate for the ongoing medical expenses incurred when you have cancer. While they are relatively inexpensive, they have a very high deductible, such as $10,000. One good thing, however, is that once you reach that level, even if your major medical policy is footing the bill, the catastrophic policy pays everything thereafter.

Make sure any catastrophic policy you consider has language in it that says the deductible will come from any sources—including your dedicated account or your major medical policy if you have one. Avoid policies with language that applies the deductible only to your out-of-pocket expenses.

Long-term care insurance

Long-tem care policies are limited policies covering home care and/or in-home nursing. They also pay a set amount each day if you need to go into a nursing home. You choose the number of years of coverage you want and the amount of money you want to pay for nursing home care each day. Premiums go up as the term gets longer and the amount per day increases. Some of these policies also have an automatic inflation factor if you choose to pay for that.

If you have already been diagnosed with cancer, you likely will not be eligible for this kind of policy, unless one is offered at group rates with no medical exam required. One other option for coverage is to ask your children and their spouses if their employers offer such a policy for parents or in-laws as well as employees. This recent trend in employment benefits offerings is an attempt to recognize the increasing responsibilities that families face in caring for older relatives while trying to work outside the home.

The following story in favor of such policies comes from a chronic leukemia survivor, who looks at his world in very practical terms:

> Based on my experience, I recommend that you get long-term care insurance, so long as the premium doesn't devastate you. My mother died in a rest home (convalescent hospital) three years ago after a three-year stay. She was totally paralyzed for the last half of her stay due to a stroke. I was very close to her healthcare situation and visited her almost daily. It cost $4,000 per month to maintain Mom in that convalescent hospital.
>
> The convalescent hospital was comfortable, but by no means a fancy or ritzy place. I am very, very lucky that my parents planned ahead for their demise. Without their thoughtfulness, I would now be bankrupt.
>
> Medicare and other plans, like Medi-Cal, don't cover everything and can lead to a poor quality of care in an already bad situation. Chronic leukemia doesn't necessarily mean you will die a quick death. You are subject to other conditions, such as strokes, which can be totally debilitating.
>
> I have long-term care coverage with built-in inflation protection at a cost of $116 per month. I feel I am lucky to have this. It's worth every penny to me, knowing that my children will not have to mortgage their future and that I will not cause a significant financial burden upon my family should I become an invalid.
>
> Your other option is to sign a contract with Dr. Kavorkian.

Hospital indemnity policies

Hospital indemnity policies are handy extras. They pay a set amount for every day that you are hospitalized. They are a welcome source of extra cash at a time when you have large expenses but less income than normal. The American Association of Retired Persons will sell such policies to anyone over 50 with only a three-month pre-existing condition exclusion.

Financial issues

Financial issues cannot be addressed adequately in one chapter of a medical consumer book. Nonetheless, we've included a few issues in this section to inform you, rather than advise you, regarding problems you may encounter.

Major points

Here's an encapsulation of some fairly prominent issues:

- Determine if it is worthwhile to refinance your home mortgage for a lower interest rate. If the current market rate for mortgages is significantly lower than yours, refinancing may reduce monthly payments, increase equity more rapidly, and ultimately, reduce debt.

- Contact the Social Security Administration to see if you, your spouse, or your children are eligible for Supplemental Security Income. Visit *http://www.ssa.gov* on the Web or call (800) 772-1213. (SSI differs from SSDI, Social Security Disability Income.)

- Fundraising in your community or your place of employment can be a very effective way to address debts related to medical care. The Organ Transplant Fund, for example, provides sound help with raising funds for bone marrow or stem cell transplantation. See Appendix A for a list of other organizations that can help with financial issues, such as fundraising.

- Estate planning should always be considered, even for seemingly small estates. Some options, such as a supportive care trust or purchase of a whole-life insurance policy, may preserve some assets for yourself, your spouse, or your children—but may interfere seriously with your eligibility for Medicaid. Estate planning is especially important if your spouse or a child also has serious health problems of his/her own, requiring long-term financial support.

- A debt consolidation or home equity loan may be a useful tool for consolidating debt.

Bankruptcy

The two leading reasons for declaring bankruptcy are excessive medical expenses and credit card debt.

Declaring bankruptcy has changed from being viewed as a last-ditch, unethical, and humiliating way to escape obligation, to an honorable, if humble, effort to restructure or reschedule debt payment. Of the three forms of bankruptcy that individuals (as opposed to businesses and farmers) may use, only one, Chapter 7 bankruptcy, discharges the debtor of all debt. The others, Chapters 11 and 13, provide for a repayment plan in a hierarchical and agreed-upon way, eliminating or postponing foreclosure on your home or repossession of your car. Moreover, once you have declared bankruptcy, your creditors are forbidden by law from harassing or suing you.

Nonetheless, declaring bankruptcy still should be considered as a last resort for resolving financial problems and should always be done under the guidance of a professional financial advisor or bankruptcy attorney.

Disability income

Several means are available to provide you with income while you are disabled.

Social Security Disability Income (SSDI)

The Social Security Administration may grant disability benefits under the Social Security Disability Income (SSDI) plan to replace lost income for an adult with leukemia. If you are unable to work because of your leukemia, you may choose to go through the paperwork jungle that is required to apply for this income. For information about coverage and starting the application process, call (800) 772-1213 or visit *http://www.ssa.gov* on the Web. To smooth the process of applying for Social Security Disability Income, bring all medical records with you, and let your doctors know you're applying, as they will need to give substantiating evidence.

If SSDI is denied—and frequently it is on the first application—ask for Publication No. 05-10041, *The Appeals Process*. Sometimes just a request to have your case reviewed by the SSA's physicians will speed an approval.

The following survivor shares her experience qualifying for Social Security Disability Income on the first try:

> I was approved for Disability upon my first application. I can give two significant reasons why I think I was approved:
>
> 1. My oncologist was very helpful. He not only completed the paperwork, but he talked with the Social Security caseworker (upon my request).
>
> 2. I acted as my own advocate because I had the expertise, and had extensive and on-going communication with the caseworker. This was in addition to all the paperwork, which I completed.

I basically made a strong case for myself as to why I was no longer able to work. My caseworker then acted as my advocate with the medical director, who ultimately made the determination for disability. I did not fall neatly into the rule book criteria, but there were other medical factors to be considered and I made sure that they were!

There are two federal programs under which you might qualify through your Social Security office. Social Security Disability Income, or SSDI, is for adults who have a physical and/or mental problem that keeps them from working at any job for at least twelve months or that is expected to result in death. Supplemental Security Insurance (SSI) is a program for those people aged 65 or older or who are disabled or blind, who have limited income and resources.

In some cases, it's possible to return to work and still continue to collect SSDI benefits. This is possible owing to special incentives the Social Security Administration provides to rehabilitate the disabled. The formula used to compute disability benefits while working is complex, but in general, you may attempt a trial work period of nine months, not necessarily consecutively, during which benefits do not change. If the trial does not succeed, benefits may continue. Ask the Social Security Administration for the publication called *Working While Disabled How We Can Help* (Publication No. 05-10095).

There is another program under which you might qualify for income payments. State Disability Insurance (SDI) is a state disability program that is handled in many states by the people who service unemployment insurance claims. The benefit amounts, paycheck days (every two weeks), and waiting period are all similar to those for unemployment benefits. You must have had earnings from a job during the period that runs from 18 months before you apply to about 6 months before you apply.

Criteria for the state program, SDI, appears to be much less stringent than for the federal program, SSDI. You must be out of work because of your medical condition, but not unable to do any kind of work or permanently disabled, as the federal program, SSDI, requires. SDI lasts for only a matter of months, so it isn't like Social Security disability. But if you will be out of work during the time needed for a particular treatment or for a limited period of time, SDI may help you to meet your financial needs. You may apply for both SDI and Social Security disability. If you are approved for

Social Security, you'll receive SDI during the 5-month waiting period. Check with your state's SDI office to be sure that this information is correct for the state in which you live.

Private long-term disability income

Disability insurance is usually an employee benefit or self-purchased policy. It pays a cash amount, which is a percentage of your earnings, if you are unable to work because of illness.

If you don't have a long-term disability insurance policy, it is wise to consider buying one. For those under age 65, the likelihood of long-term or permanent disability is far greater than the risk of death, especially for leukemia survivors who, owing to improvements in treatment, now face an illness that is shifting from fatal to chronic. For leukemia survivors who face repeated treatment and continuing aftercare, the need for disability insurance is greater when treatment leaves you unable to work.

However, be careful in researching these policies. You want one that has a short elimination period (preferably from one to three months), a lifetime benefit period, or up to age 65 or older, if you will be eligible for Social Security payments after age 65. You want the policy to be noncancelable, guaranteed renewable, with benefits for partial disability. Disability should be defined as inability to perform the major tasks of your occupation. Income should be non- or partially taxable and the policy should have no pre-existing condition exclusion.

Note that almost all private long-term disability policies reduce your monthly benefits if you receive other income, including disability benefits from the Social Security Administration. Most of the long-term disability policy insurers encourage you to apply for SSDI. Here's one patient's story that explains why:

> Generally, long-term disability plans work like this: they make sure that if you become disabled you will receive some percentage, such as 60 percent, of your current salary. But this amount includes your Social Security benefits. So, if your pre-disability income is $1000/month and Social Security pays $400/month, long-term disability would pay $200/month to bring your total income to $600/month (60 percent of your pay).

If you have long-term disability insurance, the insurance company
will take care of all of the Social Security paperwork for you. They will
apply, hire lawyers to appeal, whatever it takes. They want you to get this
money so they don't have to pay it. But you will not get any additional
money as a result of owning the policy.

Military (VA) disability income

You can receive partial VA disability benefits while working full time. Note
that if you initially refuse veterans' disability benefits from a sense of pride, it
will be almost impossible to reopen your claim later. For instance, if you suffer a heart attack years after being treated with radiotherapy or Adriamycin
(doxorubicin), and your doctors are convinced your heart was damaged by
these drugs, you will not be permitted by the VA to reopen your case and
collect benefits. As damage from treatment may develop years after it's
administered, it's best not to refuse a VA settlement if it's offered, no matter
how well you feel nor how capable of working you may be.

Employment issues

Having and being treated for leukemia can impact your job attendance and
performance. If you're very lucky, you'll have managers and coworkers who
accommodate your ups and downs. Sometimes they may even hold fundraisers for you, or donate their own unused sick or vacation time for your
use. Many people are not this lucky.

As with finance and insurance issues, you have certain protections under the
law. You should verify the details of these laws, as they may change over
time:

- The Americans with Disabilities Act (ADA) recognizes cancer as a temporary or permanent disability for which you cannot be penalized by
  demotion or dismissal. It's also illegal to deny a qualified candidate a job
  simply because of a disability, but it's difficult to prove this kind of dis-
  crimination unless you know intimately every other job applicant and
  all of their qualifications.

- The Family and Medical Leave Act (FMLA) guarantees you twelve weeks
  of leave annually for your own healthcare or to attend to a sick family

member. During these twelve weeks, your job, or a very similar one, must be held open for you and your benefits must be maintained. The FMLA applies only to companies with 50 or more employees. Violations of this law should be reported to the U.S. Department of Labor.

- Worker's Compensation for the development of any cancer is rare because few direct causes of cancer are known, much less those resulting directly from risky job responsibilities. Consult an attorney who specializes in workplace and Worker's Compensation issues.

Some employers sponsor Employee Assistance Programs (EAP) to counsel employees who are having problems that affect their job performance. A subset of these employers may require participation in their EAP in order to approve benefits payment for counseling.

Record-keeping

The value of record-keeping cannot be overemphasized. Evidence in writing that supports your position is indispensable, should disputes or questions arise. Records should be obtained for all treatment, employment, and financial matters, and should be maintained in some organized way in a place safe from fire, theft, or flood.

Establish a record trail

Simple though it may sound, getting copies of all medical information, including films, and getting written copies of all tangential records related to employment, insurance, and finance is sometimes overlooked. Here are some tips for obtaining records:

- Request and keep copies of all medical records and bills as you go through diagnosis, monitoring, and treatment. This will establish with the doctor's staff your expectations and set a tone of efficiency, and will permit you instant access to material if you need it for second opinions. Having copies made and mailed after the fact can add five or more days—even weeks—to the time needed to collect records.

- If you're requesting records that must in turn be forwarded to another health center, make a copy for yourself before forwarding the material.

- If you're hospitalized, or if your treatments are given in the hospital on an outpatient basis, ask for itemized copies of bills. General or summarized hospital bills can be astonishingly obtuse, and even an itemized bill can be unclear. Most errors in hospital billing are found in an itemized bill's relative clarity.

- Always address financial, employment, or insurance disputes in writing, and keep copies of what you've written.

- Keep a detailed phone log of all calls made to insurance companies, mortgage companies, and so on.

- Any decision reached verbally to correct errors should be followed by a written confirmation from the company. Ask for this, and if they won't furnish a written reply, write your own reply, stating, "Based on our phone conversation of the given date, it is my understanding that the following will happen," listing what you perceive to be true.

- Keep a calendar of your medical and treatment appointments. Do not discard it at the end of the year. Keep it as a permanent part of your medical and financial files.

- If space permits, your calendar can double as a log for phone calls, changes in medications or symptoms, blood test results, and so on. Otherwise, school exercise books or blank journals, the kind from which pages cannot be easily torn, may serve well.

- Record and copy outgoing correspondence. Send all correspondence that's even remotely important by certified mail, using the return receipt option. Unlike registered mail, which is logged at each stop in the postal system, certified mail does not travel more slowly than regular mail, and isn't much more expensive than regular mail. When the return receipt arrives, staple it to your copy of the correspondence: it is your proof that the mail arrived at its destination. Use fax transmission for speed when needed, but follow up with certified mail. Some examples of uses for certified mail:

  - Correspondence sent to insurance companies that require 30 days' advance notice in order to review and approve treatment plans such as bone marrow transplantation

  - All correspondence with the IRS

  - All correspondence with collection agencies, mortgage companies, or automobile loan holders

  - All correspondence with the Social Security Administration

- Have copies of all original CT and MRI films made for your own files if a review is pending. While copies of the reports that describe and analyze these films are useful, access to films is mandatory for certain kinds of review and decision-making.

- If the original CT or MRI films are loaned to other doctors for second opinions, follow up to be sure they are returned to the central film library or original office.

Organizing the record trail

How little or how much you choose to organize will depend in some measure on your overall energy level, and on your record-keeping habits in general. Don't be surprised if you find yourself, normally a well-organized person, suddenly without sufficient energy to file medical reimbursement forms. Others, though, may find themselves becoming more organized as a coping mechanism.

You may find that record-keeping is a task you can delegate to a family member, friend, or neighbor who would love to help you but doesn't know quite what to offer. Although you may not care to have someone outside your family making phone calls to correct billing mistakes, having someone sort and file bills and receipts on a weekly basis may help you. Sorting mail into stacks for filing is a task that a child might enjoy; scanning and storing documents on a PC might be something that a computer-literate relative might want to do.

Whatever method suits your current needs, do attempt, at the very least, to store medical and payment records in some organized way. A minimal technique is to put all records in one place, such as in one or more grocery bags, in case you need to access them in a hurry. If you or your volunteers have the time and energy to do so, you may lean toward a fairly elaborate system of organization that gives you instant access to items by topic, health center, or date.

Traveling for care

When the time comes for a second opinion, for you to participate in a clinical trial, or to have treatment at another location, you encounter the financial hardships travel may entail. Some health insurance policies cover airfare, but not lodging; some pay *per diem* for food and lodging, but do not cover airfare. Some pay for neither and still others pay only mileage for travel. So the first step is to verify what your own policy will or will not cover. Clearly, if airfare isn't covered by your policy but mileage is, you'll want to drive unless you are not up to it. Lodging for family members who accompany you is another expense, and the cost of food is an additional consideration. You'll also have to arrange for relatives or friends to step in and care for school-aged children while you are gone, or take the children out of school to go with you.

Fortunately, there are some resources open to you to ease these financial burdens. See Appendix A.

Air travel

If you need to fly to your destination, there are charitable groups that will fly you to your destination free of charge. Some of these groups require that the patient embark and disembark from the plane without airline assistance, or that support equipment be manageable without airline intervention. See Appendix A for a comprehensive listing of air travel resources.

Additional assistance

- **The Leukemia and Lymphoma Society (LLS).** This society will pay up to $750 for patients who have registered with them for travel to treatment. That means it will pay airfare or mileage from your home to the treatment center. That same total amount of money may also be used for reimbursement for specific drugs, blood transfusions, or X-rays. Use it where you need it most! Contact your local chapter of the Leukemia and Lymphoma Society or call (800) 955-4572. Only bills incurred after registration with your local chapter are eligible for reimbursement. In addition, it can help with travel arrangements if needed.

- **The American Cancer Society.** Its regional offices in many cities have volunteers who can provide transportation by car to and from your treatment center.

- **Traveler's Aid Society.** This organization provides emergency travel and lodging for those in dire financial need. Your local phone book will have contact information, or use the public library for phone books at your destination.

Lodging

Contact the social services department of the institution to which you are traveling. They will have up-to-the-minute listings of free or relatively inexpensive lodgings for patients and families. Some lodgings have shared kitchens for you to use, which helps with the cost of food. Some facilities, like the National Cancer Institute, permit family members of patients to share their rooms overnight. Many hospitals and medical centers have arrangements with hotels in close proximity to provide lodging for patients at reduced rates. Find out by checking with the social services department. Specific resources for lodging may be found in Appendix A.

CHAPTER 16

After Treatment

After treatment, patients have conflicted feelings. Some are frightened at leaving the structure of the treatment setting, with the frequent blood tests, the caring nurses wanting to know how they are, and the check-ins with the doctor. Others are relieved that the stressful time is over and they can try to get back to a normal routine. Survivors look at friends and relatives with different eyes, and may find it difficult to return to old roles in the family. The workplace may feel strange to survivors who have been gone for long-term treatment. For example, someone else might be doing the survivor's job and might or might not want to give the job back.

Problems such as these must be worked through. The leukemia experience doesn't end when treatment ends. It now requires adjustments and a new kind of normality.

If survivors are lucky, they can stop making leukemia the center of the universe and can attempt to resume normal life. During this process, however, they can expect to feel disorientation and the need to reassess who and what they are. Survivors are likely to feel somewhat different physically, psychologically, and physiologically than they did before diagnosis and treatment.

In this chapter, we discuss the emotional and practical considerations survivors encounter at the end of the treatment phase. We look at medical monitoring, physical and mental fitness, social and professional changes, and getting back into the social world and the world of work. In "Late effects and complications," we cover those problems that may follow certain treatments, and what, if anything, can be done about them.

Leaving the world of treatment

You've had your last course of chemotherapy and your doctor has said those wonderful words, "You're in remission!" You feel a huge surge of relief and know you should want to rush to pick up the strings of your life again, but you also may feel hesitant. Suddenly though you are free of treatment and in control of your life again, you also may be leery about your ability to deal with things as you did before.

Some survivors reassimilate easily into their old lives. However, many others feel ambivalent at the end of treatment, frightened of being without moment-to-moment back up, fearful of leaving the familiar life of a patient. For those survivors, it is hard to break away from the pattern of medical surveillance. The hospital staff isn't there to answer questions as soon as they arise. You might have built up a psychological dependence on the staff and even on the experience of being treated with chemotherapy. You might worry about missing some warning signal that relapse is occurring. You might be terrified that a runny nose or a cough is a symptom of a return of your leukemia.

If you are ambivalent about the end of treatment, know that these feelings are normal and that they should gradually fade away.

Moving on

Thirty years ago, this chapter wouldn't have been included in this book. Many leukemia patients would not have survived to read it. Because of the enormous improvements in treatments and understanding of the disease process, today increasing numbers of patients are alive to be concerned about their post-treatment options. Now survivors talk about quality of life issues that no one would have thought of then.

The medical community and survivors don't always see problems from the same perspective. The physician treats the disease to bring the patient into remission. The survivor needs to look at what kind of quality of life can be expected after that treatment.

The medical community is becoming more aware of survivors' problems and how important they are. Oncologists seek treatments that are less toxic, that do less overall damage to the patient as a whole being, and that allow the patient to enjoy a reasonable quality of life after achieving remission.

If the chemotherapy treatment or bone marrow transplant that saved your life leaves you with chronic problems, you must be vigilant about keeping up with medical monitoring. Survivors need to be aware that the treatments they have received to put them into remission may also require that they be medically monitored throughout their lives. You may be cancer free, but you are not free of the aftermath of cancer treatment. Find out when you are to schedule follow-up visits, and discuss with your doctor which member of your healthcare team to call with questions or problems. Write down information about immediate after effects and late effects of treatment that you may encounter.

After treatment, the doctor-patient relationship changes again. Again, communication is key. Both doctor and patient need to clear the air and create a new pattern for the aftermath of treatment and continuing care. Your doctor is apt to step back and be less involved than before.

If you and your oncologist have differing views of how to handle follow-up care, you need to get things out on the table immediately and discuss these differences. For example, some patients think they are "cured" and don't want to follow the doctor's recommendations for follow-up care. If you and your physician do not concur, and you refuse the additional or different follow-up treatment suggested, recognize that you are creating a situation for which you are responsible. If your doctor seriously disagrees with your decision, and communication fails, you are likely going to have to find another physician who is more in tune with the way you are thinking at this time.

Here's an example of a doctor-patient relationship that was fine during the active treatment phase, but not so good during follow-up:

> I was so thankful when treatment was finished and the doctor said those lovely words, "You are in complete remission." All things considered, treatment could have been worse, but my doctor was there for me all the time, and the hospital staff had been wonderful.
>
> Things began to change when I came back for my first follow-up visit. I expected to be told to come back periodically to check-in, and was looking forward to a long break from hospitals and chemotherapy, but instead the doctor was suggesting further treatment to make sure the remission held.
>
> First of all, this was not what he had led me to expect at any time during the treatment phase. Second of all, I had never read or heard about treatment to maintain a remission. Third of all, we had planned to take a long vacation at our summer home in New England and I knew no medical practitioners in the vicinity. Psychologically this hit me all wrong.

I was utterly unprepared for this eventuality and I needed a break from treatment. So I said, "No. I'm willing to think about starting maintenance therapy when I return in two months, but I can't even begin to think about it now."

My doctor started to pressure me. Instead of the accepting attitude I had come to expect from him, he was pushing for me to have experimental treatment with a drug I didn't know about, hadn't researched, and wasn't comfortable considering. When I asked him, "Why the pressure?" He really couldn't answer. When I asked if I could hold off for a psychological break, he didn't respond at all. It was devastating because my whole relationship with him was breaking apart and I was frightened.

Ultimately, I took the break I needed, and when I returned I asked about the experimental maintenance therapy. He brushed it off casually and I'm not on it, but I fear that our relationship will never be the same, and I'm seeking a new doctor.

Emotional responses

Almost everyone looks forward to the end of treatment with joy, relief, and celebration. After all, side effects will diminish, energy will return, the cancer is in remission, and expectations of a period of freedom from thinking about leukemia are realistic. Some people fear the end of treatment because of a feeling of abandonment. They feel that the chemotherapy and other treatments are all that stands between them and leukemia. Matter-of-fact actions by the medical staff may seem brusque or uncaring to the survivor. There is no fanfare, not even a "good-bye and good luck" in many cases, because the patient will be back for monitoring in a few weeks or a month. The end of treatment is an emotionally charged, high point for the survivor, but just business as usual for the treatment team.

Michele Stevens, a leukemia survivor being treated at the NCI, describes her ambivalent feelings about the end of treatment. She hadn't achieved a complete remission according to the bone marrow biopsy, although her blood work looked good:

Completing treatment was somewhat of a letdown for me. I somehow thought I'd be "the one" who was actually cured by chemotherapy, or at least would achieve a full remission. I didn't like to know that the cancer cells were still infiltrating two thirds of my marrow, no matter how "lightly" the doctors claimed. I felt as if I had this malevolent presence inside my bones, building up forces, until it could make its escape back into my bloodstream and lymphatic system.

I dreaded going to my oncologist for the blood work, knowing it was just a matter of time before it wouldn't be normal anymore. In a sense, it was almost a relief when the numbers started climbing again. The other shoe had finally dropped.

Worries of being abandoned by my doctors at the NIH were alleviated even before I'd finished treatment. I was assured I'd be brought back every three months for check-ups, and that when I needed more treatment, most assuredly something would be in place in which I could participate.

Some patients report that they feel nothing at all when treatment ends. They have been so emotionally drained by all they have experienced that they cannot yet look forward to the future. Others fear that remission is too good to be true and worry that they will relapse. In fact, most leukemia survivors live with fear of relapse, felt occasionally or often. Some survivors can push those fears to the back of their minds for months at a time, feeling fear only before a scheduled check-up or when an odd pain manifests itself. Ordinary aches and pains become much more significant to cancer survivors. Survivors wonder if a symptom is something to call the doctor about. Is it important or just one of those things that "everyone" has? Most of the time, an ache or pain is nothing, but as a survivor, you need to monitor your body. That doesn't make you a hypochondriac—just careful.

Some people may experience insomnia, nightmares about cancer, fear, or a need to avoid doctors and hospitals. Others report feeling jumpy and uncomfortable in everyday interactions with hospital personnel for things like flu injections. They bring back all the feelings endured during treatment. Still others experience extreme anger or sadness when hearing about someone else with cancer. Some report having post-traumatic stress syndrome experiences after treatment ends. Fortunately, with newer and less toxic treatments, fewer people have to deal with such severe reactions.

Social and professional after-effects

Those people around you who have never had cancer, or had to deal with it in their families, are usually totally unaware of the mixture of emotions that cancer patients and families are feeling. You are picking up the pieces of your life and trying to put them together again. You are learning to cope with controlling all aspects of life's activities again. Family members need to find ways to be protective without making the survivor feel under surveillance. Family and work relationships need to be forged again in the face of the survivor's changed outlook on life.

Fitting in again at work

With the end of treatment come practical considerations. Your energy will return and the leave you took from work may come to an end. You need to make several important decisions at this time. If you have been working throughout the period of treatment, these problems will be easier to solve because you haven't been out of the loop at work for any length of time, and you know more or less what is happening.

Problems may arise when you return to work and you're not yet able to put in a full day. That's not a problem in a supportive work environment with helpful coworkers, but it can pose problems if your colleagues expect to have you back at full speed the day you return. You, on the other hand, may well feel like it's the day after the Super Bowl game, and you are the losing quarterback. Be sure to make it clear that you simply can't come back that quickly, and that you will need a period of time to phase back into a full workday.

If you had to take an extended leave from work, you might encounter special problems. You will need to speak with colleagues and bosses to make sure that you find answers to the following possible problems:

- Can you return to the job you left and deal with the physical and psychological demands it places on you?

- Can you handle the travel schedule that was expected of you before you became ill?

- Can you deal with the problems associated with trying to resume duties that others have assumed in your absence?

- How do you deal with your colleagues' present and long-term perceptions that you are no longer able to deal with the pressures of your job?
- Will you be considered fairly for promotion in the future?

Family relationships

On the social front, you might meet similar problems. Your close family and friends who have seen you throughout your treatment have probably adjusted to the new you and the emotional and physical upheaval with which you've been dealing. Nevertheless, as you come to the end of treatment, you may find that some family members and friends expect that you will instantly become just as healthy and energetic as you were before.

Leukemia survivor Michele tells what she experienced after therapy was over. Fortunately, not everyone is faced with the kind of expectations that she encountered:

> I once sat with my husband and made him read an article explaining about leukemia, about the treatment I was undergoing, and the possible consequences of both. His only comment afterwards was, "Interesting!" He somehow didn't appear to associate any of it with his wife, or the possibility of his lifestyle changing drastically.

> When treatment was completed, my husband expected me to return to a state of "Damn the torpedoes, full speed ahead." This expectation didn't surprise me, because all during my treatment I remained the caregiver, chief cook, and bottle washer. I had chosen treatment 1,200 miles from home because I knew it would be the only way I would get some rest while undergoing chemotherapy. Upon returning home between therapy rounds, I was always greeted with piles of laundry (he did learn to wash his own clothes when needed), a house that needed cleaning, and an empty pantry that needed filling.

> Once I achieved partial remission, there was no "excuse" for me to take a nap in the middle of the day if I needed to. My husband was convinced that everyone else was sicker than I was, no matter what kind of cancer they had, or where they were in their treatment. When I came out of the partial remission less than eight months after completing therapy, my husband out-and-out told me, in front of everyone at the support group I had decided to try, that there was nothing wrong with me.

He commented that I only had a cold, and that I was "too ornery to die." I
never went back to that group.

Some family members and loved ones have feelings of anger and frustration that they suppressed while you were in treatment. These feelings may now emerge. Candid discussions are needed, and if the feelings persist, family counseling may be helpful.

Sometimes a spouse or partner decides that it is time to end a relationship after treatment ends. This is most likely to happen if there were problems in the relationship before diagnosis and treatment. Sometimes counseling helps in these situations, and sometimes there is no way to hold a relationship together.

Similarly, children who lack coping skills may still remain distressed and fearful about the possibility of the patient's death. They may need support with social, psychological, or academic issues. Occasionally, psychotherapy may be needed.

Friends and neighbors may well expect that you'll be the same old person they knew in the past. But diagnosis and treatment have changed you and your outlook on life, so it may take a while to rebuild these relationships.

Judit had a brother who developed leukemia, and then her husband was diagnosed and treated for CLL. Her brother and husband each responded differently to the end of treatment. Judit tells of her brother's pessimism based on his own life experience:

> *My brother just kept on hoping for a little more respite between one treatment and the next. He never celebrated or dared to rejoice at the end of any of them.*

> *Treatment or no treatment, he never stopped coming to our house and using the computer to get the support list news first thing in the morning after my husband left for work. We played four hands on the piano when we were stressed out, and it usually helped him to get through the day. It helped both of us.*

> *In spite of the times he had between treatments, he never stopped being afraid, and never hoped for much. His pessimistic attitude came from the time he lost his wife and 21-year-old son in a mammoth car accident. I think this was about the time when he started to develop*

leukemia, and not really eight years ago when he was diagnosed. I was always the only one hoping for good things for him.

In comparison, Judit's husband—with different past experiences and outlook, but the same diagnosis—celebrated remission:

> *My husband is a different story. When he went into remission six years ago, he immediately made plans to travel and to have some fun. My daughters organized a huge surprise 70th birthday party for him, and he celebrated with us without any fear or second thoughts. We went to Puerto Rico right afterwards, and he spent every night gambling in the casino, even though gambling bored me to tears.*

> *He asked me several times what I would have done if he had succumbed to the heavy chemo he'd had. I told him that I'd have buried him, and would have had a face-lift after I had finished mourning, and then would have started a new life. He liked my answer so very much that he promised to stay in remission indefinitely. I do hope he keeps this promise!*

Lingering symptoms and side effects

In general, the lingering side effects and delayed effects you may have experienced during treatment should fade away in the months following treatment. However, certain side effects take much longer to disappear. For example, those patients treated with Vincristine report that the tingling in their hands and feet (peripheral neuropathy) often takes months or years to dissipate. The return of supple veins after prolonged chemotherapy, when peripheral veins were used for treatment, happens over a long time, and some patients never recover. They live with veins that hide, roll, or are so fine that the veins cannot easily be tapped—even for blood draws. Blood counts are often slow to recover. Survivors report that old allergies may be better or worse, but that new allergies often develop to things you were never allergic to previously.

Beth is a CLL survivor. During her treatment with a standard dose of fludarabine she had minor side effects, including some headaches and a bout of shingles, following six cycles of treatment. During four standard Rituxan infusions, she noticed only a slight fever. However, after chemotherapy ended, she noted an unusual effect. This story illustrates the allergic variations that can occur among patients:

Now, having said that the side effects were minimal, I have to tell you about a major change that I have experienced since chemo that may have to be considered a side effect.

Since chemo, I have developed allergies to almost all of the foods that I normally ate. My diet is severely restricted to just a few foods—ones that I didn't use to eat much. The allergy symptom was a nasty skin rash, all over my body, that was not diagnosed by a dermatologist, even after five skin biopsies. I had elevated eosinophils and high IgE levels both caused by new food allergies. However, I seem to have lost respiratory allergies that I used to have. I have not responded to any of the air-borne allergens that used to keep me congested and sneezing (cats, dust, dust mites).

Following the Rituxan treatment, my lymphocytes were not detectable at all (either T or B cells) in my peripheral blood for several months. The cells that repopulated my peripheral blood were of a different composition than before, I guess. Long-term use of Inteferon, among other drugs, can have depressive effects on the psyche and some people will be dealing with chronic depression even after treatment is complete.

If you've had a bone marrow transplant and have chronic graft-versus-host disease, you can expect continuing health problems to monitor and to deal with. Even if you didn't have an allogeneic transplant, you may experience late effects. See Chapter 9, *Transplantation*.

Late effects and complications

It would be improbable to expect that the toxic treatments used to kill leukemic cells would not also affect normal cells and indeed, research shows that this is the case. Usually the side effects caused by treatment are temporary and disappear in days and weeks. A few of the effects of treatment, however, last longer in some people, and some complications do not emerge until years after treatment.

Most people never encounter delayed effects and, unless they relapse, go on to live more or less healthily ever after. The "more or less" is important. It means that leukemia's effect on survivors' lives doesn't end with the period immediately after treatment. If you're a survivor who has just finished treatment, and you're having a bad day, please put this section of the chapter down and come back to it, or ask a loved one to read it for you. The idea of late effects is not a cheery one for survivors.

What are late effects? Side effects happen within days and weeks of treatment. Delayed effects occur weeks and months after treatment ends. Late effects will occur months or years after treatment. Some side effects continue, and become delayed or late side effects—for example, unremitting diarrhea caused by abdominal irradiation. The medical community also distinguishes between effects that are expected, and complications, which are somewhat unexpected.

Sometimes symptoms are just annoying, and sometimes they can be life-threatening. Ask your doctor what late effects you might experience, based on your treatment and health history. Ask what symptoms should be reported. You will probably err on the side of caution, especially at first, while you are still learning what the "new normal" feels like. Report what is worrisome to you.

What symptoms might be late effects and which are a sign of a relapse? Be aware of your body, tell your doctor about symptoms that are occurring, and follow through on recommended tests and monitoring. Your doctor will help you sort out late effects from signs that might indicate a return of disease. Eventually, you'll be less likely to jump to the conclusion that any physical change means a return of the disease.

One bone marrow survivor explains her feelings about the late effects and complications that she encountered after her bone marrow transplant. The first several effects she tells about were somewhat expected or predicted, although they still required some adjustment:

> I was warned when I was preparing for transplant that my fingernails and toenails would fall out and would grow back. I accepted that, but no one told me that my fingernails would be permanently striated with white lines and black lines that look terrible. Thank goodness I'm female and can wear nail polish. The bonus is that they're stronger and longer than ever before. I'll celebrate that.
>
> I was warned that my hair would temporarily come in with different texture and color. In fact, I was hoping for that—a little color and lots of texture. What did I get? The same old baby-fine, straight-as-a-stick, can't-do-a-thing-with-it hair. To add insult to injury, it's more white than

black, and I'm not sure I'm ready to be this old looking. I'm alive to get older though, so I sure can't complain, and I do have hair, even if I'll never look like the prom queen again.

I was also warned that I could expect radiation cataracts eventually. Oh joy! When they arrived, two-and-a-half years after the transplant, I wrote to my doctor saying, "Did you have to be so right about everything? I would happily have done without this."

In fact, cataract surgery was a breeze for me, and I had distance lenses implanted, so now I only have to wear reading glasses, and I can actually see the clock across the room without glasses.

My eyelids continue to flake, but I control that with prescription cortisone ointment.

She also experienced an effect on her digestive system that hadn't been predicted and she hadn't been expecting:

The other thing that nobody told me was that I'd have irritable bowel syndrome (IBS) three years after the transplant. That was not an expected occurrence. I thought I was having gall bladder trouble and went to see a surgeon, but after the scan showed nothing, he figured that I had been through so much that it was probably IBS, and gave me medicine to try to see if that would help. Fortunately it did, but I still can't eat the salads I used to love.

The following sections briefly describe some of the major late effects that can occur for leukemia survivors. However, there isn't room to cover every possible effect that might happen after treatment.

Bone and joint pain

After receiving chemotherapy treatment patients often complain of consistent bone and joint pain. It is hard for the medical community to distinguish whether the problem is related to arthritis, since so many leukemia patients are elderly, or whether it is treatment-related. Treatment for arthritis is usually effective in either case.

Cognitive and memory problems

Many leukemia survivors of heavy-duty chemotherapy, irradiation therapy, and bone marrow transplants report that memory, concentration, reasoning, and associative skills no longer seem as sharp as they once did. This is especially true of those who have had cranial irradiation, intrathecal methotrexate, or full protocol BMTs. Specific problems mentioned include short-term memory loss, word retrieval problems, reduced math skills and ability to do word problems, spelling confusion (especially involving homonyms), moodiness, shortened attention span, and sometimes depression.

Many oncologists have discounted reports of lasting cognitive effects because those effects had not been quantitatively documented in medical literature. However, some studies are beginning to focus on memory and cognition as one possible long-term effect. For example, the results of a study at Dartmouth Medical School found that people who get standard chemotherapy are twice as likely to score poorly on certain intelligence tests than cancer patients who did not receive that treatment.[1] While this is one of the first formal studies of the problem, the results are unlikely to surprise many cancer patients who have been complaining for years about memory loss.[2]

No known solutions exist for these problems, although studies are in progress of hyperbaric oxygen treatments to try to reverse the effects of radiation on the blood supply to the brain.

A survivor used to thinking on her feet recounts problems with word recall after treatment:

> I was speaking at a professional conference as a member of a panel. I had no notes, because we were responding to questions from the audience. Someone asked me about prescription drugs and patients. Normally I handle questions like that with no stress, but this time I could not make the association that I needed to find the word for the list of drugs approved by an insurance company. I answered the question by talking all around the term I needed and hoping that I was communicating with my audience. Finally the answer was complete and, of course, that was when the word finally popped into my head. So I turned to the audience and said, "I've been talking all this time using circumlocutions for one basic term. That term finally decided to surface. The term we have been needing throughout this discussion was 'formulary.'"
>
> This was a true incident of what I can only describe as the frustrating experience of "chemo brain."

Diabetes

Diabetes can arise temporarily or permanently as a result of treatment with Prednisone, a synthetic copy of the natural adrenal hormone hydrocortisone, or following radiation therapy of the abdomen or brain. Look for increased thirst, weight loss, increased episodes of fungal infections, changed eyesight, wounds slow to heal, increased urination, mental confusion, or faintness. If these symptoms are present, ask to be tested for diabetes.

Eyes

Radiotherapy or steroid therapy can cause cataracts, which can be surgically corrected. Radiotherapy can also cause "dry eye," and flaking of the eyelids. Dry eye is treated with eye drops or prescription drugs, and flaking can be treated with prescription cortisone creams.

Immune-suppressed survivors need to be alert for the cytomegalovirus or herpes zoster (shingles), which can negatively affect eyesight. Your doctor will treat these promptly with antiviral drugs such as acyclovir or valacyclovir hydrochloride (Valtrex).

Fatigue

Fatigue is one of the most reported and most debilitating long-term symptoms associated with leukemia treatment. For a long time, when blood work didn't show anemia, survivors were told that they had no reason to feel fatigued. Nowadays, the medical community is listening, but they still have no way to explain the continuing fatigue some people endure. Long term treatment with inteferon can cause fatigue, as can cranial irradiation; heart, liver, or kidney damage; chronic pain; or the worry associated with cancer. Plenty of rest, good nutrition, moderate exercise, a carefully balanced workload, and emotional support are the best ways to avoid chronic fatigue.

Graft-versus-host disease

Patients who have had an allogeneic bone marrow or peripheral blood stem cell transplant may have graft-versus-host disease as a result of the transplant. Problems may be temporary or may continue for long periods of time. Watch for a rash that may occur anywhere on the body, and for liver, intestinal, or stomach problems. See Chapter 9 for a full discussion of this problem.

Hair loss (alopecia)

Radiotherapy and chemotherapy can cause a patient to lose hair during treatment. However, the after effects of radiation therapy to the head, groin, or armpits, or treatment with the chemical agent busulfan can result in permanent hair loss. Hair loss is most common with those suffering from graft-versus-host disease or among females who have had irradiation therapy to the head. Sometimes the hair loss is not evident for months.

Heart and vascular damage

Heart and vascular damage may emerge years after treatment with no previous warning symptoms. Doxorubicin (adriamycin), vincristine (oncovin), and ifosfamide are known to cause cardiovascular damage. If you have had radiation to the chest, you are also at risk. Watch for chest pain or tightness, swollen arms or legs, numbness in your extremities, dizziness, difficulty breathing, or shortness of breath. See your doctor for cardiac testing.

Kidney or bladder problems

Ifosfamide, methotrexate, cisplatin, or cyclophosphamide (Cytoxan) can cause damage to the urinary tract. However, Mesna is now used to protect the bladder and allopurinol is used to protect the kidneys from the toxins of dying cells. Both are given prior to treatment and sometimes during treatment as well.

Liver damage

Permanent liver damage following chemotherapy is rare, but if you've had a bone marrow transplant, be alert. If you're fatigued, nauseated, or your skin turns yellow and you look as if you're permanently suntanned, get to your doctor immediately. Blood tests can detect liver function. Dietary changes or modification of medicines and dosages may alleviate the problem.

Low blood counts

Low or low-normal blood counts can persist for years following treatment. Some drugs such as fludarabine can suppress the marrow's ability to regenerate different kinds of blood cells over the long term. If you have low red counts, you may be given erythropoietin (Epogen) to stimulate the growth of red blood cells. Either of the granulocyte colony stimulating factors, GCSF or GMCSF, may be given to build white cell production. Studies are underway on new platelet stimulating factors, called recombinant thrombopoietins. So far the medical community has not been enthusiastic about any of the thrombopoietins that have been introduced.

The blood cell stimulating factors are successful only if the bone marrow is still capable of producing these cells. Transfusions of red cells and platelets are common for leukemia patients. If you have had a transplant, be sure the medical staff uses filtered, irradiated cells. However, transfusion of white cells from a donor is not recommended unless you are on immunosuppressive drugs, because very likely the donor's white cells will attack your tissue, and your white cells will attack the donated cells.

Lung damage

Radiotherapy and the chemotherapeutic agents busulfan, cyclophosphamide, melphelan, bleomycin, or methotrexate can cause lung damage. Despite care taken to shield the lungs during prolonged radiation, problems can still occur. Watch for chest pain, coughing, difficulty breathing, or odd swellings under your skin near the chest, stomach, or arms. Call your doctor as soon as possible because such symptoms might be indicative of pulmonary damage caused by previous treatment.

Mouth, teeth, and throat

Persistent dry mouth, resulting from radiation or chemotherapy, may cause many transient side effects. But the dry mouth that continues long after treatment ends can cause serious dental health problems because the saliva's infection-fighting properties are missing. Patients report that it is wise to carry a water bottle at all times and keep the mouth area lubricated. Sucking on sugarless candy also helps. Watch for redness or swelling in your mouth, or cracked, discolored teeth, even if you have no pain. If you've had lots of problems with vomiting, see a dentist often. Teeth tend to develop cavities if you have too much acid in your mouth.

Numbness, tingling, dizziness, paralysis, deafness

Numbness, tingling, or pain in the hands and feet (peripheral neuropathy) may persist for months or years following treatment. Vincristine and cisplatin are two of the drugs associated with this condition. Pain management techniques are used for control.

Some of the major antibiotics, such as vancomycin, used for infections associated with leukemia treatment, can cause permanent or temporary hearing loss, vertigo, dizziness, or tinnitus (ringing in the ears). Surgery, drugs, rehabilitation exercises, or noise blocking devices can help.

Pain

Pain in various parts of the body such as the joints, back, and legs, can result from various chemotherapy drugs and from the cell growth factors as well. The good news is that it is usually temporary. The bad news is that if the pain doesn't fade away in a few weeks or months, it's likely to be a long-term condition. Don't ignore pain! Report it to your doctor, because untreated, it can become chronic.

Persistent pain of any magnitude might well lead you to a consultation with a pain specialist or clinic for a multi-modal approach. This might include pain medication, surgery, behavior modification, implantable pain control devices, ultrasound treatments, or relaxation training. For a lengthy, detailed, excellent discussion of pain and pain management, see Dr. Wendy Harpham's book *After Cancer: A Guide to Your New Life*.

Recall sensitivity

Certain body tissues are affected permanently by chemotherapy or radiotherapy. They become permanently sensitized, and may react with swelling, itching, or soreness if chemotherapy is readministered months or years later. This is called *recall sensitivity* and it is a physical, not a psychological, phenomenon. For example, if chemotherapy happens accidentally to leak from an arm vein during infusion, the skin may swell and hurt if chemotherapy is administered again—even if it is administered years later, and in the other arm.

A three-year leukemia survivor talks about what she is still experiencing:

> I've been finished with treatment for three years and I'm still cancer free. Blood work every three months or so is all I have and that's done in my upper arm. No more peripheral IV needles have been used in my

right arm, but I get up every morning itching on the right side of my right wrist. I scratch a few times and the situation abates.

All I can think is that this is recall sensitivity from all the peripheral IV sticks that I received during and after my BMT. Since my Hickman catheter became infected on day 20 and had to be removed, all the rest of my treatment was done using peripheral IV needles in my hands and wrists.

Secondary cancers

One of the more serious risks of treatment for leukemias is the risk of developing a second cancer. Sometimes chronic leukemias move into the acute stage, and sometimes leukemias can move into another cancer, such as non-Hodgkin's lymphoma or multiple myeloma.[3] As a natural progression of leukemia and treatment, the development of other malignancies is always a possibility. Chemotherapy with alkylating agents or radiation may also lead to second malignancies.

Sexuality and fertility

Issues of sexuality after treatment are common and treatable. Chemotherapy can damage fertility and affect sexuality. In men, noted difficulties include sterility or inability to sustain an erection. In women, difficulties include failed ovulation, failed conception, irregular menses, or painful intercourse. Be sure to bring these problems to your doctor's attention in order to receive medical and/or psychological help. Chemotherapy may affect childbearing ability, so make any plans and decisions about children before you are treated.

One couple realized too late that they should have taken more seriously the recommendation by the husband's doctor to visit a sperm bank. The wife describes her regrets:

My husband refused to believe that chemotherapy would affect his potency. He was firmly convinced that since everyone said there were few problems with this drug, he would have no difficulty later. When the oncologist strongly suggested a visit to the sperm bank before he had chemo, he simply ignored the advice and never mentioned it to me.

*The end result is that we'll have to adopt if we're going to have chil-
dren together. I'm really upset that he didn't share the information with
me, or give me a chance to make my feelings known.*

Shingles

Everyone who had chicken pox as a child, and leukemia survivors who
receive marrow from a donor who had chicken pox, harbor within their
nerve cells a herpesvirus called varicella-zoster, the virus that causes chicken
pox and shingles, two manifestations of the same disease. When the immune
system is depressed, zoster may re-emerge, causing terrible pain and blisters
called shingles. The virus can affect any or all nerve endings in the body, but
is most likely to appear on one side of the face, neck, arm, or torso.
Although 10 to 20 percent of those with shingles will never have the blisters, they will experience the pain and/or itching. Blisters tend to appear in a
line following a nerve. Shingles in the eye can cause temporary or permanent blindness.

As soon as symptoms appear, see your doctor for an antiviral, such as acyclovir or valacyclovir hydrochloride (Valtrex), and perhaps pain medicine as
well. It is not unusual to require codeine or morphine briefly for severe cases
of shingles. The virus usually clears up in four to six weeks, but sometimes
the pain lingers for years. In that case, a nerve or glycerin block can be performed by a neurosurgeon, which will last for several months and can be
repeated if needed.

Skeletal damage

Long term use of high-dose steroid therapy, with drugs like prednisone, can
damage bone, causing avascular necrosis of bone, a painful condition that
can be treated with joint replacement. Aredia (pamidronate), a drug used to
treat multiple myeloma, may also be used to treat future bone damage
caused by steroid treatment.

Skin

All kinds of skin problems are reported following leukemia treatment. Dry
skin and flaking skin, skin discoloration, and rarely, even scarring may follow treatment with chemotherapy and/or radiation. Other problems include

reactivation of psoriasis in those who have had it previously, and skin related GVHD in those who have had transplants. If you can't find relief, ask your doctor for a referral to a dermatologist who has experience treating cancer survivors.

Skin cancer in CLL deserves special attention. There are some studies that show CLL cells infiltrating the skin, causing skin lesions in a small subset of patients.[4] Further research has shown a two-to threefold increase in the incidence of skin cancer among patients with CLL.[5] Chronic lymphoid leukemia is associated with a high incidence of skin carcinomas. The immunosupression inherent in the hematologic disease would appear to favor aggressive skin cancers. The skin cancer can be either single, multiple, or recurrent, and the histologic type may be either Bowen's disease, squamous cell, or basal cell carcinoma. An increased risk of skin cancer has also been reported in hairy cell leukemia and AML.

Stomach and intestinal distress

Radiotherapy for those who have had splenectomy or total body irradiation for a BMT or peripheral blood stem cell transplant (PSCT) may cause persistent diarrhea or constipation from narrowed, tightened intestines or damaged nerves.[6] Constipation from immobility or from pain medicine may also be a lingering problem. Irritable bowel syndrome (IBS) is also seen in many post-transplant and high-dose chemotherapy patients. Pain and constipation is also seen in patients who have had Vincristine that has damaged their nerve cells. Medicine can usually control the diarrhea and IBS, while stool softeners and roughage may alleviate constipation. Do not suffer these side effects without asking for help from your doctor.

Thyroid dysfunction

The thyroid gland is a butterfly-shaped organ that wraps around the trachea. After chemotherapy, biological therapy with drugs like inteferon, and/ or radiation, the thyroid may become under-active (hypothyroidism), over-active (hyperthyroidism), or cancerous.

Symptoms of an underactive thyroid may include: lethargy, dry skin, numbness of the hands or feet, weight gain, mental slowness, sleepiness, depression, immune suppression, inability to tolerate cold, and loss of hair or altered hair quality. These are all side effects of cancer treatments as well, but thyroid blood levels can be tested to distinguish low thyroid function from treatment side effects. The problem of an underactive thyroid can usually be solved quickly by using medicines like thyroxine or synthroid to replace the missing thyroid hormones as long as no tumor is present.

Symptoms of an overactive thyroid may include: weight loss, excessive appetite that may result in temporary weight gain, irritability, inability to tolerate heat, insomnia, rapid heartbeat, high blood pressure, and protruding eyes. Loss of hair and altered hair quality may also occur. These symptoms are similar to those experienced by prednisone users, but thyroid blood levels can be tested to distinguish between an overactive thyroid and transient side effects of prednisone use.

Hyperthyroidism, not caused by a tumor, can be treated with drugs, such as Tapazole, that block thyroid hormone activity. High blood pressure medicine can control those symptoms temporarily. Injections of radioactive iodine 131 can be used to destroy overactive thyroid tissue.

The presence of a malignant tumor in the thyroid can cause a mixture of the symptoms of the two types of thyroid disease. Surgical removal of part, or all, of the thyroid cures this problem. The surgery is very safe, and is successful in over 95 percent of cases, depending on tumor stage and histological subtype.

CHAPTER 17

Recurrence

Acute leukemia offers the possibility of cure, while chronic leukemia, up to this point, is considered incurable. Leukemia can be put into remission, but it often returns. While doctors talk about curative therapy, not all patients are cured. Many live with the constant, nagging worry that the cancer will recur.

Recurrence is every patient's worse nightmare. It ranks right up there with diagnosis! When leukemia does recur, patients ask themselves if this recurrence is a death sentence. Most likely it is not.

Relapse is made somewhat easier if medical personnel have explained the likelihood of relapse and discussed practical ways to handle it. Even then, patients want to believe that it won't happen. It is wise, however, to be emotionally and intellectually prepared for the possibility.

This chapter defines recurrence and how it is detected. It next discusses the possible transformation into another subtype of leukemia or another cancer altogether. Then it covers treatment options, the emotional issues that come with recurrence, and ways of coping.

Recurrence defined

Recurrence, or relapse, is defined as the return of disease to a patient who has been in remission for a period of 30 days or more following treatment. The criteria for remission are different with each type of leukemia, but it generally means there are fewer than 10 percent leukemic cells in the patient's body as determined by flow cytometry and/or bone marrow biopsy. If the patient has never achieved remission, we don't speak of recurrence, but instead speak of disease progression.

One patient's reaction to relapse is described in these few words:

> *The call finally came through. I was biting my nails by that time. My doctor says the marrow is 95 percent involved. He wants to start me on*

something as soon as Monday. I tell him my house is torn apart and I'm using my nervous energy in painting. "Sorry," he says.

Monday he will start me on some kind of chemo. I guess I am numb and just can't believe it. All this treatment all over again. Do I have the strength to go through this again? What can I hope for this time?

Causes for recurrence

Recurrence may be caused when there is a failure to get rid of all the leukemic cells in the body. The cells may remain quiescent for weeks, months, or years, and then they begin their rapid growth again. Some scientists suggest that continued exposure to toxic substances in the atmosphere, or electrical waves may be the culprit. Most of the time, the reasons for recurrence are simply unknown.

Leukemic cells sometimes become resistant to chemotherapy drugs. Usually this happens when the cells turn on genes that block the cellular intake of certain drugs and others related to them. This phenomenon is known as multiple drug resistance (MDR).

What to look for

Clinical relapse is defined as the time when symptoms are seen by the patient, family members, or the doctor. Watch for the return of fatigue, night sweats, and other symptoms that you have had before. However, recurrence often is announced by the presence of new symptoms that have not previously been encountered. This is when the expression, "Listen to what your body is telling you" becomes really important. When things simply don't feel right, it's time to return to your oncologist for a check up.

It is important not to confuse the symptoms of late effects of treatment with recurrence of the disease.

Cytogenic relapse occurs when the disease returns, with or without symptoms, and can be seen in the blood work. In this instance, no symptoms need be present, but routine blood work or marrow biopsy shows a return of disease. Tests, similar to those done previous to diagnosis, will likely be done again, to find out the status of the disease.

The following patient describes her reaction to her cytogenic relapse. Tests show cancer, although she feels fine, physically:

> I saw my doctor yesterday and he is working to figure out what chemotherapy he will put me on next week. I guess this relapse thing still gets me. I feel fine. I just finished an hour of hard workout. I am constantly keeping busy, and I am full of cancer. I don't get it. It just doesn't make sense.

> My doctor has me starting Ara-C tomorrow. Yes, he told me the reasoning for it, but I have been tuning people out lately in an alarming manner.

> I am getting more scared about what the next year will bring. I sometimes just get so tired of all of this that I need to look into my little boys' faces and remember why I am going through this. This is consuming my life, and it's getting harder and harder.

When am I safe from fears of relapse?

There are no guarantees. "Continued remission" is the term used when speaking of leukemias; the word "cure" is seldom used. Nevertheless, 30 years of data in the International Bone Marrow Transplant Registry indicate that the likelihood of a cure after an allogeneic bone marrow transplant (BMT) for acute lymphocytic leukemia or acute myelogenous leukemia is high, if the transplant is followed by a two-year disease-free interval.

Chronic leukemia patients are warned to expect relapses and are told that relapse is not a death sentence in most instances. If you deal with any of the chronic leukemias, you're already aware that there is no cure, and that you will always be monitoring yourself or your loved one, for relapse. With CML it is said that the only possible cure is an allogeneic bone marrow transplant. Statistics about BMT are now being collected and will be evaluated over time.

Treatment options

The method of treatment after your relapse depends, in part, upon the treatment you had previously. If you responded extremely well to a drug protocol and it appears that it will work again, your doctor may use it this time also. The doctor may think it best to combine it with other drugs that may work synergistically to do a better job for you.

Often your doctor will choose other treatment options, because if the drugs given previously were effective you wouldn't have relapsed; or because your leukemia cells have become refractory to a drug, so you no longer respond to it. Some of the more toxic drugs may only be taken for a certain period of time before they can harm your organs, so other choices must be made. New drugs for all the leukemias are in development and new clinical trials open almost weekly. This is definitely the right time to look closely at the possibilities offered by clinical trials. See Chapter 7, *Treatment Options*, Chapter 9, *Transplantation*, and Chapter 10, *Clinical Trials and Beyond*, for more information about treatment options.

Transformations

Relapse is sometimes associated with a transformation from one form of leukemia to another. For example, when chronic myelogenous leukemia cells change into acute leukemia. Usually CML becomes AML, but occasionally CML changes into ALL. CLL cells sometimes develop into larger cells called prolymphocytes, which are indicative of prolymphocytic leukemia. Other times, the leukemia transforms into another form of cancer altogether. Examples of this are also seen in chronic lymphocytic leukemia. CLL seldom turns into ALL, but sometimes transforms into Richter's syndrome, a form of non-Hodgkin's lymphoma.

The following patient went through Richter's transformation from CLL. She also faced relapse when feeling physically well:

> When I got to the doctor's office, he sat down next to me. Right then I knew he had bad news from my bone marrow biopsy and the CT scan. I know him so well now that I know the tone of his voice and his body language. He said the CT scan report had just been received and he wanted my husband in the office with us.
>
> All I could see was the word "transforming" on the report. He said the lymph nodes have grown as well as the spleen, and the marrow showed the same 80 percent or more involvement, but that the cells appeared to be changing into lymphoma cells.

*Basically, the next step is a lymph node biopsy that they want imme-
diately. From that, they will see how advanced the cancer is and what
treatment may work for me.*

Emotional responses

When there is recurrence, there is worry, fear, and concern on the part of the
patient, family members, and the doctor. No one is happy about relapse.

A leukemia survivor facing relapse explains how awful she felt on hearing
the news:

> *I felt like I did when I was first diagnosed, and what a horrible, ach-
> ing feeling that is. My doctor says he has treatment options and refuses to
> give up or let me give up hope. He consulted with Dr. John Gribben at the
> Dana-Farber Cancer Institute for additional ideas. He also advised us of
> his suggested opinion about treatment. So it's now something I must think
> about immediately.*

> *I feel fine! This disease just doesn't make sense. You think that you're
> doing so well. You try so hard to keep thinking positively. You follow all
> the rules you are given, yet you still get awful news. I must admit I am
> really starting to loose faith, heart, and hope. This battle is going on too
> long, and I just want it to resolve. My husband says we must stay positive
> and we are in this together. This is just so hard to bear!*

Patients and family members have described their emotional responses as
extreme:

- Terror is one response to the news of relapse. No matter how good the
  prognosis for returning to a period of remission following recurrence,
  you can still be terrified that this time there is no hope. It really requires
  an enormous amount of will to keep hope alive. However, as relapses
  continue to occur in some patients, they become more comfortable with
  the idea that relapses are to be expected, and are treatable.

- Extreme anger is another response. You fought hard for the remission
  you have just lost. You certainly didn't expect this relapse and consider
  it very unfair. Anger may smolder covertly, or it may come out openly in
  behavior that can be hurtful to family and friends.

- Grief is almost a universal response. It is experienced from the time of the initial diagnosis by both the patient and family. Life has been turned upside down. Hopes and dreams are put on hold because of this damnable disease and its impact. With relapse, you can feel that you are facing death again and it is hard to overcome those feelings.

- Despair is yet another response. A patient and family that approached the first few treatment regimens with hope and willingness to do what had to be done, may find it harder to sustain that attitude. It's easy to become tired of the constant battle, and feel that there is no point to continuing, no matter how good your chances may be if you achieve a solid second remission.

- Loss of trust in the medical system often accompanies recurrence. This is when some people turn to questionable, and sometimes downright fraudulent, means of treatment. People sometimes appear to be grasping at straws to hold on to hope. Such patients tend to regard additional treatment suggestions from their doctors with skepticism or negative feelings.

- Feelings of spiritual abandonment are common. Many patients become angry and feel abandoned by their God. You might feel that you have fought hard, did what you had to do, kept your faith, and now feel forsaken. This can become an extremely difficult feeling for spiritual people to overcome.

Mobilizing for treatment again

It's not always easy to get into the mind-set needed to deal with another round of treatment, especially if your first experience was difficult. There is added discouragement knowing that though you've already been treated, you relapsed, and now you must submit to it again. This frustration is particularly true if you've had a long remission. Nevertheless, more than ever, this is the time when you must maintain active participation, taking your share of responsibility for battling the disease.

Here is the experience of a survivor when she encountered her first relapse:

> Even though I had been prepared for needing periodic treatment
> cycles for the rest of my life, when it first happened my instinctive

reaction was, "Oh $%#&!" I couldn't really begin to express my disappointment and anger. I was also frightened. I knew what I needed to do— get back in treatment. But after five years of remission, I wasn't happy at the prospect.

Nevertheless, I insisted on restarting treatment that day, because despite my frustration, I knew, deep down, that there was no point in delaying the inevitable. I had been having some clinical symptoms, but there had been nothing in my bone marrow six months earlier, and there was nothing in my blood counts to suggest that this day would be coming so soon. So this really came as a huge shock, even though the symptoms were there.

Today, four years later, I'm back on treatment again, but this time I am more accepting and less panicked when remission ends, and just as determined to live.

This is the time to gather up all your spirit, heart, and hope. Use your support resources. Research to find the latest therapy, so that you can fight the good fight again. Maintaining your quality of life and reviving your fighting spirit is a very important part of healing.

Adjusting to treatment again

There is huge variation in treatments for leukemia. There is also a great diversity of patients in terms of personal and social characteristics as well as economic and educational differences. So it is not unexpected that survivors will react in different ways to news of relapse, and that they will adapt to the need for additional treatment in disparate ways. Strong spousal and family support are key elements in fighting relapse.

A number of studies have indicated that there is a remarkable resiliency in many cancer survivors' marriages, helping them withstand the considerable stress of their disease. On the other hand, if a marriage is shaky, relapse is only going to add to the stresses and strains of the relationship. This is a good time to get psychological help or marriage counseling if the situation at home is rocky. The emotional roller coaster of dealing with relapse is likely to cause subtle changes in marital adjustment all over again.

Cancer patients dealing with relapse also find that friends and colleagues are less supportive over time, and that this is the single most distressing hardship they encounter. This is particularly true of those who have had transplants. Family members and friends may not understand what survivors experience. Some lack ease in discussing cancer, wishing not to offend or distress the patient. The fear of the disease and the specter of death raised by relapse get in the way of family members and friends giving support. Often it is the cancer survivor who is better able to deal with relapse than others.

What family and friends can do

Common sense responses and thoughtful gestures are really appreciated at this time:

- **Send a card.** Don't be afraid to be witty. If the patient has a sense of humor, it will be very much appreciated. Cancer patients share some of the wryest humor heard anywhere.

- **Call to say hello.** Focus on the person, not on the disease. It doesn't have to be a long call, just touch base and make the patient and family aware that you're thinking of them.

- **Stop in for short visits.** Share humorous incidents in the neighborhood, at work, or about the children, just as you would at any other time.

- **Bring a meal.** You don't even have to cook it yourself for it to be appreciated. A precooked chicken and salad will be most welcome. It's not only the caring thought, it's the planning and food preparation time that you spare the family.

- **Offer child care.** Pick up or drop off children, care for them when the patient has medical appointments, take them on an outing with yours, or offer to help with homework. Children's needs often are overlooked due to the stress of cancer treatment. Your offer will ease the stress and take major concerns off the family agenda.

- **Provide transportation and be a buddy.** If you are comfortable doing it, drive the patient to a chemotherapy session and be there to talk, to fetch anything needed, and to make sure the patient's concerns are addressed when asked to do so.

- **Run errands.** Do some food shopping, drive a carpool, wash a load of laundry, or even pick up the dry cleaning if that's what's needed.

- **Listen.** Sometimes the best thing you can do is simply listen when a patient or family member really needs to talk. A pat on the hand or a quick hug is sometimes all the response that's needed.

- **Help with fund raising.** If there is treatment needed that insurance won't pay for, or if there is no insurance coverage, financial help may be needed. Fundraising efforts need to be done with family cooperation, and funds raised need to go into a charitable fund. If that's the route you desire, talk with your banker or lawyer to find out how to create a charitable entity for that purpose.

What the patient can do

It is easy to become engulfed in treatment routines once more and neglect yourself as a whole individual. Quality of life issues need to be addressed and so do spiritual needs. Take some time to know yourself and what is really important to you.

Complementary therapies

This is a time when patients often look to alternative or complementary therapies, even if they haven't tried them before. The important thing is not to use alternative therapies in place of western medicine, but to talk with your doctor and find things that can complement conventional therapies. Even the medical traditions of the east—Ayurvedic (from India), Chinese, and Tibetan medicine—clearly acknowledge that they are unable to do very much once the disease process has become firmly established.

Distinguish between herbal medicines that are used to treat illness and vitamin and enzyme supplements used to boost body systems. If you find something that makes you feel better, and that won't stimulate the development of the cells that are active in your leukemia subtype or work against the treatment you are having, tell your doctor about it. Most of the time there will be no reason to stop using it.

Overcoming fear

It is important to deal with the fear that recurrence unleashes. Do not permit it to control you. Recognize that fear is a perfectly normal reaction. Every patient feels it, but can also overcome it. Be open to new ideas and to the help that others offer. Don't shut people out because fear overwhelms you. Take the time you need to replace fear with knowledge. Keep fear in perspective by changing your focus and use the emotions that make you fearful in positive ways. Take action to change the thing you fear.

Keeping faith

Faith in a deity, in yourself, or in a treatment or medical system means that you have the general expectation that, whatever happens, "it will be all right."

Have faith in yourself; take your time in making decisions. Don't be rushed into treatment. Wait until you find out what will be involved, and what you can expect from these treatments. Seek out the information you need about treatments and care, but also allow time for rest, relaxation, and thinking. Don't judge yourself and what you feel. Accept that you have the right to your feelings. Similarly, give yourself the opportunity to feel comfortable with your decisions.

Maintaining your quality of life

Try not to let treatment take over your life after recurrence. There is more to you than the leukemia. You need to take care of all your needs, not just those of the body. Try to keep to your usual routine, continue to exercise, eat healthy foods, and keep in contact with friends. The more positive your attitude, the better off you are. Most importantly, do things you enjoy or that you have always wanted to do. If you are a spiritual person, make use of the clergy or your spiritual community. Take time to do what you feel necessary to enhance your spiritual harmony.

Seeking and using support resources

Join a support group if you haven't before. Make use of every opportunity to share information with other patients and learn what they have to offer. Sometimes the most basic suggestion is the one that makes the biggest difference. Build confidence by finding people who have relapsed and are doing well again. Help others who have not yet been in treatment by sharing your experiences in a healthy way. Your family cannot always be the ones with whom you do that—sharing experiences with other patients eases the emotional turmoil, and studies have shown that it prolongs survival as well.

For further information about coping, see Chapter 13, *Stress and the Immune System* and Chapter 14, *Getting Support*.

CHAPTER 18

If All Treatments Have Failed

Ultimately, the time comes for all of us to leave this life. Recently, we have learned more about how to help those who can no longer be treated. Restrictions on support for cancer pain have been made more realistic. We understand better how to provide comfort for the patient and family. Nevertheless, everything we know about dying comes from the words of the living.

This chapter assumes that there are no more treatment options available or that the patient has decided not to continue with treatment for whatever reason. This is a chapter that you may choose not to read now, if you have just begun to fight your leukemia, because you may not need it for many years. If you find it upsetting at present, wait to read it. However, the information may be immediately helpful if you have an elderly family member, with or without leukemia, who faces end-of-life issues.

This chapter focuses on the patient's needs rather than the needs of family and others. Much has been written for those who must deal with grief, but here we provide pragmatic and helpful information to make things easier for the patient. Our approach starts with practical things that should be done and ends with emotional issues.

Setting new goals

When curative treatment is no longer pursued, there are still many other goals that may be achieved. This is the time when goals such as attaining comfort, reconciling with family members, gaining time to express love, or participating in such events as marriages or the arrival of grandchildren need to be met. Living life fully, creating memories, searching for life's meaning, or taking steps to care for the family allow you to tie up the loose ends of life and meet emotional needs.

If you're well enough, take the vacation you've always wanted and revisit places that have happy memories. After all, if you don't do it now, you probably won't. Ask your family and friends to slow down and take time to relax with you. There may not be a great deal of time, but there is enough time to do what you wish to do. Tell your family how you feel about them. Record your childhood experiences and the changes in the world that you have seen. Later, these may become their most cherished memories of you.

Deciding when to terminate curative treatments can be difficult. Rosemary Bradford writes about the decision that she and her husband Tony made to end Tony's chemotherapy treatments:

> I'm trying to write this for Tony, because he's still not fit enough to write himself. He's had a rough time recently, spending most of the New Year in the hospital suffering from another chemotherapy-induced infection, which was very difficult to overcome. Since his return home, we have spent much time heart-searching with our two daughters, and we have had long discussion with the consultant.
>
> Together we have come to the conclusion that further chemo would be too risky for Tony. The likelihood of it affecting the leukemia is minimal, and the chances of it causing further infection and more febrile episodes, which would be fatal, are very high. We have decided that is not the road we want to take, and although this has been a very difficult decision, we all feel that it is the correct one for Tony. He will now have palliative care only, including radiation treatment on three large nodes in his neck that have appeared over the last few weeks.

Rosemary and Tony have set new goals:

> We are all trying to enjoy our time together to the fullest. We are getting a lot of support from friends, and from family. The other support services here are proving invaluable. Tony attends the local hospice one day a week at the moment, and already they have given him a sense of peace and security we would not have believed possible a few weeks ago. We expect this care and help to increase as time goes on.
>
> I hope this letter does not depress fellow sufferers. We felt it important to tell the truth. Neither do we want to give the impression of doom and gloom here. We have not given up the fight! We have short-term goals, which we will extend ad infinitum. Your positive thoughts can only help!

When there are no more options, and they have been offered only palliative care, many patients feel that there are loose ends they need to tie up. One irony of finding out about terminal illness is that the patient may feel quite well at the time. Nevertheless, there are things that must be done.

Gloria, a leukemia patient, shared some of the anguish that ensued as she prepared for death:

> When the doctor told me that treatment had failed, I was devastated. What other options were left to try? There were none. I knew it, my husband knew it, and the doctor knew it also.
>
> The doctor talked about palliative care and hospice. We had no idea what that would mean. Sure we had heard the words, but this was real, and we didn't have a clue. We were also in shock again. So many high hopes for this last clinical trial had gone up in smoke.
>
> Things left undone crowded my head. I needed to call my boss and tell him that I'd never be back to work. I needed to deal with bank accounts and bills. Where was the insurance information? Had we talked about funeral arrangements? This couldn't be real! How could it be happening to me? Life was chaos!

Accepting help

Most comfort during this time will likely come from immediate family, but don't be surprised if a cousin, aunt, or sibling also makes huge sacrifices to help you. Some friends and family members will behave differently around you. That usually indicates that they don't know what to say or do, and they may be coming face to face with their own mortality for the first time. Psychologists say that treating them the same way you have previously usually helps them get over the awkwardness.

No matter how independent you have been all your life, this is the time to allow yourself to accept gifts and services from friends and family. It helps you, it makes your life easier, and you might receive something you will really treasure. You should also ask for assistance freely. It helps others feel they are doing something useful and raises their comfort level. On the other hand, don't be afraid to ask for time alone to enjoy the beauties of the world around you, to contemplate, or to read a book. Take time for yourself when you need it. Listen to your own feelings and ideas. Well-meaning people may try to tell you what to do. Consider the alternatives, keep your own counsel, and do what seems best for you.

Patients who need to be monitored 24 hours a day can begin to feel that they are burdening their family members because of their unrelenting needs. Hospital care, home healthcare, hospice care, or part-time nursing assistance can help, but that adds to the financial drain. Check your insurance policy to see which of these services it covers—and to what extent.

Following the patient's wishes

If you're the kind of person who needs to know what is happening to you, ask your doctor and family members for honesty. You have to be able to trust that you are getting accurate and necessary information about your condition. Explain your feelings about this to everyone so that there is no mistaking your desire to be informed. On the other hand, if you don't wish to be told about what comes next, tell that to your doctor and family. The patient's wishes are primary.

Most physicians and caregivers have problems communicating with patients and families about death. They are much more efficient at organizing heroic efforts to prolong life. But often prolonging life isn't what the patient wants, and making life more comfortable would be preferred.

Caring for a terminally ill patient is always difficult for loved ones as well as physicians. Families often feel confused and helpless, dependent on the healthcare team. They may question the healthcare team's intentions. It is most important that the team meets the patient's needs, and that can be very difficult if the family has different ideas.

The insurance maze

As if it were not enough being critically ill, you also have to deal with insurance matters. More people are treated in hospitals these days, and terminally ill patients must thread their way through bureaucratic mazes to get the care they want and need. It is best if you can assign one family member to deal with insurance claims. It helps tremendously if someone can find a continuing contact person to deal with at the insurance company. Then when questions arise, as they invariably will, your situation is known to the contact person, so things may be expedited.

Find out if your insurance coverage includes home healthcare, home health appliances like a hospital bed or oxygen, and hospice care. May injectable medicines be given at home and are they covered when given that way? May family members be trained to provide needed care? Your family needs to know these things, so that everyone may help meet your needs and keep you comfortable.

Work with the social services department of your hospital to find out the resources available for you in the community. Remember to have someone check with the insurance company to make sure that the services are covered when you choose to use them. See Chapter 14, *Getting Support*, for more information.

Suzanne described the blitz of medical bills for her mother's treatment, the unceasing influx of bills with which many families have to deal:

> *The bills began coming in waves. It started with a few the first week, and it soon turned into an ocean. The dining room table was piled with bills separated by where they came from: hospitals, doctors, or home healthcare providers.*
>
> *Each bill had to have been through Medicare, through Medigap, and then be submitted to her private insurance carrier. What a nightmare! I am young, well educated, and healthy. Can you imagine what it must be like for a sick or elderly person dealing with all that paperwork?*

Legal issues

It is smart to have a will. This is particularly true when you have a life-threatening disease. Writing and updating a will, however, may be a source of psychological stress. The need to think of finances at this time can be depressing and appear crass, but it must be done. Dealing with legal questions can be especially difficult if you are the primary family breadwinner. How will your family survive? What are the long-term financial implications for the family? Are there sufficient life insurance policies to make things work? How far into debt will the family be driven by your illness? These legitimate questions add to the patient's concerns for the family. Consult with a good lawyer and maintain open communication with all the involved family members wherever possible.

If the patient has also been the money manager, a surrogate must be selected. This person needs to be instructed about family finances, financial institutions that hold the money, and where important records are kept. It really helps to maintain continuity if bank and brokerage signature cards are signed early on and arrangements are made in advance for access to safety deposit boxes. With these matters in place, the new family financial manager can take over as the patient's illness progresses. Prepare a power of attorney document in advance to ensure the transfer of financial authority to someone who is qualified to act on your behalf. Further explain to this individual about any work benefits or insurance policies, and where they are located. It is often wise to meet with a tax accountant so that your financial surrogate can be fully informed of what to expect.

Some people may wish to establish a memorial or donate sizeable funds to a charitable organization. In that case, speak with the organization's bequest department to be sure that the necessary paperwork is done in the proper way.

Advance directives

Most people feel strongly about when they want medical treatment stopped. A living will, or advance directive, is a document that states your preferences for continuing medical treatment if you are terminally ill or near death. With this document, you are able to communicate your wishes to your doctors and family even if you cannot speak. The latest forms have checklists that can help you describe what you want. Each state has a form, specific to the laws of the state, that you can modify to address your particular concerns.

However, a living will by itself is very limited. It usually covers only a small number of conditions and treatments. It contains your written instructions, which are expected to stand on their own. No one is identified to interpret your wishes.

A more powerful document for most people is the healthcare power of attorney or healthcare proxy. These advance directives describe your wishes and say who should speak for you if you cannot. You also can indicate in your healthcare power of attorney the kinds of treatments or situations you do, or do not, want.

If you haven't already completed advance directives (or haven't reviewed them recently), now is a good time to do so. Have you signed a living will? Is it in your hospital records? Does your physician know how you feel about being resuscitated or put on life support? If you haven't discussed it, do so now, and put it in writing for hospital files. You need to sort out your desires, make them known to the doctor and your family, and make sure they are noted. You have the right to stop seeking a miracle and to face the inevitability of death.

One cancer survivor included a personal note in her medical power of attorney form that could be referred back to:

> Thank you for helping me carry out my medical wishes. I want you to know that I don't expect you to come up with miracles and that there might not be one "right" answer. I don't want you to experience any guilt, afterwards, about any decisions. You'll do the best you can, with the information you have at the time.

> I was diagnosed with cancer in March of 1995. Since that time I have been more aware, not only of mortality, but also that my dying might happen before I have attained a "ripe old age." I have given a lot of thought to death-and-dying issues and have been working to have my emotional and financial affairs in order. My aim is to be "ready" whenever the end occurs.

> I do want to live to be an opinionated old lady. I will care proactively for my health and follow medical advice to attain that end, if possible.

> If I am battling a terminal condition, my priorities will be to live a meaningful life for those days I have left, to balance comfort (e.g., pain medication) with clarity of mind, and to die in as human a setting as possible. It is much more important to me to be able to hold someone's hand at the end, or to look out a window framing tree branches, than to have a medical procedure that will extend my life for only a few hours or days.

> If at all possible, I would like to die either at home or in a hospice setting. I want to be able to focus on my spiritual journey and on saying good-bye to people, not on medical procedures. Thank you for any help you can give me to achieve these goals.

Caring for the patient at home

Terminally ill patients have good days and bad days. Some good days are wonderful and hope for life may be rekindled. Unfortunately, such days are few, and a downward trend is more usual. When the family tries to decide what to do, home healthcare is usually the first choice. It gives the patient more time in familiar surroundings at home.

In the book *Fading Away: The Experience of Transition in Families with Terminal Illness,* Dr. Betty Davis and her co-authors list four factors needed for success with home care for the terminally ill patient. The factors are:

- **An able and available caregiver.** One or more family members care for the patient 24 hours a day.

- **Reliable and well-trained family members.** The caregiver must know how to operate all medical equipment, administer all medications, and care for all personal hygiene equipment needed by the patient. A visiting nurse service should be used at least once a week and for emergencies.

- **Patient in reasonable physical condition.** If the patient is too ill, the caregiver will be overwhelmed and unable to meet physical and emotional needs.

- **Suitable physical environment in the home.** The home must have a place for the patient with a bathroom on the same floor. If a hospital bed or other equipment is needed, there must be room to accommodate it. Stairs and dropped floors are hazardous.

While caring for the terminal patient at home sounds wonderful, and many people manage to care for the patient to the very end, the toll on the caregiver can be staggering in terms of isolation, physical and emotional exhaustion, and loss of freedom. Most people cannot live up to this high standard of care and feel guilty when they need to turn to others, but in truth, there is no need to feel guilty. Loved ones do what they are capable of doing.

Hospitals

Fewer people die at home these days, but those who do are usually under hospice care. Home care becomes more difficult over time. Not all families can be there for the patient 24 hours a day, plus deal with emergencies as well. Therefore, many terminally ill people spend their last days in the hospital or hospice.

Choose a house doctor or nurse or some such contact person, and keep them apprised of what is going on. This gives you someone on whom to rely and who can assist you with needs while you or your family member is in the hospital.

Make it a point to learn the hospital rules dealing with terminally ill patients. Hospitals and medical centers have written rules and procedures that outline how they will deal with such patients. Hospitals are obligated and usually more than willing to share this information with patients and their families. The information should cover how the hospital will handle "no extraordinary measures" or "no resuscitation" directives.

Contact the Chaplain's office. Every hospital has someone for patients to talk with about spiritual and religious needs, and at life's end, these concerns may become paramount for patients and family members. Make use of hospital psychological and financial counseling services, and any insurance form assistance programs that are available. The social services department will have referral options for hospice and home healthcare services as well as lodging for patient families from out of town.

Your family insurance handler may wish to meet with the financial professionals for assistance in dealing with the bills. The services are there to help.

Hospice

Modern hospice concentrates on caring for terminally ill cancer and heart patients. It attempts to provide comfortable maintenance care in a pleasant setting for patients in the final stages of their disease. Hospices depend on family presence for support as well. Perhaps for the first time, patients will meet others going through the same personal end-of-life crisis and feel a sense of community that is calming and reassuring. Hospice is a final destination, and should be understood as a necessary and concluding phase of your life. Sometimes painkilling drugs keep the patient only dimly aware of what is happening. Hospices provide peace and dignity for the patient and the family.

Hospices will also work with families providing care at home. They send people into the home to work with the patient and the caregiver to help deal with end-of-life issues. Hospice nurses visit daily or stay in the home to administer pain medication and, in some cases, to help the caregivers with certain household chores. They are trained to recognize the signs of impending death, and can help the family with the arrangements that are necessary just after a death in the home has occurred. Their focus includes the physical and emotional comfort of the patient, and the well-being of the surviving family members after death.

Some hospice services charge little or nothing for those who cannot afford the service. In some cases, a doctor's statement stating that the patient has less than six months to live is necessary in order for that patient to be eligible for hospice care.

Bettina describes what happened when she and her husband Philip decided to call in hospice:

> We had been dealing with home care nurses and they were not very effective at all. Our basic home is on one floor, and the bathroom is in the bedroom, so the situation was perfect, but one nurse was grossly obese and couldn't lift my husband, even with the hospital bed we rented. Another one smoked. Can you imagine doing such a thing around a dying cancer patient?
>
> Finally, our doctor said that it was time to get hospice involved.

Bettina recalls the relief that hospice provided for her and Philip:

> They came each day and made a huge difference in the way Phil felt and in convincing us that we were doing the right thing. They gave him his pain patches and showed me how to give the pain killing shots. What a difference they made. I'm very grateful.

After Philip's death, hospice continued to help his wife:

> The night he died, I called 911, but I knew he was dead. The police arrived with the ambulance. I called my friend, Barb, to come stay with me, because I didn't want to be alone. She called hospice for me and arranged for the funeral home to come get the body as hospice recommended. Hospice also assured the police that Phil had been their patient so there was no foul play involved in his death. Such a possibility had never occurred to me. I was so grateful for all they did.

Emotional concerns

How do we prepare to die? Spiritually and philosophically preparing for death is not much different than preparing to live, yet it is a unique phenomenon that everyone will experience. Some people will weaken slowly; some will have profound and unrelenting physical pain and discomfort. Some will go quickly; some will linger. Some will welcome death, tired of life's battles; some will fight to their last breath.

Much of what we know about death and dying was written 30 years ago by Dr. Elisabeth Kubler-Ross. In her book, *On Death and Dying*, she described five mental stages: denial and isolation, anger, bargaining, depression, and acceptance. These stages are not necessarily sequential and discrete. For instance, you don't necessarily feel anger until it's spent and only then move on to bargaining. The stages often overlap or occur simultaneously. While Kubler-Ross' stages are not universally accepted, and not all patients go through them all, they do provide a general road map of what to expect.

A death that is anticipated gives family and friends a chance to say good-bye. It gives the patient a chance to say farewells and to pull together the threads of life. In the US, death is often difficult to speak of and frequently shrouded in euphemisms because it is feared and represents the unknown. However, there are many choices that can make a difference in you and your family's experience, if you are willing to think and talk about them.

Difficult family issues

While approaching death, we often need to deal not only with our own feelings but with those of our loved ones. This can be made even more difficult if their experiences with loss and grief are out of phase with our own. Our relatives' denial that we are dying is not the only issue that may sadden our final days. They may grieve earlier than we do, anticipating our death before we ourselves have accepted it—or indeed, perhaps before we're dying at all. They may lag behind us in the stages of acceptance, continuing to bargain with medical personnel for life-support measures when we're ready to let go. Or perhaps the family will express anger when we ask questions about dying, railing against any sign that we've given up.

You may ease your family's acceptance of your death by reassuring them that they will be taken care of and telling them that you love them. Explain that you're weary of the battle and you welcome death. Try saying good-bye in loving ways, both overtly and symbolically.

Leaving a loving legacy

The hardest thing for dying patients to deal with is the fear that they will be forgotten. Many accept death, but want to be reassured that they will be remembered. Various suggestions have been made to ease that fear:

- Take the time to keep a journal as you look back over your life. Write down things that have been important to you. Put together for your family a picture of what you have believed in and what you have stood for and accomplished in life. Some patients describe this as writing their own eulogy. It often becomes a treasured family document that gives peace to family members after you've gone.

- Decide what religious beliefs, if any, have sustained you in life, and share them in your journal. Recognize that spirituality does not necessitate religiosity, so try not to get caught up with religious baggage that you may have accumulated during life. Now is the time to think about what you really believe, and state it as honestly as you can. Write about your fears, about the course of your illness, and about your hopes for the future. Express your feelings. Leave loved ones with good memories, shared stories, and positive thoughts.

- Tell your children and grandchildren over and over that you love them, and that you would not leave them if you had a choice. Write it, so they have your statement to keep. Record it so they can hear you saying it again and again. Videotape it or put in on a DVD so it becomes a treasured memory of your love. One mother, wanting to ensure that her young child didn't forget her, bought and wrapped gifts for her daughter's birthdays until she reached twenty-one years of age. She arranged with her husband to give them to her daughter each year. That child knew how much she was loved and felt her mother was with her throughout life.

What to tell young children

Children need unique reassurances that they will be loved and well cared for after you're no longer available to love and help them. Of course, by now you've most likely done your best to arrange loving care for them, and they probably know of these arrangements.

Fortunately, there are many good books you can use to help your child understand death, in particular *I'm with You Now* by M. Catherine Ray (see Appendix A, *Resources*). It is wise to give children as much honest and pointed information as possible, in terms appropriate for their age. For instance, it may be upsetting for your child to hear you say that you're in pain and are taking medicine for pain. It's likely to be much more damaging if the child sees you suffering, wasn't prepared to see this, and thinks your suffering cannot be relieved.

Make it clear to your children that your illness was not caused by anything they did. Children are egocentric, and need repeated reassurance that their thoughts and actions did not cause your illness. Explain, as well, that your spouse and the child's siblings are not to blame.

Expect that children will be openly or secretly angry with you for leaving them. Spurts of this anger are natural and inevitable. They may also understand that it's not acceptable to blame you for dying. This leaves the anger with nowhere to go. So if they cannot blame you, and the burden of anger and self-blame is too great to carry alone, they may blame the surviving parent or a sibling. Make it as clear as possible that nobody is to blame, and that everybody is feeling sad and sorry about your dying.

There are specific points to be avoided, though, when talking to a child about dying. In her book *The Art of Dying*, Patricia Weenolsen suggests you avoid saying the following:

- Do not say you're simply going to sleep for a long time. Children may develop a fear of falling asleep if it's compared to dying, this phenomenon which is making all the grown-ups act so sad. They may even fear that they will never wake. If your faith includes a belief in an afterlife during which one awakens and is reunited with loved ones, try to explain by using an analogy that does not parallel the child's normal daily actions.

- Likewise, don't tell them you're going on a long trip. They may never accept that you've died, and they may never again trust others to return. Your death may raise enough issues with trust as it is; don't add to these issues by using allegorical detail with children who are too young to do anything other than take what you say literally.

- Be cautious about suggesting that your spiritual presence will remain nearby if your children believe in and act fearful of ghosts. They may become fearful of being haunted after you've died.

Forgiveness and other emotional closures

Some religions emphasize that before one dies, certain spiritual life tasks must be completed, such as forgiving those who have harmed you, forgiving yourself, and admitting what you have done wrong.

Only you need to be satisfied with the state of your inner being as you prepare to die. You may choose to adhere closely to religious beliefs, or you may decide that you wish to die peacefully without trying to meet religious goals.

Detachment

Just as we may withdraw quite naturally from friends who are unaware of the profound changes we must face after our diagnosis and bond instead with other cancer survivors, as death approaches, we may find ourselves wanting and needing to withdraw from the living. This is a natural process, partly physical, as we weaken and perhaps suffer physical pain, but partly emotional, as our needs shift to more spiritual matters.

You may sense that people who have died are trying to communicate with you. You may dream about those who have died or about places distinctly not of Earth's confining dimensions. Before dying, other people have reported such happenings, and appeared to be much comforted by them. Often these dreams and perceptions occur in the last week or so of life.

An observer might often be appalled, watching family members sitting in the dying person's room, talking among themselves as if the patient had already died. Sometimes the family members are ignoring the person's need to communicate. At other times it's a reflection of the family's tacit understanding of the person's withdrawal from the living.

Permission to die: The last gift of love

Some dying people need permission from their loved ones to let go. If you are blessed with time, you might discuss this in advance with your family. Particularly if you are in pain, try to make it clear to them that they give you a great gift when they give you permission to die. At times, a final verbal or tactile gesture of letting go by the family seems necessary in one's final moments to allow one to die.

Physical aspects of dying

Many leukemia survivors and their families ask what dying will be like.

How will I die?

Death can occur in many ways, because leukemia may occur in almost any part of the body. In general, life-threatening symptoms will be related to the failure of organs invaded by leukemia cells. Leukemia in the central nervous system may suppress the brain center that controls breathing or may cause seizures. Leukemia cells in the liver or kidney may cause toxins to accumulate, resulting in coma. Death from leukemia is often related to secondary infections or blood loss. Uncontrollable respiratory infections may cause the lungs or heart to fail. Complications that develop following marrow transplantation may also cause death. Many die from pneumonia or other viral infections resulting from suppressed immune systems.

Your oncologist is the best person to prepare you for the physical symptoms you are most likely to face, and what level of pain, if any, you may need to counter with medication. Some, but not all, leukemia deaths are accompanied by pain, which should be relieved and controlled by a hospice or a physician.

Even a death preceded by great pain and discomfort is usually, in its very last stage, peaceful and illuminated by a brief cognizance.

When will it occur?

No human knows the answer to this question: not in relation to leukemia, nor for any other form death may take. There are well-known physical signs associated with the very last stage of life, yet some people have revived after all signs of life are extinguished. Many people have rallied for months or years after feeling so ill they wished for death or after their doctors had given up all hope for survival. We can know only that our death will end our lifetime.

The final moments of life

Most people at this stage seem unaware of what is happening to their body, or they seem to drift in and out of awareness. The perception of family members looking on at this stage is that the patient is in great discomfort, but those who have had near-death experiences do not report remembering great distress at this stage. The truth is unknown to the living.

The visible physical signs seen most often just before death comprise the "agonal" stage, and may include muscle spasm, one or more large gasps for breath, breathing that starts and stops, heaving chest or shoulders, a single deep exhalation, clear or unclear vocalizations, or noisy breathing. All muscles, bowel and bladder sphincter muscles included, will relax. This might release no body waste, though, if no food was taken recently.

These signs may be visible for just an instant or may last for several minutes.

How medical staff defines death

Currently, brain death is the criterion used to ascertain that death is irrefutable. Other classic signs of death, such as cessation of heartbeat, can be misleading or can be reversed using 21st-century medical technology.

Signs of brain death include loss of all reflexes, such as the blink reflex or the pupil's response to light, failure to respond physically or verbally to urgent or painful stimuli, and the absence of electrical activity within the brain as measured by an electroencephalogram (EEG).

Can we make dying easier?

Death may be eased in many ways, including: receiving physical and emotional comfort, finalizing affairs, or perhaps forgiving oneself and others for old grudges and sins. Spiritual comfort and philosophical priorities are addressed in many fine books.

Pain control

The most pressing concern is pain control in the last stages of life. Several studies have shown that many dying cancer patients did not receive adequate medication to control pain. Medical doctors were concerned about addiction or accidental overdose. Recently, however, many physicians have become more informed about pain control for the dying cancer patient and are doing a better job of providing proper palliative care. State medical organizations are working on initiatives to ensure that physicians are correctly informed about the new rules for using pain medicine with the terminally ill. Nevertheless, patients and caregivers must remain vigilant and insist on sufficient pain medication.

Euthanasia

Unfortunately, there can be painful preludes to death for which no amount of medication is adequate. In some cases, because of horrific suffering, terminal patients and their loved ones feel the need to end life sooner than the disease would end it.

Euthanasia, the hastening of the end of life by active intervention, has always been controversial in the US. Groups such as the Hemlock Society and the American Medical Association have expressed divergent points of view. The American Medical Association states that doctor-assisted suicide violates doctors' professional ethics. The Hemlock Society publishes literature on dying and the right to die, including the book *Final Exit*.

Some doctors will privately state that they have broken the law to ease a patient's going. One geriatric neurologist stated that, among her fellow medical doctors, about half will help one of their own patients to die when medicine and technology cannot relieve suffering.

Planning your own memorial ceremony

It's an odd fact that many people who cannot bear to think of the dying process, who cannot even conceive of their mortality, are quite happy to plan their own memorial ceremony and burial. As death becomes a certainty, many people find comfort in planning how others will remember them and celebrate their life.

Some of the things you might want to consider are:

- Whether you would like to be buried or cremated, where and how you would like your remains to be preserved or honored
- What memories of your life you'd like retold at your funeral or memorial service
- If there are special poems or music you want read or played
- Whether the ceremony will be a religious one
- If your internment or the scattering of your ashes will be private

There can be a large financial saving if you preplan and prepay for your funeral—having time to look around and get competitive prices as well as arrange for desired services. This is becoming very common among survivors today.

We'll end this chapter with a story of love from Dave Palmer about his wife Ellen May:

> *This is the note no one wants to write or read.*
>
> *Ellen began a new journey this morning, with new wings, perhaps a new form—but certainly the same wonderful soul. We were not ready to start a journey in separate worlds, but God provided a path and Ellen was able to choose to follow it, with all my love and support.*
>
> *Our four-year journey was aided and comforted by dozens, if not hundreds, of others. You are a gift of immeasurable value. I will always be in your debt. Her new journey began at 7:30 a.m., very quietly and with a great deal of peace.*
>
> *A compassionate emergency room staff aided me in one of the decisions no caregiver ever wants to exercise. Our cancer support group is led by a minister and a social worker. A second hospital minister befriended us over the months. With their love and support my separate road started with prayers, compassion, and realistic support—and I am most thankful for that.*

CHAPTER 19

Researching Your Leukemia

When diagnosed with leukemia, most people have no idea what that really means. They may know that it's a form of cancer and may have heard of the Leukemia and Lymphoma Society. Unless they have had previous experience with leukemia in the family or among friends, they probably know little more.

Patients and their loved ones decide to research the disease for several reasons. Some do it because they want to know and understand their options. Some feel it is important to their survival. Others feel compelled to know about the disease and prognosis. Many seek information to corroborate that their doctors are relaying accurate and up-to-date information, even when the care they've received has been very good.

This chapter offers ways to find information about your illness, in addition to what you receive from your doctor. First, we cover a few basics about research, then we discuss using medical libraries and research journals, as well as the National Cancer Institute's Internet, phone, FAX, and clinical trials services, and hiring a search firm to do the legwork for you. We also offer methods for checking drug side effects, verifying your chemotherapy dosage, finding support groups, interpreting test results and evaluating unproven remedies.

For each type of information, we outline ways to access the source with and without a computer when it is possible to do so. For instance, the *Merck Manual* section on laboratory results is available both on paper and on the Internet. Certain unique resources, however, are found only on the Internet.

Web site addresses are called URLs, which is an acronym for universal resource locator. It is important to note that there is never any punctuation mark following a URL. So if the web address you see in the text ends with a comma or a period, do NOT include that when you type in the address.

Why researching helps

With the advent of managed care in America, HMOs constrain medical professionals from telling patients of new and expensive treatments, or turn down doctors' requests for patient care. Despite laws to the contrary, as long as HMOs get by with refusals to pay for treatment, they will persist in this behavior. To ensure that proper treatment options are made available to you, you must research your leukemia and have studies available to thrust into the maw of HMO refusals.

The growing number of patients that doctors are required to see daily and the incessant paperwork prevent even the best physicians from keeping up with the thousands of studies being done—and doctors have many diseases to be concerned about. You have only one disease to research and one life. Finding the latest information and sharing it with your doctor may well save your life.

Moreover, many people find that knowing about their disease is empowering. Research concerning stress and cancer indicates that having a proactive attitude contributes to length of survival. Patients can feel more in control of situations that could otherwise easily lead to dependence. For many people, the more they learn, the more comfortable and relaxed they are in dealing with leukemia.

Some people can't deal with the information they find. The statistics and prognoses can be very frightening. The results of studies and side effects reported can cause patients or loved ones to worry needlessly. For those folks, researching may not be a good idea, and they should not feel badly about choosing to take a different route to healing.

People's responses to leukemia and whether or not they want to research the disease varies by individual. Here are the stories of several people who, when confronted with a frightening diagnosis, chose to respond by researching the disease.

Art, a patient with CLL, notes that researching helped him put the disease in perspective:

> Like most people, when I'm sick I see my doctor, expect him to provide a solution, and don't feel a need to go any further. In many cases, that works well. With CLL, that is not the case. It is considered incurable and there is no one treatment plan. It's a condition I'll be dealing with for a long time, and there is no "cookbook" answer.

> To deal with the emotional stress of having an incurable leukemia, I find that being informed helps me put the disease in perspective. It cuts it down to size. And staying informed allows me to participate with my doctors in my treatment plan. This gives me a feeling of some control over what is happening to me, and that is a comfort too.

Another patient with CLL was a hospital social worker. Her familiarity with a medical library helped her get started in researching:

> When I was diagnosed in 1992, I didn't even own a computer. However, I was determined to learn everything I could about chronic lymphocytic leukemia. As a hospital social worker, I had access to the hospital's medical library, where I was able to research the disease and available treatments. My anxiety lessened as knowledge replaced "fear of the unknown."
>
> Armed with information, I felt more in control; rather than putting myself in my doctor's hands, I prepared myself to be an educated partner with my doctor. I was able to share current articles and news of clinical trials.
>
> Today, the Internet and my desktop computer allow me to read studies from major cancer centers as soon as they are published. Research articles from all over the world are open to doctors and their patients, and I feel as though I am privy to the same information as my doctor.
>
> The "unknown" is a lot less frightening now, and I can dispel the nagging fear that there is "something else out there" that might have been missed. As a result of my research, I feel confident that the decisions I reach are well-informed and reasoned.

Another patient responded to a diagnosis of leukemia—and her need for information and connection—by going to the top medical web sites on the Internet:

> What was this disease that was being linked with me? I knew nothing about it. Well, that was about to change and rapidly. First I went to the National Cancer Institute's web site and looked into the Physicians Data Query to find out what the disease was and how it was treated. Then I went to the National Library of Medicine web site to learn more about who was working on this disease at what institutions.

Finally, I went on to the broader web and found patient sites and sto-
ries. "GrannyBarb and Art's Leukemia Links" was a wonderful place to
find places for research, and the patient stories gave me hope that there
really would be life after cancer.

Another patient, Hazel, describes how her research helped lessen her fear
and regain a sense of control:

Once my head stopped reeling from the impact of the oncologist's
words, "You have leukemia," it was time to take stock. I realized that
other than identifying leukemia as a cancer that children get, I knew
almost nothing about it. Researching the leukemia is serving a number of
purposes. The information that I have collected has enabled me to:

- *Find answers to many questions*
- *Lessen the fear of the unknown*
- *Become a more knowledgeable patient when interacting with my*
  doctor
- *Regain some sense of control over my life*
- *Focus my energies on fighting this disease*

The familiar statement "Knowledge is Power" has developed added
significance for me now.

What you'll need to begin

If you are researching your disease, it doesn't matter how much education
you have or how long it has been since you did research in school. You have
a unique motivation this time. You want to live. So you need to know and
understand the information. You're not too old. The fastest growing segment of Internet users is over 65. You may struggle with the vocabulary and
jargon at first, but you'll soon become acclimated. Ask for help. Persist. Your
doctor's nurse is a good resource, and your local librarian is another. If
there's a medical school in town, ask the medical librarian.

Make sure of facts

Before you start, you need to know a few specific facts about your diagnosis
to make searching more fruitful. You also will benefit by knowing what to
avoid, and what to insulate yourself against.

You'll need four things before you start:

- The exact name of your leukemia and its subtype, if there is one
- The stage of your disease
- The classification system(s) used in diagnosis
- A medical dictionary

If you don't know your precise diagnosis, you'll waste a lot of time and precious energy reading the wrong material. You may even frighten yourself unnecessarily with information that doesn't pertain to you.

Your pathology report will tell the precise type of leukemia you have. If you haven't been in the habit of requesting copies of pathology reports, begin right now. Purchase a medical dictionary to help you with the terminology you will encounter, which becomes increasingly easy to understand with greater exposure. Appendix A, *Resources* list several reasonably priced medical dictionaries. One of the most useful is *The Cancer Dictionary*, by Altman and Sarg. A helpful general medical dictionary is *Taber's Cyclopedic Medical Dictionary*, edited by F. A. Davis. Appendix D, *FAB Staging of Acute Leukemia*, lists the French-American-British (FAB) classification of the acute leukemias.

Clarify what you want to learn

When you're researching something, be specific about what you want to know. When you ask for help, do the same thing. Clarifying what you're seeking makes the entire job easier. Start with the basics. If you're reading a medical journal article, read the abstracts first. Then go the next step and read the entire paper. The latter is most important, because often the abstract is written before the research is complete, and it may not accurately report what the entire paper says. The abstract is the summary of the full paper that follows. Read the abstract to be sure that the article is relevant and then read on.

Once you've read and understood the information, always verify it with your oncologist. It's important that you and your doctor have the same perspective about a possible treatment option. If you have more than one research paper to discuss, it is diplomatic to make a separate appointment with your oncologist and beforehand, provide him with the references you are using so the appointment time can be useful to you both. Giving him the references in advance lets him prepare for your meeting as well. It is not fair to your doctor or to other patients to try to use office visit time for long discussions of possible treatment options you've turned up, so schedule separate appointments in advance for that. This also avoids putting your doctor on the defensive if he's been too busy to keep up with the latest papers in his field. See Nancy Keene's book, *Working With Your Doctor*, and Nancy Oster, et al., *Making Informed Medical Decisions*, for more information.

You have a right to your doctor's respect for your efforts. When you share what you've learned in a special appointment made for that purpose, if the response you receive from your doctor is cavalier or condescending, it may be necessary to discuss this attitude with him or to find a new doctor.

One survivor tells about how she first chose a doctor who was open to her research style:

> First I went doctor hunting. I needed to find someone who would understand my need to know about my disease. I cope by gathering information. The doctor had to be open to discussion of the latest treatment options and clinical trials that I would be bringing periodically. My first oncologist couldn't deal with my research and questions. So I was determined I would find an oncologist who kept up with his field and who encouraged his patients to do that also. A large order, you say? Yes it was! But I found him, and what a difference it has made in the way I feel about leukemia, treatments, and follow-up.

This survivor tells how she shares information ahead of time and makes an appointment for a focused discussion:

> We have an agreement. I email him the web addresses of the articles I'm researching, and then every three months or so I make a separate appointment to talk about what I'm finding. Since he knows what I'm researching and has access to the same papers, when we meet he's as prepared as I am. Sometimes he even shares articles with me that he's found. Meetings are short and to the point, and I've learned so much from his willingness to work with me. It's extremely reassuring, and I know I'm with the right oncologist.

Ways to find information

There are several possible methods for obtaining information about leukemia. The next few sections describe the following methods in detail:

- If you have computer access, you can find an almost limitless amount of information about leukemia on the Internet, some of which is highly accurate, some of which is of lesser quality. The highly reliable information at the National Cancer Institute's CancerNet site and the latest medical research papers from CANCERLIT, an ongoing source of information should be your starting points.

- If you have siblings, children, or grandchildren with computer access and you don't feel like starting from scratch using a computer amidst your worries about cancer—and who would blame you?—ask them to do Internet searches for you. Make sure you tell them the specifics of your diagnosis, and what you're looking for: treatment options, complementary therapies, stories of other patients, clinical trials, and so on.

- If you're friends with a doctor, nurse, or librarian, ask them to do searches of various resources, such as the National Library of Medicine's MEDLINE database and the NCI's Physician's Data Query (PDQ).

- Pay a commercial firm to do a search for you.

- Visit an academic or medical library to research the medical journals in the periodicals section and their medical texts.

- Ask your doctor for help getting copies of research papers from medical journals, but offer to pay for any photocopying that's needed.

- Contact the Leukemia and Lymphoma Society, the Chronic Lymphocytic Leukemia Foundation, or the American Cancer Society and ask for information that can be mailed to you.

- Call the National Cancer Institute at (800) 4-CANCER and ask for information, or ask for help using their CancerFax service.

Getting started

An excellent place to start researching your disease is *Cancer Guide*, a web site at *http://www.cancerguide.org* written by Steve Dunn, a cancer survivor. Read his article called *The Pros and Cons of Researching Your Own Cancer.* Also on that site, read Stephen Jay Gould's, *The Median Isn't the Message*. You'll leave this site with good information and a positive attitude.

Phone or fax

The first place to go for leukemia information is the National Cancer Institute's Cancer Information Service (800) 4-CANCER. The information on cancer amassed and maintained by the National Cancer Institute, a division of NIH, constitutes the grandmother of all cancer databases and should be your starting point for learning the basics about leukemia. It's accurate, current, and free.

You will be asked the specific type of leukemia you have and the stage you are in. Tell them to send you the PDQ (Physicians Data Query) for patients with your leukemia. That is a general article giving basic information about the disease, how it's staged, and first-line standard treatments for each stage. Also ask for any additional information they can provide about this disease.

Once you have read and understood the patient's version, call again and ask them to send you the information for professionals. It's far more complete, although the prognosis statistics may be unsettling. You may have to tell them your doctor is asking for you to have that information.

You can also ask for all clinical trials for your disease. Be sure to tell the staff member that you want clinical trials from all over the country, not just in your area, so you know what is available throughout the US. Always ask for the full information on clinical trails, not the summaries. If you ask friends for help or hire a search firm to do a medical search, the same considerations apply.

Computer access

If you have Internet access, getting the information is easier still. Go to the NCI's CancerNet website at *http://cancernet.nci.nih.gov*. Once you are at their home page, click on "leukemia" and go from there. If you have only email access, send an email to: *cancernet@icicc.nci.nih.gov* with the word HELP as the only thing in the body of the message. That will bring you a list of everything available by email from CancerNet. Follow the simple directions to get the PDQ for patients or for professionals.

You can also get listings of current research abstracts from the NCI CAN-CERLIT section at *http://cnetdb.nci.nih.gov/overview.html.*

Next, go to the Leukemia and Lymphoma Society (formerly the Leukemia Society of America) at *http://www.leukemia-lymphoma.org,* where you'll find all kinds of leukemia articles written for patients. You'll also find out about the patient assistance plans and leukemia support groups. A call to (800) 955-4LSA or (800) 955-4572 will also get the information sent by US mail.

"GrannyBarb and Art's Leukemia Links" at *http://www.acor.org/leukemia* will provide loads of places to go for further leukemia information. Check out the patient stories also.

Research papers from medical journals

Reviewing the research papers published in medical journals is the best way for a leukemia survivor to get the most current information. Textbooks are out of date almost as soon as they're printed. NCI's PDQ information is a good foundation, but it doesn't reflect every emerging trend still in the test phase.

Reading medical research papers is arguably the most difficult part of learning about progress against leukemia, as well as the best way to keep abreast of progress. A medical dictionary will serve you well in this effort, and you should ask your doctor about parts that are unclear. Usually the abstract (summary) of a paper will suffice, as abstracts of cancer research studies normally contain conclusions, but at times obtaining the full text of the paper will be necessary.

If you use the full text of a paper, don't try to understand the whole thing at first. Just read the introduction, the conclusions, and the discussion. The middle sections deal with scientific methodology that's important in verifying that the research was performed to strict scientific standards, but this part has been peer-reviewed by other scientists and the editors of the journal. This material is usually, but not always, less important to a patient trying to find good prospects for care. As you become more comfortable reading research papers and their terminology, occasionally you may want to read the remaining sections as well.

Medical journals that tend to have many articles on the leukemias are *Blood*, *Transplantation*, *Leukemia and Lymphoma*, *Journal of Clinical Oncology*, *The British Journal of Haematology*, *The American Journal of Hematology*, *Bone Marrow Transplantation*, *The European Journal of Haematology*, *Seminars in Haematology*, *Haematologica*, *The Annals of Hematology*, *Leukemia Research*, *Current Opinions in Hematology*, *Leukemia; Cytokines and Molecular Therapy*, *Hematology and Oncology Clinics of North America*, and *The Journal of the National Cancer Institute*.

If you like to read about basic cancer research that's years away from becoming treatment, the journals *Science*, *Cell*, and *Nature Biotechnology* are good choices.

Many medical journals are now on the Web, including *Blood*, *Bone Marrow Transplantation*, *Science*, *The Journal of the American Medical Association*, *The American Journal of Hematology*, and *The Journal of the National Cancer Institute*. Some of these cannot be viewed online unless you're a subscriber to the standard paper edition. An excellent resource for journal articles is available online at *http://www.amedeo.com*.

Journal subscriptions

Subscription costs for some of these journals often start at about $100 per year and can go much higher. The disadvantage of subscribing to individual journals, besides the accumulation of hard-to-index paper copy, is that good research articles on leukemia are spread among these journals, and subscribing to several becomes prohibitively expensive.

Using MEDLINE

An absolutely indispensable resource—some say the most important resource—is MEDLINE, maintained by the US National Library of Medicine (NLM). Various free MEDLINE database search engines are available on the Internet, giving you access to the 9 million medical research papers in the National Library of Medicine.

If you don't have computer access, ask a friend or relative who does to do a search for you. Alternately, a nurse or someone affiliated with a hospital, your local cancer center, or public library will likely have MEDLINE access. The National Library of Medicine's MEDLINE web address is *http://www.ncbi. nlm.nih.gov/entrez/query.fcgi?db=PubMed*.

If you're using a computer, at most MEDLINE sites you'll generally find a search engine that accepts keywords and returns summaries of the medical research publications that match your keywords. For example, if you type the terms "AML, treatment, PAME" and click on the search button, you'll receive in return the titles of the studies regarding treating AML with PAME. Clicking the mouse on each title will display the summary (abstract) of the study's results on your screen. You'll note that the latest studies appear first. After you've read a number of these studies, the terminology becomes familiar, and you can repeat the search using new keywords.

Almost all of the web-based MEDLINE search engines use an organizational hierarchy called Medical Subject Headings (MeSH). MeSH terms group references by category so that you'll get more research papers returned for your searching efforts, even if you're not familiar with the right medical terms or if you slightly misspell a word. Some MEDLINE search tools invoke MeSH terms behind the scenes when you enter a keyword; others, like Paper-Chase, prompt you to pick a MeSH term from a list that they produce that is associated with the keyword you entered. Still others have advanced searches that you invoke using MeSH terms explicitly.

Here is a partial list of MeSH terms that might be used behind the scenes or offered to you as a choice when you use the word "lymphocyte" as the keyword in a MEDLINE search:

- LYMPHOCYTE COOPERATION
- LYMPHOCYTE COUNT
- LYMPHOCYTE COUNT, CD4
- LYMPHOCYTE CULTURE TEST, MIXED
- LYMPHOCYTE DEPLETION
- LYMPHOCYTE DIFFERENTIATION ANTIGENS, B
- LYMPHOCYTE DIFFERENTIATION ANTIGENS, T
- LYMPHOCYTE EPITOPES, B

A good way to get background information on any medical topic is to seek out the review articles in MEDLINE. Enter various phrases, like:

- immune, leukemia, review
- leukocytes, immune, review
- dendritic, immune, review

These will retrieve the abstracts of review articles that are geared to physicians who might not be specialists, and articles appearing in more generalized publications such as *Family Practitioner* or *Nature*, which contain more explanatory material and make fewer assumptions.

If you need help searching, call the National Library of Medicine at (800) 272-4787 or (301) 496-6308.

If the MEDLINE summaries (abstracts) you read are more tantalizing than edifying, you can order the full text of any research paper from companies that specialize in this service. Some of these companies, such as Infotrieve, are web-based; others can be found by calling a medical school library and getting recommendations from a librarian. Unfortunately, at the time of this writing, the National Library of Medicine's service does not offer full text retrieval to those articles and journals not associated with an academic library. Those who are, however, can use the Loansome Doc service to order full text of papers. On the Internet, the MEDLINE service providers Biomednet, HealthGate, Medscape, Helix, PDRnet.Com, Infotrieve, PaperChase, and others offer full-text services for a fee.

The National Library of Medicine now has begun to put complete books online. Visit *http://www.ncbi.nlm.nih.gov/books/mboc/bookshelp/bookover.html* for their book section.

Using medical libraries

Another way to find articles in medical journals is to visit a medical or university library and examine their journals and recent texts, borrowing or photocopying what you find most useful. Copyright law permits photocopying one copy of a journal article if it's for your own immediate use. Avoid using textbooks that were published more than two years ago, as the time it takes to bring a text to print makes the source material used to prepare a text out of date.

Note that some university and medical libraries restrict entry to those affiliated with the institution in some way. You can find the nearest medical library open to the public by calling the National Network of Libraries of Medicine at (800) 338-7657. You can often make arrangements to use a medical library at a local college through your doctor.

Local hospitals also may have medical libraries. To find articles in medical journals, ask the main information desk where periodicals are stored and how to search them by subject. There's some variety in how different libraries store, search, and retrieve journal articles. Some academic libraries have all periodicals stored on CD-ROM, for example, but others are still stored as paper copy in the stacks. Regardless of these differences, there's always a way to search by subject, and this is how you should. The library you visit may also have access to MEDLINE or Index Medicus.

Often the periodicals section of a medical or academic library will have staff devoted to helping you. All should have material you can read at your leisure, describing how to search their collection. Don't be shy about asking for help. Most librarians are proud of their ability to root out obscure references and are in that career because they want to connect people to information. Use the cancer information center nurses as resources to find the information for you.

Arrive prepared to pay for photocopy fees and with coins for photocopy machines.

Hiring a search firm

Before hiring a commercial firm to do a search of the medical literature, you might want to call the National Library of Medicine's Management Desk at (800) 638-8480 and ask for whatever help they can provide.

You might choose to pay a search fee to one of a number of companies who provide this service. Tell them what topic you're interested in, but keep in mind that the more specific you can be, the better—for instance, treatments for AML with 6-hydroxymethylacylfulvene. The search firm will locate copies of articles from medical journals and mail them to you.

Here's a partial list of such commercial search companies. A listing here does not imply endorsement of their services:

- The Health Resource, Inc. Phone: (800) 949-0090 or in Arkansas (501) 329-5272; email: *moreinfo@thehealthresource.com*; web site: *http://www. TheHealthResource.com*

- Can Help. Phone: (800) 565-1732 or in Washington (360) 437-2291; email: *canhelp@olympus.net*; web site: *http://www.canhelp.com*

- Schine On-Line Services. Phone: (800) FIND-CURE (346-3287); email: *schine@findcure.org*; web site: *http://www.findcure.com*

How to obtain medical textbooks

Texts on cancer, immunology, hematology, and leukemia can provide you with the foundation for understanding more timely sources, such as the papers published in medical journals. In general, the more recent the text, the better.

A source of background information might be an immunology text aimed at pre-med college students or first-year medical students. The terminology might be a notch higher than many people are comfortable with, but not nearly as difficult as that found in medical journals, and definitely geared to providing broad, fundamental information. Textbooks probably range in price from $40 to $200, but it's fairly easy to get used copies at college and university bookstores.

Using the list of books in Appendix A as a guide to reliable texts, visit your local public library, academic library, or a medical bookstore.

Medical bookstores are usually found near medical schools. Some of the largest well-known bookstore chains also carry hard-to-find textbooks, or they can order them for you. Several bookstores have web sites that greatly facilitate ordering books, especially if you're not feeling well enough to drive, park, browse, and lug heavy texts home. Medscape has an excellent online medical bookstore at *http://medscape.medbookstore.com.*

Because of the high cost of textbooks, most people prefer to borrow texts.

If you haven't used a public library lately to search for holdings, you might be pleasantly surprised to find that, in many cases, the old card catalogs are gone, replaced by fast and easy-to-use computer workstations. Their databases can tell you within a few minutes how many copies of a book exist in their system, which branches of the library own the book, whether another borrower has taken it out, and when it's due back.

If your public library is in a large urban area, the materials you need may be readily accessible, but if not, your library system may be able to borrow the materials you need even if they're not in their holdings. As with searching for medical research papers, it pays to ask for help. You may have to wait longer for an interlibrary loan, but it can save you the cost of an expensive text.

One book, *The Wisdom of the Body*, has a chapter on blood and the immune system. It might not be as complete as some would like, but it's readily available in many public libraries.

Finding clinical trials

New and possibly better treatments are available to leukemia patients in carefully controlled settings called clinical trials, which are described in depth in Chapter 10, *Clinical Trials and Beyond*. You should become familiar with the trials that are available before you need one, for trials are frequently needed when events have reached crisis level and time is running low.

In order to choose the best from among several clinical trials, it's necessary to be familiar with the track record, if any, of the agents being used in each trial. Each of the drug names appearing in a trial's title can be used as a keyword to search medical journals (as described earlier in "Research papers from medical journals") for any previous research studies published. This is a daunting task; do not expect to finish it in one sitting or even in a few days. Once it's done, though, you only need to search for new drugs or substances as they first appear in the clinical trials database or among your other sources of information.

You can use several methods to find clinical trials, including the following.

Ask your oncologist

If your oncologist is affiliated with a teaching hospital, there will be a list of clinical trials being done at that institution. Ask your oncologist which trials would suit your medical circumstances. This method has its advantages and disadvantages. An advantage is that you need do very little except trust. A disadvantage is that trials at other institutions may not be considered.

Call the National Cancer Institute

Call the NCI at (800) 4-CANCER and ask about trials for your subtype of leukemia. Specify whether you're willing to travel—otherwise they'll send you local trials only—and be sure to ask for the full document, not the summary.

Use a personal computer

You can use a computer to research US and international clinical trials at the NCI's web site, *http://cancertrials.nci.nih.gov*. This, in conjunction with learning to use MEDLINE, is by far the most comprehensive way to check on new treatments being tested. The NCI now provides this tool free of charge over the Internet. We strongly suggest that you examine all trials available for your kind of leukemia—not just those in your geographical area.

When you visit this site, you'll be presented with a form of choices for finding trials by cancer type, phase of trial, status of trial (is it open or full and closed), and so on. Fill in the form by clicking on the pull-down menu next to the section header, and then scroll down and click on the disease for which you're seeking trials. For example, choose something like:

- chronic myeloid leukemia, adult
- acute lymphocytic leukemia, adult

If you're using this search engine for the first time, it's a good idea to view all leukemia trials of your type available for adults. Use the down arrow next to Trial Type to select the word "treatment," then click the search button. The result will be a large list of all trials for leukemia that focus on treatment.

You can repeat the search using the City and State fields to see trials in your own area, or with the phase field to see only phase I, phase II, or phase III trials, which are explained in Chapter 10.

If you're interested in a particular kind of drug or method, you can use the Modality field to select only trials using this technology, such as monoclonal antibodies, which are categorized as such and also as antibody therapy.

Other means of finding clinical trials include:

- CenterWatch's site on the Internet to track new cancer treatment trials. Find them at *http://www.centerwatch.com*.
- Commercial Internet service providers such as America Online (AOL) receive email press releases from pharmaceutical companies concerning new products in development.

How to find support groups

Local hospitals, a local branch of the national Wellness Community, the Leukemia and Lymphoma Society, the American Cancer Society, and the Internet offer solid information and access to others who have been through what you're going through. The American Cancer Society can be reached at (800) ACS-2345; ask for their "I Can Cope" program. The Wellness Community in your area is listed in the phone book.

The Association of Cancer Online Resources (ACOR) has pointers to many of the Internet hematologic cancer email discussion groups as well as a handy automatic subscription feature at *http://www.acor.org*. There are lists for each of the leukemias and one list for general discussion of all the hematologic malignancies. See Chapter 14, *Getting Support*.

How to verify drug information

Pharmaceutical information tools are useful for finding drug side effects, mode of action, and marketing names. Find more information through your pharmacist, library, bookstore, computer, or the FDA can be sources of information.

You can call your pharmacist for information about drugs, or ask for the foldout paper of small print that comes from the drug manufacturer but that is seldom included with your prescription unless you ask for it.

The Physician's Desk Reference (PDR), a compendium of information about drugs, is now reprinted in versions that are easier for the general public to understand, but you might appreciate the learning experience gained from reading the original PDR. In addition to the PDR, many other drug encyclopedias are available to the general public.

The Food and Drug Administration can also verify drug information. Call (888) 332-4543, (800) 532-4440, or visit its web site at *http://www.fda.gov*.

You can report adverse effects of drugs to the FDA, too, or use their Med-Watch web site: *http://www.fda.gov/medwatch/how.htm*.

The following sites have search engines requiring only a drug name:

- RXList: *http://www.rxlist.com*
- Clinical Pharmacology Online: *http://www.cponline.gsm.com*
- PharmInfoNet: *http://pharminfo.com/drg_mnu.html*
- DrugInfoNet: *http://www.druginfonet.com/*
- HealthTouch: *http://www.healthtouch.com/level1/p_dri.htm*

Verifying your chemotherapy dose

You can use the general formula for calculating dosages of your chemotherapy drugs and compare it to the amount recommended to you in your medical records. Keep in mind, though, that your doctor may be using a different dose for very good reasons.

Medicine Online's DoseCalc site deserves special mention as a user-friendly research site because it's a great help in verifying your chemotherapy dosage. Go to *http://www.meds.com/DChome.html* and enter your height, weight, and a drug name. Behind the scenes, it calculates your square feet per meter (yes, square, not cubic, feet per meter—the basis for most chemotherapy dosages) and gives you the standard dose administered for a person your size.

You can also do this calculation using your body surface area and the standard recommended dose for your body surface area. Appendix C, *Body Surface Area in Square Meters*, contains a chart of heights, weights, and body surface areas. Appendix C also lists other methods and sources for calculating body surface area.

Once you've calculated your body surface area, you need to know the recommended dose per square meter for each of the drugs you're getting. You can ask your doctor's staff for this information or use Medicine Online's site, as discussed previously. If you notice a substantial difference between the calculated and actual dose given, ask your doctor why. Often there are very good reasons for differences, though.

How to interpret test results

Your doctor is generally the best person to tell you how to interpret test results, but there are several references available for comparing your test results to normal values (please note that a value outside of the normal range does not always indicate a problem):

- Appendix B, *Normal Blood and Marrow Test Values*, lists the normal adult values for a variety of blood tests.

- The *Merck Manual*, either the paper version or the version on their web site, has a section devoted to laboratory pathology. Many public libraries have a copy of the *Merck Manual* in their noncirculating reference section. At Merck's web site, just enter the test name and click on the search button. You can find the search facility at *http://www.merck.com*.

- The American Society for Clinical Laboratory Science has a very informative page explaining what blood tests are and what they measure at *http://ascls.org/labtesting/index.htm*. Normal ranges are not included.

Each of the following web sites also has a search engine for finding the normal values of various test results:

- The University of Michigan Pathology Laboratories Handbook. Allows you to search by test name at *http://po.path.med.umich.edu/handbook*.

- The Lupus Lab Tests web site. Has tests commonly done for lupus, but many of these are also done for hematologic cancers such as leukemia. See *http://www.mtio.com/mclfa/lfalt1.htm*.

How to assess unproven remedies

If your treatment isn't giving you good results, you may become vulnerable to the claims for a quick cure made by certain practitioners. While some of these treatments may have merit, others are simply the means by which charlatans realize financial gain. How can you separate treatments that may have unrecognized medical potential from those that have been tried and discarded by reputable researchers and those that are, or were, the focus of legal action? Try using the following:

- If you're considering using any alternative or complementary medicine supplements, it is wise to visit the National Center for Complementary and Alternative Medicine at their Internet web site: *http://nccam.nih.gov*.

- QuackWatch on the Internet gives the medical scientist's evaluation of those unusual remedies you've been hearing about at *http://www.quackwatch.com*.

- The National Cancer Institute publishes a great deal of information on untested remedies. Call (800) 4-CANCER or visit *http://cancernet.nci.nih.gov*.

- The American Cancer Society has a list of questions you should ask before becoming involved with unusual remedies. Call (800) ACS-2345, or visit its web site at *http://www.cancer.org*.

- The Consumer Health Information Research Institute provides an integrity index and a credibility of publication index, including one that rates cancer books. Call (816) 228-4595.

Other unique web resources

If you don't have a personal computer yet, or if your kids won't let you near it, this section may convince you how easily and quickly you can get the answers you've been looking for despite your inexperience.

Please note that web sites may be inaccessible on occasional days owing to data reorganization or maintenance, and that web site addresses can change:

- **The Atlas of Hematology.** Offers photographs of microscopic slides of normal and diseased blood at *http://pathy.med.nagoya-u.ac.jp/atlas/doc*, with accompanying text.

- **The American Medical Association.** Provides a doctor locator and other useful features: *http://www.ama-assn.org*.

- **Oncolink.** A highly reliable source of cancer information: *http://www.oncolink.org*.

- **The Merck Manual online.** An indispensable source of medical information: *http://www.merck.com*.

- **Cancer News.** Includes links to several sites containing press releases: *http://www.cancernews.com*.

- **Mid-South Therapeutics, Inc.** Hosts a web site with information for patients about tests and procedures: *http://www.msit.com/patients.htm*.

- **HealthAnswers.** A web site with a search engine that can supply information about how to prepare for tests, and so on: *http://www.health-answers.com*.

- **The Thrive Health Library.** A good general site for questions and answers: *http://www.thriveonline.com*.

What next?

Think of researching your condition as a cyclical activity. Although you can accumulate and absorb the basic facts about your leukemia in a burst of initial activity, certain parts of the literature search process should be repeated about once a month in order to stay in touch with improvements in care. Several areas in particular should be revisited on a regular schedule:

- The National Cancer Institute updates the physician's state-of-the-art treatment statement as new standards of care are chosen. If the treatise on your leukemia is modified, the NCI can notify you via email, or you can call the NCI at (800) 4-CANCER each month and ask them to check the date of last update on the NCI PDQ physician's statement for your type of leukemia. The NCI classifies changes to these documents as either substantial or editorial. Editorial changes might include replacing one citation with a better one.

- Every month, medical journals publish new research papers about leukemia, the summaries (abstracts) of which are collected in MEDLINE and in CANCERLIT, which is a subset of MEDLINE consisting only of cancer literature. See *http://cnetdb.nci.nih.gov/cancerlit.shtml*.

- New clinical trials for treatment are added to the NCI database every month. See *http://cancernet.nci.nih.gov/trialsrch.shtml*.

- Amedeo, *http://www.amedeo.com*, will search a series of medical journals for you and set up a special page to list all the articles it culls for you. The Amedeo listing of new articles comes directly to your email weekly.

Resources

This section gathers together resources that we have mentioned in previous chapters of the book and additional listings that you may find helpful. All entries in each category are listed in alphabetical order, not by importance.

Key leukemia resources

This first category includes resources you're likely to use most often, the richest sources of leukemia-specific information.

Organizations

Chronic Lymphocytic Leukemia (CLL) Foundation
c/o William D. Hoops, Esq.
1415 Louisiana Suite 3625
Houston, TX 77002
(713) 752-2350
http://www.cllfoundation.org

Funds research to fight chronic lymphocytic leukemia.

CLL Research Consortium
c/o Dr. Thomas Kipps
9500 Gilman Drive, 0940
La Jolla, CA 92093-0940
http://cll.ucsd.edu
(858) 657-8242
fax (858) 532-5620
cllrc@ucsd.edu

GrannyBarb and Art's Leukemia Links
http://www.acor.org/leukemia

An award winning compendium of places to go to research your leukemia, and read patient stories. The web site is run by GrannyBarb Lackritz and Arthur Flatau, two leukemia survivors.

Leukemia and Lymphoma Society
600 Third Avenue
New York, New York, 10016
(212) 573-8484
Information Resource Line (800) 955-4572
http://www.leukemia-lymphoma.org
infocenter@leukemia-lymphoma.org

Offers information, peer-support via local chapters, and a $750 grant for registered patients for drugs, travel, etc. Fundraising for leukemia research projects as well. Local chapters with support groups.

Leukemia Research Foundation
820 Davis Street, Suite 420
Evanston, IL 60201
(847) 424-0600
fax (847) 424-0606
http://www.leukemiaresearch.org

Founded in Chicago in 1946, the Leukemia Research Foundation recently celebrated its 50th anniversary. Research and quality of life assistance for leukemia patients.

Internet support groups

A list of leukemia-related Internet support groups follows. Because the Internet is a dynamic resource, this list may not be comprehensive. The number of subscribers given was approximate at the time of writing and will vary over time. The Association of Cancer Online Resources (ACOR) has pointers to all of the hematologic cancer email discussion groups. ACOR offers a handy automatic subscription feature for these and more than one hundred other discussion mailing lists it hosts, at *http://listserv.acor.org*.

- ALL-L. This list offers medical discussion and emotional support for all acute lymphocytic leukemia survivors. ALL-L has about 200 subscribers concerned with both adult and childhood ALL.

- AML. Run by Arthur Flatau, this offers medical discussion and emotional support for all acute myelogenous leukemia survivors. AML has about 325 subscribers concerned with both adult and childhood AML.

- BMT-TALK. Medical discussion and emotional support for those who will be having or who have had bone marrow transplantation for any cancer. Several oncologists subscribe to this list, which has 1,200 subscribers.

- CANCER-HOSPICE. Another new list for those patients and caregivers dealing with hospice needs.

- CANCER-PARENTS. A brand new list for those concerned with parenting issues of cancer patients. After only a few weeks of existence, this list had 45 subscribers.

- CLL. Run by GrannyBarb Lackritz, this list offers medical discussion and emotional support for chronic lymphocytic leukemia and small-cell lymphocytic lymphoma (SLL). The list is a virtual community of patients, caregivers, and professionals, with about 1,830 subscribers.

- CLL-CN. For those dealing with the Canadian medical system, this supplements the information on the full CLL list. Begun in late 1999, this list has about 64 subscribers.

- CML. Medical discussion and emotional support for chronic myelogenous leukemia with about 450 subscribers.

- HAIRY-CELL. Medical discussion and emotional support for hairy cell leukemia with about 50 subscribers.

- HEM-ONC. The grandmother of the hematological malignancy lists offers medical discussion and emotional support for all hematologic malignancies, including all of the leukemias. Several very helpful oncologists subscribe to this list of about 725.

- MPD-NET. This list offers medical and support services for those with myeloproliferative disorders, including CML. Almost 1,650 subscribers create lively discussions about clinical trials and the latest treatment options.

Additional ACOR lists include Cancer-Depression, Cancer-Fatigue, Cancer-Pain, Cancer-Sexuality, and a Long-Term Survivors (LT-Survivors) list.

Telephone support

If you have the desire to talk with a patient who has been where you are likely to have to go in the future, there are many resources for talking with a counterpart.

Leukemia and Lymphoma Society—First Connection
(800) 955-4572
http://leukemia-lymphoma.org

A leukemia survivor in remission who has your disease and the treatment you anticipate will call and chat for approximately an hour.

The Anderson Network
(800) 345-6324
http://www.mdacc.tmc.edu/~andnet.

A member of a group of patients and former patients of the M. D. Anderson Cancer Center in Houston is available to speak with other patients who are matched for disease and treatment. This service is available to anyone, regardless of where they live or where they receive treatment. In addition, the same service is available for caregivers, family members, or even a patient's friend.

The Blood and Marrow Transplant Infonet "Patient-to-Survivor"
http://www.bmtinfonet.org/survivor.html
(847) 433-3313 (Chicago area)
(888) 597-7674 (toll free)

Telephone link for bone marrow and/or stem cell transplant patients. This program matches survivors to patients by disease and kind of BMT.

National Bone Marrow Transplant Link (BMT Link)
(800) Link-BMT (546-5268) (National Bone Transplant Link program)
(248) 358-1886 (in Southfield, Michigan)
fax (248) 358-1889
http://comnet.org/nbmtlink

This service provides you with phone contact with a patient who has gone through the same type of bone marrow transplant you are facing.

The Cancer Hot Line, R. A. Bloch Cancer Foundation
http://www.blochcancer.org
(800) 433-0464

Offers the opportunity to talk with a survivor with your type of cancer.

Dana-Farber Cancer Institute (DFCI) One to One—The Cancer Connection
(617) 632-4880

Helps arrange for you to talk with a present or former DFCI patient who is matched to you by disease and treatment. You do not have to be a DFCI patient to take advantage of this service.

Basic reading and reference material

Taber's Cyclopedic Medical Dictionary, by F. A. Davis Company is illustrated in full color and has concise, helpful information. It is used by nurses as a standard reference.

The Cancer Dictionary, by Robert Altman and Michael Sarg, is a good medical dictionary specifically for cancer survivors.

Steadman's Medical Dictionary, published by Williams and Wilkins, is another excellent reference. It uses a categorical organization that is very helpful.

Leukemia, by Edward S. Henderson, MD, et al. (Philadelphia: W.B. Saunders Company, 1996) is an excellent text for general information about the leukemias.

Leukaemia and Related Disorders, by J. A. Whittaker and J. A. Holmes (Oxford: Blackwell Science, 1998) This text, written by two of Great Britain's foremost oncologists, is broad-based and full of information.

The National Library of Medicine's MEDLINE database
http://www.ncbi.nlm.nih.gov/entrez/query.fcgi

The best place to find the published results of studies on cancer treatment and care, it houses more than nine million research papers. If you need help searching, you can call the National Library of Medicine at (800) 272-4787 or (301) 496-6308.

The U.S. National Cancer Institute (NCI)
Bethesda, MD 20892
(800) 4-CANCER
http://cancernet.nci.nih.gov

A division of the National Institutes of Health, the NCI has a hotline to help cancer survivors with a variety of issues, such as physician referrals, and maintains an enormous web site and numerous tracts, statements, booklets, and books about cancer treatment and care. Many of the statements about cancer come from the Physicians Data Query (PDQ) in two versions, patient's and physician's. You might prefer to start with the patient's version, but it's likely that, as you learn more, the physician's statements will provide better, more detailed answers to your questions.

Document Retrieval Services can fax or mail you the full text of any published research paper. On the Internet, the Medline service providers Biomednet, Health-Gate, Medscape, Helix, PDRnet.Com, Infotrieve, PaperChase, and others offer full-text services for a fee. Do a Web search for any of these names.

Other companies that will do medical information searches for you for a fee include:

The Health Resource, Inc.
(501) 329-5272

Can Help
(360) 437-2291

Schine On-Line Services
(800) FIND-CURE

General cancer resources

The following resources, while not specific for leukemia, are varied and numerous, and are likely to offer you aid and services suited to your needs.

Organizations

Agency for Health Care Policy and Research
P.O. Box 8547
Silver Spring, MD 20907-8547
(800) 358-9295

American Cancer Society (ACS) National Office
1599 Clifton Road NE
Atlanta, GA 30329-4251
(800) ACS-2345
http://www.cancer.org

The American Cancer Society has many national and local programs to help cancer survivors with problems such as travel, lodging, and emotional support. ACS publishes an excellent book, *Informed Decisions: The Complete Book of Cancer Diagnosis, Treatment and Recovery.* This hefty book is a comprehensive guide to care and treatment for all aspects of all cancers. ACS also offers a 24-hour support line for both English- and Spanish-speaking cancer survivors. Check your local phone directory for the office nearest you or contact the national office. ACS also hosts the Cancer Survivors Network web site.

American Red Cross
430 17th Street NW
Washington, DC 20006
(202) 737-8300

The American Self-Help Clearinghouse
25 Pocono Road
Denville, NJ 07834
(973) 625-7101

Publishes a national directory of self-help groups.

American Institute of Stress
124 Park Avenue
Yonkers, NY 10703
(914) 963-1200
fax (914) 965-6267
http://www.stress.org
stress124@earthlink.net

The institute publishes a monthly newsletter, *Health and Stress.*

Bloch, R. A. Cancer Foundation
4400 Main Street
Kansas City, MO 64111
(800) 433-0460
(816) 932-8453

Offers a variety of services to cancer patients and survivors, such as books, telephone-based second medical opinions, and one-on-one phone contact between cancer survivors.

Burger King Cancer Caring Center
4117 Liberty Avenue
Pittsburgh, PA 15224
(412) 622-1212

Provides counseling and a hotline service for those with cancer.

Cancer Care, Inc.
275 Seventh Avenue
New York, NY 10001
(212) 302-2400 or (800) 813-HOPE
fax (212) 719-0263
info@cancercare.org
http://www.cancercare.org

Provides information, teleconferences, and support for those affected by cancer.

Cancer Family Care
7162 Reading Road, Suite 1050
Cincinnati, OH 45237
(513) 731-3346

Offers counseling to families affected by cancer.

Cancer Research Institute
681 Fifth Avenue
New York, NY 10022
(800) 99-CANCER

Offers services such as PDQ searches for clinical trials and free literature on cancer.

Cancervive
6500 Wilshire Boulevard, Suite 500
Los Angeles, CA 90048
(213) 655-3758

Offers many services to cancer survivors.

Center for Medical Consumers
237 Thompson Street
New York, NY 10012
(212) 674-7105

Provides information referrals to other organizations and maintains a medical consumer's library.

Consumer Health Information Research Institute
300 East Pink Hill Road
Independence, MO 64057
(816) 228-4595
http://www.reutershealth.com

Provides an integrity index and a credibility of publication index, including one that rates cancer books.

Hereditary Cancer Institute
2500 California Plaza
Omaha, NE 68178
(402) 280-1746 or (402) 280-2942

Evaluates families for risk and furnishes educational material to families with hereditary cancers.

International CANCER Alliance/I Care
48653 Cordell Ave, Suite 11
Bethesda, MD 20814
(800) I CARE 61
http://www.icare.org

Provides newsletter *Cancer Breakthroughs*, educational information, and cancer treatment reviews.

Make Today Count
1235 East Cherokee
Springfield, MO 65804
(800) 432-2273

Offers peer support via local chapters for those with life-threatening illnesses.

Mautamar Project for Lesbians with Cancer
1707 L Street NW, Suite 1060
Washington, DC 20036
(202) 332-5536

Offers support to lesbians and their families.

National Coalition for Cancer Research
426 C Street NE
Washington, DC 20002
(202) 544-1880

An activist group that monitors government spending on cancer.

National Coalition for Cancer Survivorship
1010 Wayne Avenue, 5th Floor
Silver Spring, MD 20910
(301) 650-8868
http://www.cansurvive.org

Formed by cancer survivors to offer support and to effect change in progress against cancer through legislative efforts. It has published the *Cancer Survivor's Almanac*, a good reference for any cancer survivor.

National Family Caregivers Association
9621 East Bexhill Drive
Kensington, MD 20895
(800)-896-3650

Provides a variety of services to caregivers.

National Patient Advocate Foundation
735 Thimble Shoals Boulevard, Suite A
Newport News, VA 23606
(757) 873-0438
fax (757) 873-1082
http://www.npaf.org
action@npaf.org

A national network for healthcare reform, provides assistance in dealing with problems encountered with managed care providers.

People Living Through Cancer, Inc.
323 Eighth Street, SW
Albuquerque, NM 87102
(505) 242-3263
cancerhope@aol.com

Offers many services to cancer survivors.

Well Spouse Foundation
610 Lexington Avenue, Suite 814
New York, NY 10022
(800) 838-0879

Offers support to those whose spouses are chronically ill.

Wellness Community
2716 Ocean Park Boulevard, Suite 1040
Santa Monica, CA 90405
(310) 314-2555

Branches are located throughout the US. Check your local phone book for the chapter nearest you. Provides support groups, and activity programs for cancer survivors.

Books about cancer

The Alpha Book on Cancer and Living. Alameda, California: The Alpha Institute, 1993.

Brenner, David J., and Eric Hall. *Making the Radiation Therapy Decision.* RGA Publishing Group, 1996.

Cancer Rates and Risks, 2000. The National Cancer Institute, (800) 4-CANCER.

Crane, Judy B. *How to Survive Your Hospital Stay.* Westlake Village, California: The Center Press, 1997.

Cukier, Daniel, and Virginia McCullough. *Coping with Radiation Therapy: A Ray of Hope.* Los Angeles: Lowell House, 1996.

Dollinger, M., E. Rosenbaum, and G. Cable, editors. *Everyone's Guide to Cancer Therapy.* Andrews & McMeel, 1998.

Drum, D. *Making the Chemotherapy Decision.* Lowell House, 1997.

Dunn, Steve. *CancerGuide. http://www.cancerguide.org/sdunn_story.html.*

Finn, Robert. *Cancer Clinical Trials: Experimental Treatments and How They Can Help You.* Sebastopol, CA: O'Reilly and Associates, 1999.

Friedman, A., T. Klein, and H. Friedman. *Psychoneuroimmunology, Stress, and Infection.* New York: CRC Press, 1996.

Glaser, Ronald, and Janice Kiecolt-Glaser. *Handbook of Human Stress and Immunity.* New York: Academic Press, 1994.

Harpham, Wendy Schlessel. *After Cancer: A Guide to Your New Life.* New York: W.W. Norton, 1994.

Harpham, Wendy Schlessel. *Diagnosis: Cancer.* New York: W.W. Norton, 1998.

Harpham, Wendy Schlessel. *When a Parent Has Cancer: A Guide to Caring for Your Children*. HarperCollins, 1997.

Hoffman, Barbara, ed., The National Coalition for Cancer Survivorship. *A Cancer Survivor's Almanac*. Minneapolis: Chronimed, 1996.

Inlander, Charles B., ed. *People's Medical Society Health Desk Reference: Information Your Doctor Can't or Won't Tell You*. New York: Hyperion, 1996.

Johnson, J., and L. Klein. *I Can Cope: Staying Healthy with Cancer*. Minneapolis: Chronimed, 1994.

Keene, Nancy. *Working with Your Doctor: Getting the Healthcare You Deserve*. Sebastopol, CA: O'Reilly & Associates, 1998.

Lerner, Michael. *Choices in Healing: Integrating the Best of Conventional and Complementary Approaches to Cancer*. Cambridge: MIT Press, 1996.

Lee, G. Richard, MD, et al., *Wintrobe's Clinical Hematology*. Baltimore: Lippincott Williams & Wilkins, 1999. Medical information on all phases of hematology. This is the book used by professionals, and patients may find it hard to navigate to find material scattered throughout the book.

McKay, J., N. Hirano, and M. Lampenfeld. *The Chemotherapy and Radiation Therapy Survival Guide*. New Harbinger Publications, 1998.

The Merck Manual. Mark H. Beers, MD and Robert Berkow, MD. Merck Research Laboratories: Whitehouse Satation, NJ, 1999. Available in either the paper version or in the Home version at the web site (*http://www.merck.com*), a vast resource. Many public libraries have a copy of the Merck Manual in their non-circulating reference section.

Murphy, G., L. Morris, and D. Lange, editors. *Informed Decisions: The Complete Book of Cancer Diagnosis, Treatment and Recovery*. The American Cancer Society. New York: Viking Press, 1997.

PDQ Treatment Statements for Patients or Professionals. The National Cancer Institute. Covers ALL, AML, CLL, CML, and HCL. *http://cancernet.nci.nih.gov/pdq/pdq-treatment.shtml*

Olson, Kaye, R.N. *Surgery and Recovery: How to Reduce Anxiety and Promote Healthy Healing*. Traverse City, Michigan: Rhodes and Easton, 1998.

Radiation Therapy and You, a 50-page booklet available from the U.S. National Cancer Institute by calling (800) 4-CANCER.

Schover, L. *Sexuality and Fertility After Cancer*. New York: John Wiley & Sons, 1997.

Theodosakis, Jason, MD and Feinberg, David T., MD. *Don't Let your HMO Kill You*. New York: Rutledge, 1999.

Zakarian, Beverly. *The Activist Cancer Patient*. New York: John Wiley & Sons, 1996.

Zukerman, Eugenia, and Julie Ingelfinger. *Coping with Prednisone (and other cortisone-related medicines)*. New York: St. Martin's Press, 1997.

Magazines dealing with cancer

Cancer Communication
Published by PAACT
Patient Advocates for Advanced Cancer Treatments
1143 Parmelee Northwest
Grand Rapids, MI 49504
(616) 453-1477

Coping
P.O. Box 682268
Franklin, TN 37068
(615) 790-2400

Living Through Cancer
323 Eighth Street, SW
Albuquerque, NM 87102
(505) 242-3263

Medical resources

Medical information targeted to special topics is available through the resources listed in these categories.

Organizations that provide information about doctor and hospital credentials

The American College of Surgeons
633 North Saint Clair Street
Chicago, IL 60611
(312) 202-5000

Can verify whether your surgeon is board certified in a surgical specialty.

Center for Medical Consumers
237 Thompson Street
New York, NY 10012
(212) 674-7105

Provides information referrals to other organizations and maintains a medical consumer's library.

College of American Pathologists
325 Waukegan Road
Northfield, IL 60093-2750
(800) 323-4040

The Consumer Health Information Research Institute
(816) 228-4595
http://www.reutershealth.com

Provides an integrity index and a credibility of publication index.

Foundation for Accreditation of Hematopoietic Cell Therapy (FACHT)
Linda Miller, MPA
FAHCT Administration Office
University of Nebraska Medical Center
986065 Nebraska Medical Center
Omaha, NE 68198-6065
fax (402)595-1144.
http://www.unmc.edu/Community/fahct/accredi.htm

Organization that gives accreditation to transplant centers. This web site lists the accredited hematopoietic cell therapy (BMT/PSCT) centers. Each center will have to provide you with its own statistics for transplantation.

The Joint Commission on Accreditation of Health Care Organizations (JCAHO)
1 Renaissance Boulevard
Oakbrook Terrace, IL 60181
(630) 792-5800

National Council Against Health Fraud
P.O. Box 1276
Loma Linda, CA 92354
(909) 824-4690

Books about doctors and hospitals

American Medical Association Directory of Physicians in the US, published by the American Medical Association, provides a means to verify your doctor's credentials. The AMA's *Physician Select* web site (*http://www.ama-assn.org/aps/amahg.html*) is an excellent means to check your doctor's education and board certification.

The Official ABMS Directory of Board Certified Medical Specialists 1998, 1997. Also, Marquis' *Who's Who*. This is a directory of board certified physicians who have chosen to specialize in a particular area of medicine.

US News and World Report's annual "Best Hospitals" edition. Write to 2400 N Street NW Washington, DC 20037-1196, or call (202) 955-2000.

Web sites concerning doctors and hospitals

QuackWatch
http://www.quackwatch.com

QuackWatch gives the medical scientist's evaluation of those unusual remedies you've been hearing about.

American Board of Medical Specialties
http://www.abms.org

Gives data about a doctor's education, license.

HealthGrades
http://www.healthgrades.com

Provides healthcare report cards for all areas of healthcare.

Other helpful Web sites include:

http://www.searchpointe.com/
http://www.certifieddoctor.org/
http://www.certifieddoctor.org/verify.html
http://www.docboard.org

Bone marrow transplantation

This expensive and lengthy treatment procedure is addressed by the following publications and support groups.

Donor registries

The Blood and Marrow Transplant Information Network
(847) 433-3313 or (888) 597-7674
http://www.bmtinfonet.org
Maintains a list of facilities that accept donations of cord blood for public use.

The Caitlin Raymond Registry
(800) 726-2824 or (508) 792-8969
fax (508) 792-8972
Info@CRIR.org
http://www.crir.org)
Provides cord blood referrals.

The National Marrow Donor Program
(800) MARROW2
Office of Patient Advocacy telephone (888) 999-6743
http//www.marrow.org
Provides cord blood referrals.

**American Bone Marrow Donor Registry Search Coordinating Center,
Patient Search Information**
(800) 7-A-MATCH or (800) 726-2824

Transplant centers

The Blood and Marrow Transplant Newsletter
(847) 433-3313
http://www.bmtinfonet.org
Contains useful information for choosing a cancer center.

Oncology Nursing Society (ONS)
(412) 921-7373

Every two years, the ONS publishes an extensive guide to transplant centers. There is a minimal charge for the booklet.

The National Marrow Donor Program
800) 654-1247 or (800) 526-7809

Publishes a booklet on transplantation using an unrelated donor.

GrannyBarb and Art's Leukemia Links
http://www.acor.org/leukemia/bmtctrs.html.

Contains a current list of cancer centers.

Reading material for transplantation

Bone Marrow Transplantation and Peripheral Blood Stem Cell Transplantation. The National Cancer Institute offers this treatise on marrow or stem cell transplantation. On the web at *http://cancernet.nci.nih.gov* or call (800) 4-CANCER.

Martin, Paul, MD (member, Fred Hutchinson Cancer Research Center; professor of medicine, University of Washington.) *A Short Primer on HLA and Bone Marrow Transplantation.* On the web at *http://www.giftoflife.com/articles.htm.*

Stewart, Susan L. *Autologous Stem Cell Transplants: A Handbook for Patients.* Highland Park, Illinois: Blood and Marrow Transplant Information Network, 2000. *http://www.bmtinfonet.org.*

Stewart, Susan L. *Bone Marrow Transplants: A Book of Basics for Patients.* Highland Park, Illinois: BMT Newsletter, 1992. *http://www.bmtinfonet.org.*

Transplant Center Access Directory. National Marrow Donor Program. Call (800) 526-7809; or on the Web at *http://www.marrow.org* and *http://www.bmtinfo.org.*

Reading material for finding a donor

"Tissue Typing for Beginners": *http://www.umds.ac.uk/tissue/what1.html.*

HLA Gene and Haplotype Frequencies in the North American Population: The National Marrow Donor Program Donor Registry: *http://www.swmed.edu/home_pages/ASHI/prepr/Motomi.htm.*

Haplotype searching: *http://www.swmed.edu/home_pages/ASHI/prepr/ mori_abd.htm.*

Histocompatibility: Interpretation and Correlation of HLA Typing for Bone Marrow Transplantation: *http://www.bmtinfo.org/bmt/topics/htm/type_b.htm.*

HLA Class I and II Sequence Alignments: *http://www.anthonynolan.com/HIG/data.html.*

Transplant advocacy and support groups

Blood and Marrow Transplant Information Network
2900 Skokie Valley Road, Suite B
Highland Park, IL 60035
(847) 433-3313, toll free (888) 597-7674
http://www.bmtinfonet.org

Offers support, publications, and guidance to legal aid for those getting transplants.

Bone Marrow Transplant Family Support Network
P.O. Box 845
Avon, CT 06001
(800) 826-9376

Offers counseling and support for those going through a transplant.

Living Bank
4545 Post Oak Place, Suite 315
Houston, TX 77027
(800) 528-2971

Motivates and facilitates organ donor commitment.

National Bone Marrow Transplant Link
29209 Northwestern Highway, No. 624
Southfield, MI 48034
(800) LINK-BMT
http://comnet.org/nbmtlink

Offers peer support and a variety of services for those being transplanted.

National Marrow Donor Program
3433 Broadway Street, NE, Suite 400
Minneapolis, MN 55413
(800) MARROW-2

Coordinates national and international testing and matching of marrow donors and recipients.

Organ Transplant Fund
1027 South Yates
Memphis, TN 38119
(800) 489-3863

Provides a variety of services, including financial services, to those receiving transplants.

Drug and dosage information

Organizations

U.S. Food and Drug Administration (FDA)
5600 Fishers Lane
Rockville, MD 20857
(301) 827-4420
(888) 332-4543
(800) 532-4440
http://www.fda.gov

You can report adverse effects of drugs to the FDA, too, or use their MedWatch web site: *http://www.fda.gov/medwatch/how.htm*.

Books

The Physician's Desk Reference (PDR), a compendium of information about drugs, is now reprinted in versions that are easier for the general public to understand, but you might appreciate the learning experience gained from reading the original PDR. In addition to PDR, many other drug encyclopedias are available as well for the general public.

Web sites for pharmaceutical companies

Clinical Pharmacology Online
http://www.cponline.gsm.com

DrugInfoNet
http://www.druginfonet.com

Glaxo's DoseCalc
http://www.meds.com/DChome.htm

HealthTouch
http://www.healthtouch.com/level1/p_dri.htm

PharmInfoNet
http://pharminfo.com

RxList
http://www.rxlist.com

Calculating body surface area

Cornell University
http://www-users.med.cornell.edu/~spon/picu/bsacalc.htm

Martindale's HS Guide
http://www-sci.lib.uci.edu/HSG/Pharmacy.html

Medical College of Wisconsin
http://www.intmed.mcw.edu/clincalc/body.html

Pain and other side effects

The American Cancer Society has many programs to help cancer survivors with problems such as pain. Call (800) ACS-2345 or check your local phone directory for the office nearest you.

American Society of Anesthesiologists
515 Busse Highway
Park Ridge, IL 60068
(847) 825-5586

American Society of Clinical Hypnosis
2200 East Vine Avenue, Suite 291
Des Plaines, IL 60018
(847) 297-3317

National Lymphedema Network
2211 Post Street, Suite 404
San Francisco, CA 94115
(800) 541-3259
Provides information on swollen limbs, which may occur soon or many years after treatment.

Pain-management web sites

All of the States in the USA have Cancer Pain Initiatives. Many have web sites, so do a web search to see if your state has a Cancer Pain Initiative site.

Cancer Care's web site about Cancer Pain: Let's Talk about it.
http://www.cancercare.org/clinical/page1.htm
Discusses causes, assessment, treatment, side-effects, myths, etc.

Cancer-pain.org
http://www.cancer-pain.org
A web page created by the *Association of Cancer Online Resources* (ACOR) with input and advice from patients, caregivers and an Advisory Board of health care professionals dedicated to providing the most advanced cancer pain relief.

Talaria
http://www.talaria.org
Talaria, a resource for healthcare professionals, addresses the management of pain in patients with cancer. It provides a hypermedia implementation of the *Clinical Practice Guideline on the Management of Cancer Pain*, a publication of the Agency for Health Care Policy and Research. Excellent reference for what is state of the art.

Tests and procedures

These resources can help you learn how tests are done, and what the results mean.

Information on how tests are done

Andrews, Maraca and Michael Shaw. *Everything You Need to Know About Medical Tests.* Springhouse, 1996. An excellent, comprehensive (691 pages) reference written for the patient in a readable and respectful style.

Barry, L., ed., with Peter Zaret, and Lee D. Jatlow. *The Patient's Guide to Medical Tests.* Houghton Mifflin Co., 1997.

The Biology Project. University of Arizona: *http://www.biology.arizona.edu.*

Brodin, Michael B. *The Encyclopedia of Medical Tests.* Pocket Books, 1997.

Department of Pathology, University of Washington, Seattle: *http://www.pathology.washington.edu.*

The Family Internet site at *http://familyinternet.com.*

N.L. Glifford, PhD, *Common Blood Tests.* Makes the complex subject of blood tests understandable.

HealthGate: *http://www.healthgate.com.*

Mid-South Imaging & Therapeutics, P.A.: *http://www.msit.com.*

Mosby Consumer Health Series: http://www.mosbych1.com/mhc/top/003833.htm.

Pagana, Kathleen, and Timothy Pagana, editors. *Mosby's Diagnostic and Laboratory Test Reference.* Mosby, 1992.

Shtasel, Philip. *Medical Tests and Diagnostic Procedures: A Patient's Guide to Just What the Doctor Ordered.* Harper and Row, 1990.

Stauffer, Joseph, and Joseph C. Segen. *The Patient's Guide to Medical Tests: Everything You Need to Know About the Tests Your Doctor Prescribes.* Facts on File, 1997.

ThriveOnline: *http://www.thriveonline.com.*

University of California at Los Angeles: *http://anima.crump.ucla.edu.*

Normal values for tests

The American Society for Clinical Laboratory Science
http://ascls.org/labtesting/index.htm

A page (with pictures) that explains the CBC and other laboratory blood tests.

Haematological Malignancy Diagnostic Service
http://www.hmds.org.uk/index.shtml

A page (with pictures) that explains all laboratory blood tests. Since this comes from Leeds University in the UK, the normal ranges will be expressed in European terms.

The Lupus Lab Tests
http://www.mtio.com/mclfa/lfalt1.htm

This site has tests commonly done for lupus, but many of these are also done for hematologic cancers such as leukemia, and they are easy to understand.

The University of California Division of General Internal Medicine.
http://www.oncolink.upenn.edu

Enter the test name and click.

The University of Michigan Pathology Laboratories Handbook
http://po.path.med.umich.edu/handbook

Enter the test name and click.

Understand the Immune System
http://rex.nci.nih.gov/PATIENTS/INFO_TEACHER/bookshelf/NIH_immune/index.html

This link has the simplest explanation of the blood count morphology, along with antibody expression, VJ regions, etc. The illustrations help immensely to build understanding.

HLA and the Immune Response
http://www.ama-assn.org/special/hiv/newsline/briefing/hla.htm#structure

There is a lot of information about human leukocyte antigen matching, herpesviruses (shingles), Epstein Barr virus, etc. and how they affect the immune response as well as how they might be associated with certain types of cancer.

Web resources for tests and procedures

Because the web is a constantly updated resource, home pages are offered here instead of direct URLs.

Thriveonline
http://www.thriveonline.com

To find information on many tests, this site has a search engine into which you may enter a test name.

HealthGate
http://www.healthgate.com/HealthGate/free/dph/static

Also for many tests and bone marrow aspirations

FISH: Department of Pathology, University of Washington, Seattle
http://www.pathology.washington.edu

The Biology Project, University of Arizona
http://www.biology.arizona.edu

Immunophenotyping State University of New York at Stony Brook, Department of Pathology
http://www.path.sunysb.edu/hemepath/tutorial/immuno/immuno.htm

MUGA scan: HealthAnswers
http://www.healthanswers.com

The Family Internet site
http://familyinternet.com

Mid-South Imaging & Therapeutics, P.A.
http://www.msit.com

Nuclear Medicine Tests: The University of California at Los Angeles site
http://anima.crump.ucla.edu

Clinical trials and investigational new substances

Books

The book *Intuitive Biostatistics,* by Harvey Motulsky, can help you understand published results of clinical trials, and can help you assess trial design if you're planning to enroll in a trial.

Web sites

The Food and Drug Administration
(800) 532-4440
http:///www.fda.gov

The FDA contains regulations for investigational new drugs and for importing foreign drugs for single-patient use.

The National Cancer Institute Clinical Trials web site
http://cancertrials.nci.nih.gov and the new one *http://CancerTrials.gov*

This is the most comprehensive way to locate trials of new substances and treatments.

QuackWatch
http://www.quackwatch.com

Gives the medical scientist's evaluation of those unusual remedies you've been hearing about.

Steve Dunn's Cancerguide
http://www.cancerguide.org/sdunn_story.html
dunns@h2net.net

This is an excellent resource for learning how to assess clinical trials and how to research your illness.

Complementary and alternative medicine

Share with your treating physician what alternative remedies you are using, whether it's vitamins and minerals or mushrooms. Use *www.quackwatch.com* before you act upon any recommendation for complementary and alternative treatments.

For people who have some curiosity about complementary and alternative medicines, the National Center for Complementary and Alternative Medicine (NCCAM), of the National Institutes of Health has a web site that serves both researchers and consumers who want to explore the literature available on non-Western healing modalities. The web address for this site is *http://nccam.nih.gov/nccam*.

Here you can use the NCCAM Complementary and Alternative Medicine (CAM) Citation Index (CCI) (*http://156.40.172.112*) that contains more than 175,000 bibliographic citations from 1963 to the present. These citations were extracted from the National Library of Medicine's Medline database. The citations were obtained using MeSH controlled vocabulary terms from the "alternative medicine" tree structure, and other selected MeSH terms.

There's also HerbMed(r) (*http://www.amfoundation.org/herbmed.htm*) an interactive, electronic herbal database which provides hyperlinked access to the scientific data underlying the use of herbs for health. It is an evidence-based information resource for professionals, researchers, and general public. HerbMed(r) is a project of the Alternative Medicine Foundation, Inc. (*http://www.amfoundation.org*) provided as a freely available, public resource.

Searching for information on herbal remedies here provides:

- Human Clinical Data on use (all supported by citations from the medical literature with active links to PubMed)
- Traditional and Folk Use Reports (again with links to PubMed)
- Contraindications and Adverse & Toxic Effects (again with links to citations in PubMed)

Books

N.D. Francis J. Brinker, *Herb Contraindications And Drug Interactions*. Eclectic Medical Publications: 1998. It uses data from the German Commission E Monographs, the world's most respected source of recent scientific research and traditional clinical experience.

Lucinda G. Miller and Wallace J. Murray (editors). *Herbal Medicinals: A Clinician's Guide*. Haworth, 1999.

PDR Family Guide to Natural Medicines & Healing Therapies, 1st edition (Medical Economics Company, Inc.).

PDR for Herbal Medicines. Medical Economics Company Inc., 1999. This book combines the work of Germany's Commission E, the foremost regulatory body in the world on herbal medicines, with the expertise of Jöerg Grüenwald, PhD, a world-renowned botanist and expert on herbal medicines.

Schuyler W. Lininger Jr. (editor). *The A-Z Guide to Drug-Herb and Vitamin Interactions*. Prima Publications, 1999.

Acupuncture

American Association of Oriental Medicine
433 Front Street
Catasauqua, PA 18032-2506
Phone: (610) 266-1433
Fax: (610) 264-2768
AAOM1@aol.com

National Acupuncture and Oriental Medicine Alliance
P.O. Box 77511
Seattle, WA 98177-0531
(206) 524-3511
76143.2061@compuserve.com

National Acupuncture Foundation
1718 M Street, Suite 195
Washington, D.C. 20036
(202) 332-5794

The following two web sites have useful information about acupuncture:

- *http://www.acupuncture.com/Referrals/ref2.htm*
- *http://www.acupuncture.com/StateLaws/StateLaws.htm*

Massage

American Massage Therapy Association
820 Davis Street, Suite 100
Evanston, IL 60201-4444
(847) 864-0123
fax (847) 864-1178
http://www.amtamassage.org

Also, the publication Massage just printed some articles about massage in March/April 2000 issue. There are abstracts at *http://www.massagemag.com*. The magazine says that NCI endorses the use of massage for musculoskeletal pain in cancer patients. Jacox A. et al., "Management of Cancer Pain: Adults Quick Reference Guide." There also has been a study of therapies such as massage with leukemia, Caudell, K.A., "Psychoneuroimmunology and Innovative Behavioral Interventions in Patients with Leukemia," *Oncology Nursing Forum*, 1996; 23(3):493–502.

The site *http://altmedicine.about.com/health/altmedicine/msubmssg.htm* has many helpful links to massage information as well.

Healthcare financial and legal issues

Beyond the physical aspects of cancer lie its effects on careers and finances. The following resources can offer guidance and aid.

Organizations

The Blood and Marrow Transplant Newsletter
1985 Spruce Avenue
Highland Park, IL 60035
(847) 831-1913

Offers guidance to legal aid for those seeking transplants.

The Center for Medical Consumers
237 Thompson Street
New York, NY 10012
(212) 674-7105

Provides information referrals to other organizations and maintains a medical consumer's library.

Consumer Credit Counseling
(800) 388-2227

Can provide help getting expenses under control.

The Federal Trade Commission
(202) 326-3650

Can provide information about the federal Consumer Credit Protection Act, a landmark series of laws passed in 1968 to protect debtors.

Health Care Cost Hotline
(900) 225-2500

Can furnish the median fee and range of fees charged by doctors for various services and procedures. The call is $2.00 to $4.00 per minute.

Health Insurance Association of America (HIAA)
555 13th Street NW
Washington, D.C. 20004
(202) 824-1600
http://www.hiaa.org/index.html

Has more than 250 members consisting of insurers and managed care companies. HIAA can supply booklets on disability income, health insurance, long-term care, medical savings accounts, and general insurance information, including a directory of state insurance departments.

Lexis Law Publishing
(800) 542-0957

This group can send you a copy of any law.

The Medical Information Bureau (MIB)
P.O. Box 105, Essex Station
Boston, MA 02112
(617) 424-3660

Records all entries made by insurance companies about your health, and will send a copy of this information to your physician if you request it. If you find an error in these files, you can contact the bureau for the procedures necessary to correct errors.

The Organ Transplant Fund
1027 South Yates
Memphis, TN 38119
(800) 489-3863

Provides help with fundraising to those receiving transplants.

Magazines
Health Pages reports on ranges and norms of doctor's fees. Call (212) 929-6131.
Medical Economics reports on ranges and norms of doctor's fees. Call (201) 945-9058.

Social Security Administration bulletins
The chief resource in this category is the 1997 Social Security Handbook. On the Web at *http://www.ssa.gov/OP_Home/ handbook/ssa-hbk.htm.* (2001 revision expected soon.)

Other, more specific SSA bulletins include:

Social Security: What You Need To Know When You Get Disability Benefits (6/96; Pub. No. 05-10153)

Social Security Disability Programs (5/96; Pub. No. 05-10057)

Social Security: If You Are Blind, How We Can Help (6/96; Pub. No. 05-10052)

A Guide to Social Security and SSI Disability Benefits for People with HIV Infection (6/95; Pub. No. 05-10020)

Disability Based on Drug Addiction or Alcoholism (5/96; Pub. No. 05-10047)

How We Decide If You Are Still Disabled (4/96; Pub. No. 05-10053)

How Social Security Can Help with Vocational Rehabilitation (9/94; Pub. No. 05-10050)

Working While Disabled...How We Can Help (1/96; Pub. No. 05-10095)

Red Book on Work Incentives for People with Disabilities (8/95; Pub. No. 64-030)

Insurance Links

Some helpful Web sites with information about insurance are:

> *http://www.cancercareinc.org/patients/plinksfinancial.htm*
>
> *http://www.cancercareinc.org/patients/plinks2.htm*
>
> *http://www.go.com/WebDir/Business/Management/Insurance/For_individuals/Cancer_insurance*

For an insurance-related Web site that deals specifically with cancer, go to:

> *http://www.vh.org/Patients/IHB/Cancer/NCI/FacingForward/04.html*

More insurance-related Web sites include:

A Shopper's Guide to Cancer Insurance
http://www.state.wi.us/agencies/oci/pub_list/pi-001.htm

America's Guide category of Cancer Insurance
http://www.americasguide.com/national.asp?cat=CIN
http://www.noah.cuny.edu/cancer/cancercare/library/cobra.html
Information About COBRA

Conquering Cancer, but Way Behind on the Bills
http://www.cancerinsurance.com/English/Collaterals/NY_Times_16NOV1997.html

Medical Insurance: A "Hidden Crisis" for a Growing Number of Cancer Patients
http://noah.cuny.edu/cancer/cancercare/library/crisis.html

Financial Assistance
http://noah.cuny.edu/cancer/cancercare/services/financia.html

Catholic Charities web links
http://www.ccspm.org/links.htm

United Way
http://www.unitedway.org

The Robert Wood Johnson Foundation
http://www.rwjf.org/text.html

The Medicine Program
http://www.themedicineprogram.com/info.html
http://www.cancersupportivecare.com/drug_assistance.html
Drug assistance programs from pharmaceutical companies:

National Association for the Terminally Ill
P.O. Box 368
Shelbyville, KY 40066
Free phone line: (888) 847-0390
http://www.terminallyill.org

The National Association for the Terminally Ill, gives financial assistance to the children and families of those suffering from a terminal illness whose life expectancy is five (5) years or less. Help with day-to-day living expenses such as: rent or mortgage, groceries, electric, car payments, insurance payments, etc. is provided according to the need of each family on a case-by-case basis.

Free treatment resources

The National Cancer Institute
Bethesda, Maryland
(800) 4-CANCER

They will in some cases help pay for the travel and lodging expenses of those being treated at the NCI in addition to providing free treatment.

Free travel for care—US

There are charitable groups that will fly you to treatment free of charge. Some groups require that patients be able to embark and disembark from the plane without airline assistance or that support equipment be manageable without airline intervention.

Air Care Alliance (ACA)
(888) 662-6794
(757) 318-9145
http://www.angelflightfla.org/aircareall.org/acahome.html.
Helps cancer patients travel to distant health centers for care.

Air LifeLine
(877) AIR-LIFE (toll free number)
http:// www.airlifeline.org

AirLifeLine is a national, non-profit organization that provides free air transportation to medical facilities for people who cannot afford commercial flights. AirLifeLine partners with Ronald McDonald House Charities and the American Cancer Society. It is a major humanitarian organization, with over 1,000 pilots who volunteer their time and pay for fuel and other flight expenses. See the web site or call the toll free number for eligibility requirements.

Corporate Angel Network
(914) 328-1313
http://www.corpangelnetwork.org

Helps cancer patients travel to distant health centers for care in empty seats on regularly scheduled flights. There is no financial hardship requirement. Patients must be able to fly without any form of life support or medical assistance.

The Leukemia and Lymphoma Society
(800) 955-4LSA
http://www.leukemia-lymphoma.org

Will reimburse up to $750 per year in travel/or drug expenses.

Mercy Medical Airlift
(800) 296-1191
http://www.mercymedical.org

Helps cancer patients travel to distant health centers for care. Will direct patients to best available options on Air Care Alliance (private aviation sector), Corporate Angel Network (empty seats on commercial flights), or be able to tell patients about occasional special prices or free tickets for those who need to travel for medical care, but who cannot afford full ticket prices.

The Red Cross
(202) 728-6400 or (202) 728-6401 (24 hour line)

The Red Cross provides emergency travel and communication for military personnel. Call to find the chapter nearest you or your destination.

Free travel for care—Canada

In addition to the Mission Air Transportation Network (416) 222-6335 with information listed above, the following Canadian services are available:

The Canadian Cancer Society
(604) 872-4400 or (416) 961-7223

Offers various forms of assistance. The following table lists Canadian Cancer Society resource numbers by province:

Province	Phone number
Alberta	(403) 228-4487
Manitoba	(204) 774-7493
New Brunswick	(506) 634-6272
Newfoundland and Labrador	(709) 753-6520
Nova Scotia	(902) 423-6183
Ontario	(416) 488-5400
Prince Edward Island	(902) 566-4007

Province	Phone number
Quebec	(514) 255-5151
Saskatchewan	(306) 757-4260

The British Columbia Medical Services Plan
(800) 661-2628 or (250) 387-8277

Coordinates sharing travel expenses with commercial transportation firms such as airlines or ferries. Your doctor must fill out a travel assistance form.

Hope Air
(877) 346-4673 (Canada Toll Free)

Air tickets are donated by airlines so travelers fly free; however, travelers don't find out until about 4 days before traveling whether or not there are tickets available for them. (Thanks to the Vancouver Leukemia Research Foundation for this information.)

Mission Aviation Fellowship (MAF)
(909)794-1151

Supports air ambulance services and medical assistance in 57 countries.

Lodging resources

American Cancer Society's Hope Lodge
http://www.cancer.org/frames.html

Offers free lodging in various cities for cancer patients and their families who travel to receive cancer care when the patient is being treated in nearby facilities. Their service is also available to non-US citizens traveling within the USA for medical care. Lodging is free and provided on a first-come, first-served basis, so contact the ACS for the phone number of the Hope Lodge nearest to your destination. Check your local phone book, or visit their web site.

National Association of Hospital Hospitality Houses (NAHHH)
(301) 961-3094
(317) 883-2226
(800) 542-9730
http://visit-usa.com/hhh/members.htm

Can recommend nearby hotels with reduced rates for cancer patients.

Some major cancer centers like Johns Hopkins in Baltimore and MD Anderson Cancer Center (MDACC) in Houston, Texas have hospital owned outpatient lodging run for the benefit of patients having consults, short, or long-term treatment. The one in Baltimore is mainly geared to patients having long-term treatment. The one at MDACC is run by the Marriott chain, with laundry facilities, a cancer library, an occupational therapy program, a general reading library, a hair dresser who works with wigs, plus a work-out room and swimming pool. In addition it provides a variety of bedrooms and mini-suites. Prices are not cheap, but they are affordable.

End-of-life resources

Resources for increasing comfort and serenity in the last stage of life are included in this category.

Home and hospice care

Community Health Accreditation Program, Inc.
350 Hudson Street
New York, NY 10014
(800) 669-9656

Provides a list of accredited home care organizations.

National Association for Home Care
519 C Street NE
Washington, DC 20002
(202) 547-7424

Represents all home health care agencies in the US. They offer publications on selecting home care.

National Hospice Organization
1901 North Moore Street, Suite 901
Arlington, VA 22209
(800) 658-8898

Offers information on the goals of hospice and how to choose a hospice.

Oley Foundation
214 Hun Memorial
Albany Medical Center A-23
Albany, NY 12208
(800) 776-OLEY

Offers help with parenteral or enteral nutrition—that is, feeding by IV or stomach tube.

Olsten Health Services National Resource Center
175 Broadhollow Road
Melville, NY 11747
(800) 66-NURSE

Offers help with all home health care services.

Visiting Nurse Associations of America
3801 East Florida Avenue, Suite 900
Denver, CO 80210
(800) 426-2547

Provides skilled nurses, aides, and therapists for home care.

Books—general

Basta, Lofty. *A Graceful Exit: Life and Death on Your Own Terms*. New York: Plenum Press, 1996.

Bernard, Jan, and Miriam Schneider. *The True Work of Dying*. New York: Avon, 1996.

Callanan, Maggie, and Patricia Kelley. *Final Gifts: Understanding the Special Awareness, Needs, and Communications of the Dying*. New York: Bantam Books, 1997.

Furman, Joan, and David McNabb. *The Dying Time: Practical Wisdom for the Dying*. New York: Bell Tower, 1997.

Groopman, Jerome. *The Measure of Our Days*. New York: Viking Press, 1997.

Humphry, Derek. *Final Exit: The Practicalities of Self-Deliverance and Assisted Suicide for the Dying*. The Hemlock Society, 1997.

Kramp, Erin Tierney, Douglas H. Kramp, Douglas H. and Emily P. McKhann. *Living with the End in Mind: A Practical Checklist for Living Life to the Fullest by Embracing Your Mortality*. Three Rivers Press, 1998.

Kubler-Ross, Elisabeth. *Death: The Final Stage of Growth*. New York: Simon and Schuster, 1975.

Kubler-Ross, Elisabeth. *Living with Death and Dying*. New York: Touchstone (Simon and Schuster), 1981.

Kubler-Ross, Elisabeth. *On Death and Dying*. Macmillan, 1969.

Kubler-Ross, Elisabeth. *To Live Until We Say Good-bye*. New York: Fireside (Simon and Schuster), 1978.

Lattanzi-Licht, Marcia, John Mahoney, and Galen Miller. *The Hospice Choice: In Pursuit of a Peaceful Death*. New York: Fireside (Simon and Schuster), 1998.

McPhelimy, Lynn. *In the Checklist of Life: A Working Book to Help You Live and Leave Life*. AAIP Publishing Company, 1997.

Nuland, Sherwin. *How We Die: Reflections on Life's Final Chapter*. New York: Alfred A. Knopf, 1993.

Ray, M. Catherine. *I'm with You Now: A Guide Through Incurable Illness for Patients, Families, and Friends*. New York: Bantam Books, 1997.

Weenolsen, Patricia. *The Art of Dying*. New York: St. Martin's Press, 1996.

Books for children

Buscaglia, Leo. *The Fall of Freddie the Leaf*. New York: C.B. Slack, 1982.

Hitchcock, R. *Tim's Dad: A Story About a Boy Whose Father Dies*. Human Services, Springfield, Illinois, 1998.

Holden, L.D. *Gran-Gran's Best Trick: A Story for Children Who Have Lost Someone They Love*. New York: Magination, 1989.

Krementz, Jill. *How It Feels When a Parent Dies*. New York: Alfred A. Knopf, 1981.

LeShan, Ed. *Learning to Say Good-by: When a Parent Dies*. New York: Macmillan, 1976.

O'Toole Donna. *Aarvy Aardvark Finds Hope*. Burnsville, North Carolina: Celo, 1988.

Vigna, J. *Saying Good-bye to Daddy*. Morton Grove, Illinois: Albert Whitman, 1991.

White, E.B. *Charlotte's Web*. New York: Harper & Row, 1952.

Normal Blood and Marrow Test Values

Tables B-1 through B-3 provide approximate quantitative information about certain blood test results. Test results can be influenced by many things, such as how the blood was drawn and stored, whether the patient exercised recently or was dehydrated, how tight the tourniquet was, medications taken by the patient, and so on. Moreover, your lab will display its own norms alongside your test results. These norms may differ from other sources, as each lab recalculates its norms as its data accumulates. After the tables, you will find instructions for calculating absolute lymphocyte counts and absolute neutrophil counts.

Table B-1. Complete Blood Count Values

Component	Measurement	Normal High and Low
White blood cell (WBC)	Number of WBCs in a / µL(microliter)of blood	3.9 –11.3 k/µL
Red blood cell (RBC)	Number of RBCs in a /µL of blood	4.52–5.90m/µL men 4.1–5.10m/µL women
Hemoglobin (HGB)	Number of grams per deciliter of blood	14.0–18.0g/dL men 12.3–15.3g/dL women
Hematocrit (HCT)	Percent of blood volume that is made up of red cells.	40–52 % men 36–45 % women
Mean corpuscular volume (MCV)	Volume of the average red blood cell.	80.0–100 fl
Mean corpuscular hemoglobin (MCH)	Content of hemoglobin in the average red blood cell.	26.4–34.0 pg
Mean corpuscular hemoglobin concentration (MCHC)	Average concentration of hemoglobin in a given volume of red cells; calculated from Hgb and Hct	31.0–36.0 %
Red cell distribution width (RDW)	measure of variation of red cell size	11.5–14.5 %
Platelets (PLT)	Number of platelets in a / µL of blood	140,000 –450,000 /µL

Table B-2. White Count Differential of the CBC

Cell Type	Normal Low	Normal High	Normal Absolute Numbers
Neutrophils (polys)	42 %	78 %	3,000 – 7,000/μL
Bands	0 %	4 %	
Eosinophils	0 %	7 %	50 - 400/μL
Lymphocytes	15 %	45 %	1,000-4,000/μL
Monocytes	0 %	12 %	100-600/μL
Basophils	0 %	2 %	25-100/μL
Atypical Lymphocytes	0 %	4 %	

Table B-3. Other Blood Values in Normal Adults

Test Name	Acronym	Low	High
Beta-2 Microglobulin, g/ml	B2M	0	2.5
Direct Bililrubin, mg/dl	Bili	0	0.4
Total Bilirubin, mg.dl	Bili	0	1.0
Blood urea nitrogen, mg/dl	BUN	8	25
Cholesterol		130	200
Creatinine, mg/dl	CRT	0.6	1.5
Calcium, mg/dl	Ca	8.5	10.5
Chlorine, mEq/l	Cl	95	100
Potassium, mEq/l	K	3.5	5.0
Phosphate, mg/dl	P	2.5	4.5
Sodium, mEq/l	Na	135	145
Magnesium, mEq/l	Mg	1.5	2.5
*Erythrocyte sedimentation Rate, mm/hr	ESR	0	20
Glucose, mg/dl		65	100
Immunoglobulin A, mg/dl	IgA	90	325
Immunoglobulin D, mg/dl	IgD	0.3	30
Immunoglobulin E, mg/dl	IgE	0.002	0.2
Immunoglobulin G, mg/dl	IgG	720	1500
Immunoglobulin M, mg/dl	IgM	45	150
Lactate dehydrogenase, u/l	LDH	100	190
Albumin, gm/dl	Alb	3.5	5.0
Alkaline Phosphate, u/l	AlkP	50	135
ALT, formerly SGPT, u/l		5	40
AST, formerly SGOT, u/l		10	50
Thyroid	TSH	0.5	5.0
Thyroid Free	T4	1	4
Uric acid, mg/dl		2.5	8.0

Calculating absolute lymphocyte count (ALC)

Multiply the white blood count times the percentage of lymphocytes to get the absolute lymphocyte count.

Some confusion arises because there are two systems for reporting the number of blood cells; one gives its figures in thousands, the other in small numbers. The digits are the same in both cases only one equals the other multiplied by 1000.

Your absolute lymphocyte counts using the two systems are:

- 39,170 (cells per microliter)
- 39.17 by the SI system: showing them as 39.17 x 10^9 (cells per liter). The 10^9 part which means 1,000,000,000, is usually avoided because so many digits would be required, so the count would be commonly given as a plain 39.17.

The normal range of ALC is often quoted as 1,500 - 3,500 lymphocytes /microliter, although it has been given as high as 4,000.

Calculating absolute neutrophil count (ANC)

Multiply the white blood count times the percentage of neutrophils to get the absolute neutrophil count.

The normal range for the ANC are about 1,700 - 6,100 neutrophils /microliter.

Body Surface Area in Square Meters

The chart below shows body surface area for typical heights and weights. Calculations were made using the DuBois & DuBois formula:

$$kg^{.425} \times cm^{.725} \times 0.007184$$

Weight is the horizontal axis, first in pounds, then in kilograms. Height is the vertical axis, first in inches, then in centimeters. Results are body surface areas in square meters.

If your height or weight falls between or outside the ranges of this chart, you can use one of the following web sites to calculate body surface area:

Cornell University: *http://www-users.med.cornell.edu/~spon/picu/bsacalc.htm*

Medical College of Wisconsin: *http://www.intmed.mcw.edu/clincalc/body.html*

Martindalee's HS Guide: *http://www-sci.lib.uci.edu/HSG/Pharmacy.html*

Or, try a Web search on the phrase "body surface area." Note that some of these sites use slightly different formulae, so the results will differ slightly.

In/Cm	100 Lbs/ 45 Kg	110 Lbs/ 49.5 Kg	120 Lbs/ 54 Kg	130 Lbs/ 58.5 Kg	140 Lbs/ 63 Kg	150 Lbs/ 67.5 Kg	160 Lbs/ 72 Kg	170 Lbs/ 76.5 Kg	180 Lbs/ 81 Kg
60/ 152.4	1.38	1.44	1.50	1.55	1.60	1.65	1.69	1.74	1.78
61/ 154.9	1.40	1.46	1.52	1.57	1.62	1.67	1.71	1.76	1.80
62/ 157.5	1.42	1.48	1.53	1.59	1.64	1.69	1.73	1.78	1.82
63/ 160.0	1.43	1.49	1.55	1.61	1.66	1.71	1.75	1.80	1.84
64/ 162.6	1.45	1.51	1.57	1.62	1.68	1.73	1.77	1.82	1.86
65/ 165.1	1.47	1.53	1.59	1.64	1.70	1.74	1.79	1.84	1.88
66/ 167.6	1.48	1.55	1.60	1.66	1.71	1.76	1.81	1.86	1.90
67/ 170.2	1.50	1.56	1.62	1.68	1.73	1.78	1.83	1.88	1.93
68/ 172.7	1.52	1.58	1.64	1.70	1.75	1.80	1.85	1.90	1.95
69/ 175.3	1.53	1.60	1.66	1.72	1.77	1.82	1.87	1.92	1.97
70/ 177.8	1.55	1.61	1.67	1.73	1.79	1.84	1.89	1.94	1.99
71/ 180.3	1.56	1.63	1.69	1.75	1.81	1.86	1.91	1.96	2.01
72/ 182.3	1.58	1.64	1.71	1.76	1.82	1.87	1.93	1.98	2.02
73/ 185.4	1.60	1.66	1.73	1.79	1.84	1.90	1.95	2.00	2.05
74/ 188.0	1.61	1.68	1.74	1.80	1.86	1.92	1.97	2.02	2.07
75/ 190.5	1.63	1.70	1.76	1.82	1.88	1.94	1.99	2.04	2.09
76/ 193.0	1.64	1.71	1.78	1.84	1.90	1.95	2.01	2.06	2.11
77/ 195.6	1.66	1.73	1.79	1.86	1.92	1.97	2.03	2.08	2.13
78/ 198.0	1.67	1.74	1.81	1.87	1.93	1.99	2.05	2.10	2.15
78/ 198.0	1.67	1.74	1.81	1.87	1.93	1.99	2.05	2.10	2.15

In/Cm	190 Lbs/ 85.5 Kg	200 Lbs/ 90 Kg	210 Lbs/ 94.5 Kg	220 Lbs/ 99 Kg	230 Lbs/ 103.5 Kg	240 Lbs/ 108 Kg	250 Lbs/ 112.5 Kg	260 Lbs/ 117 Kg	270 Lbs/ 121.5 Kg
60/ 152.4	1.82	1.86	1.90	1.94	1.97	2.01	2.04	2.08	2.11
61/ 154.9	1.84	1.88	1.92	1.96	2.00.	2.03	2.07	2.11	2.14
62/ 157.5	1.86	1.91	1.94	1.98	2.02	2.06	2.09	2.13	2.16
63/ 160.0	1.88	1.93	1.97	2.01	2.04	2.08	2.12	2.16	2.19
64/ 162.6	1.91	1.95	1.99	2.03	2.07	2.11	2.14	2.18	2.21
65/ 165.1	1.93	1.97	2.01	2.05	2.09	2.13	2.17	2.20	2.24
66/ 167.6	1.95	1.99	2.03	2.08	2.11	2.15	2.19	2.23	2.26
67/ 170.2	1.97	2.02	2.06	2.10	2.14	2.18	2.21	2.25	2.29
68/ 172.7	1.99	2.04	2.08	2.12	2.16	2.20	2.24	2.28	2.31
69/ 175.3	2.01	2.06	2.10	2.14	2.18	2.22	2.26	2.30	2.34
70/ 177.8	2.03	2.08	2.12	2.17	2.21	2.25	2.29	2.33	2.36
71/ 180.3	2.05	2.10	2.15	2.19	2.23	2.27	2.31	2.35	2.39
72/ 182.3	2.07	2.12	2.16	2.21	2.25	2.29	2.33	2.37	2.41
73/ 185.4	2.10	2.14	2.19	2.23	2.27	2.32	2.36	2.40	2.44
74/ 188.0	2.12	2.17	2.21	2.26	2.30	2.34	2.38	2.42	2.46
75/ 190.5	2.14	2.19	2.23	2.28	2.32	2.36	2.40	2.45	2.48
76/ 193.0	2.16	2.21	2.25	2.30	2.34	2.38	2.43	2.47	2.51
77/ 195.6	2.18	2.23	2.28	2.32	2.36	2.41	2.45	2.49	2.53
78/ 198.0	2.20	2.25	2.30	2.34	2.39	2.43	2.47	2.52	2.56
78/ 198.0	2.20	2.25	2.30	2.34	2.39	2.43	2.47	2.52	2.56

FAB Staging of Acute Leukemia

The diagnosis and staging of leukemia is made by microscopic examination of bone marrow and peripheral blood. Therefore the classification scheme is predicated on cellular morphology and histologic staging qualities, rather than the TNM classification used for solid tumors.

The French-American-British (FAB) is used universally. The leukemias are divided into acute lymphocytic leukemia (ALL) or acute nonlymphocytic leukemia (ANLL) based upon the cell type of origin (see Table D-1). Currently, there is a group trying to develop a newer classification that takes into account the microscopy, immunology (flow cytometry results), and genetic mutations seen in the leukemia. It is hoped that when completed, this classification will allow for more specific identification and treatment.

Table D-1. FAB Staging of Acute Leukemia

ALL	FAB Type	Morphology	Histology
Childhood ALL	L1	Small blasts, scant proto-plasm	PAS[a] + Peroxidase −
Adult ALL	L2	Large cells, abundant cyto-plasm, large variation in size and shape.	PAS + Peroxidase −
B-ALL	L3	Large cells, strongly baso-philic cytoplasm (associated with Burkitt's lymphoma)	PAS − Peroxidase −
Myelocytic	M0	Very undifferentiated cells, microscopic identification impossible, requires use of flow cytometry	Negative for all stains
Myelocytic	M1	Very undifferentiated cells, occasional cytoplasmic gran-ules	PAS − Peroxidase +/−
Myelocytic	M2	Granulated blasts, Auer's bodies present	PAS − Peroxidase +
Promyelocytic	M3	Hypergranular prolympho-cytes, basophilic and eosino-philic	PAS − Peroxidase +
Myelomonocytic	M4	Mixture of myelocytic or gran-ulocytic cells, elevated serum lysozyme	PAS +/− Peroxidase +

ALL	FAB Type	Morphology	Histology
Monoblastic	M5A	Large monoblasts abundant, agranular cytoplasm	PAS +/– Peroxidase +/– Esterase +
Monocytic	M5B	Twisted, folded appearance of nucleus	PAS +/– Peroxidase +/– Esterase +
Erythro-leukemic	M6	Multinucleated red cell precursors, sideroblasts present	PAS +
Megacaryocytic	M7	Megakaryocytic features and platelet antigens present	Variable

[a] PAS = Periodic acid-Schiff stain

Genetic Classification of the Lymphocytic Leukemias

Table E-1 provides genetic information pertaining to the lymphocytic leukemias, while Table E-2 defines the symbols used therein.

Table E-1. Antigens and Genetic Features of Lymphocytic Leukemias

Leukemia Type	CD Antigens	Other Antigens	Genetic Feature
B-Cell CLL **B-Cell PLL**	CD5+ CD19+ CD20+ CD23+ CD79a+ CD43+ CD10– CD11c –/+ (faint) CD22+ (in some subtypes only) CD52+	Faint SigM SigD+/– Cig +/	Ig HC and LC gene rearranged; trisomy 12 in 33% of cases; abnormality of 13q in 25%; transposition of chromosomes 11–14; bcl-1 gene rearranged
Hairy Cell	CD5–, CD10– CD11c+ (strong) CD23– CD25+ (strong) CD103+ (MLA) CD19+, CD20+ CD22+, CD79a+	Sig+ (M+/–D, G, or A) FMC7+ TRAP+ (in majority of cases)	IgHC and LC genes rearranged
T-Cell CLL **T-Cell PLL**	CD2+, CD3+ CD5+, CD7+ CD4+ /CD8– (65% of cases) CD4+/CD8+ (21% of cases) CD4– /CD8+ (rare) CD25–		TCR gene rearrangement; inversion of chromosome 14 on long arm, loci 11 to 32 in 75% of cases; trisomy 8q (three copies of long arm of chromosome 8)
Adult T-Cell Leukemia/Lymphoma	CD2+,CD3+ CD5+, CD4+ CD25+ CD8+ (rare)	Caused by HTLV-1	TCR genes rearranged; integrated HTVL-1 genome in all cases

Table E-2. Key to Understanding Table E-1

Symbol	Meaning
+	Over 90% of observed cases were positive
+/−	Over 50% of observed cases were positive
−/+	Less than 50% of observed cases were positive
−	Less than 10% of observed cases were positive
TCR	T-cell receptor gene
IgH	Immunoglobulin heavy chain gene
IgL	Immunoglobulin light chain gene
Sig	Contains surface immunoglobulin
Cig	Contains cytoplasmic immunoglobulin
CD	Cluster of differentiation
trisomy	Three copies of a chromosome or part of one.
HTLV-1	Human T-cell lymphotropic virus
TRAP	Tartrate-resistant acid phosphate

This information is an amalgamation of material from Wintrobe's Hematology, Whittaker's Leukemia, and Handin's Blood.

Progression of Cell Development

This appendix gives more details about cell development, described in Chapter 1, *What Leukemia Is*. It was written by Susan J. Leclair, MS, CLS (NCA), Professor of Medical Laboratory Science at University of Massachusetts Dartmouth.

The pluripotential stem cell is responsible for the production of all blood cells. Many texts abbreviate this cell's name to PSC.

When it is stimulated by specific hormones or hormone-like substances, this cell will commit to either the myeloid cell line or the lymphocyte cell line.

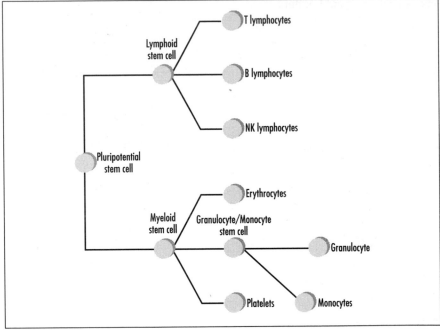

Figure F-1. Progression of cell development from stem cell to definite cell line.

The myeloid line

The term "myeloid" refers to the bone marrow or cells that originate solely from the bone marrow. The cell newly committed to the myeloid cell line is the colony-forming unit: granulocyte, erythrocyte, monocyte, and megakaryocyte or CFU-GEMM.

The erythrocyte cells will separate from the CFU-GEMM through the action of erythropoietin (EPO). The megakaryocyte cells will separate from the CFU-GEMM through the action of thrombopoietin (TBO) and produce platelets.

The white cells, granulocytes, and monocytes, have a common progenitor cell, the colony forming unit granulocyte/monocyte or CFU-GM which is under the control of a stimulating factor known as granulocyte/monocyte colony stimulating factor or GM-CSF. This cell then separates into two distinct progenitor cells, the granulocyte colony forming unit and the monocyte colony forming unit.

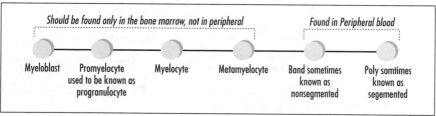

Figure F-2. Development of the myeloid cell line from myeloblast to poly

Sometimes, the term "myeloid" as in "myeloid series" will refer to only the granulocyte cells, that is the neutrophils, eosinophils, and basophils. Visible differences in the cells occur at the myelocyte stage so, for example, the full name of a cell might be basophilic myelocyte. But, because the neutrophilic cells are the dominant cell within this group, the adjective "neutrophilic" is usually dropped so, for example, the common name for the myelocyte of the neutrophilic variety is simply myelocyte.

All of the progenitor cells are morphologically alike and are in such low numbers that it is vitally important to identify them in a bone marrow or peripheral blood smear. Thus, the first recognizable cell in the granulocyte series is the myeloblast. This cell undergoes mitosis and maturation to become two promyelocytes. The promyelocyte undergoes mitotic division and maturation to become two myelocytes. The myelocyte undergoes division and maturation to become two metamyelocytes. There is no mitotic division after the myelocyte stage. The metamyelocyte matures into the band. The band is the first cell of the series to leave the marrow and enter the peripheral blood. The final stage of the cell series is the polymorphonuclear neutrophil.

The lymphoid line

The cell newly committed to the lymphoid line is more correctly defined as a progenitor cell rather than a stem cell and is called a lymphoid progenitor cell or colony-forming unit lymphocyte (CFU-L). From this cell, come T cells and B cells and the other subsets of lymphocytes (large granular, null, NK cells, etc.).

The maturation of the lymphocyte cell line is more complex to follow because, unlike the myeloid cells, these cells typically show no significant changes other than a maturation in the nucleus. The understanding of lymphocyte maturation comes

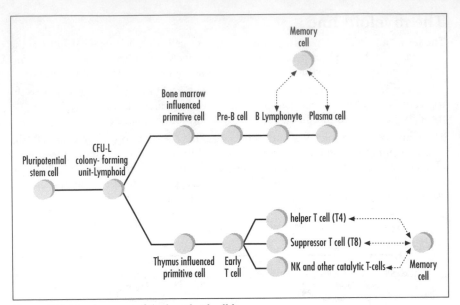

Figure F-3. Development of the lymphoid cell line

from an appreciation of the receptors and functions of the cells rather than how they look.

By proving the presence or absence of these receptors, we can separate T cells from B cells. T cells are primarily responsible for cell-to-cell interaction and response while B cells are primarily responsible for the production of antibodies. T cells are under the influence of the thymus, a gland under the breast bone. B cells are under the control of the bone marrow.

There is no way to determine the relative percentages of T cells and B cells in the routine hematology laboratory. This must be done by the use of the flow cytometer.

As a general rule, B cells are identified by the continuous increase of immunoglobulins leaving from their surface, while T cells are identified by the presence of structures built to receive substances.

Leukemia Drugs

This appendix lists drugs commonly used for treatment of leukemia. Table G-1 lists the abbreviations for different types of Leukemia, which you should use to understand the information in the subsequent tables. Table G-2 provides the trade name, common name, description, and use for various treatment substances; Table G-3 provides the same information for biological reponse modifyers.

Table G-1. Abbreviations for Different Types of Leukemia

Abbreviation	Type of Leukemia
ALL	Acute Lymphocytic Leukemia
AML	Acute Myeloid Leukemia
APL	Acute Promyelocytic leukemia
CLL	Chronic Lymphocytic Leukemia
CML	Chronic Myeloid Leukemia
HCL	Hairy Cell Leukemia
MDS	Myelodysplastic Syndromes
MLL	Meningeal Lymphocytic Leukemia
NHL	Non-Hodgkin's Lymphoma
PLL	Prolymphocytic Leukemia
PV	Polycythemia Vera

Table G-2. Treatment Substances

Generic Name	Trade Name	Common Name	Description	Use
Aldesleukin	Proleukin,	Interleukin 2, IL-2	(T-cell growth factor)cytokine biological response modifier	ALL, AML, CLL, CML
alemtuzumab	Campath-1H	Campath-1H	anti-CD52 humanized IgG1 monoclonal antibody	CLL, NHL; waiting FDA approval, in compassionate use trials

Table G-2. Treatment Substances (continued)

Generic Name	Trade Name	Common Name	Description	Use
amsacrine	Amsidine	m-AMSA, AMSA,	topoisom-erase II inhibitor	ALL, AML
arsenic trioxide	Trisenox	As2O3	orphan drug	APL
asparaginase	Elspar	L-asparaginase	Enzyme	AML, CLL, CML in lymphoid blast crisis
busulfan	Myleran	BSF	alkylating agent	CML, CLL, PV
carmustein	BiCNU	BCNU	alkylating agent	ALL
chlorambucil	Leukeran	chlorambucil	alkylating agent	CLL, HCL, NHL,
cisplatin	Platinol	cis-platinum, CDDP	heavy metal alkylating-like agent	CLL, NHL
cladribine	Leustatin	2-chlorodeoxy-adenosine, 2CdA	purine antime-tabolite	HCL, CLL, NHL
Compound 506U78	AraG	arabinosyl gua-nosine	purine analog	still in trials
cyclophospha-mide	Cytoxan	CTX	alkylating agent	ALL, AML, CLL, NHL
cytarabine	Cytosar U	Ara-C, cytosine arabinoside	antimetabolite	ALL, AML, CML, NHL
dactinomycin	Actinomycin	actinomycin D,ACT-D	antitumor anti-biotic	ALL, AML,
daunorubicin	Cerubidine	daunomycin, DNR	anthracycline antitumor anti-biotic	ALL, AML, NHL
decitabine	investigatory	5-AZA-2'-Deox-ycytadine, DAC	still in trials	CML
dexametha-sone	Decadron	DXM	adrenal corti-costeroid	CLL, NHL
doxorubicin	Adriamycin	hydroxydauno-rubicin	anthracycline antitumor anti-biotic	ALL, AML, CLL, NHL
epirubicin	Ellence	4'-epidoxo rubicin	anthracycline antitumor anti-biotic	AML, NHL
etoposide	Vepesid	VP-16	Plant alkaloid, topoisom-erase II inhibi-tor	ALL, AML, NHL
fludarabine phosphate	Fludara	FAMP	purine antime-tabolite	CLL, HCL, NHL, PLL
gemtuzumab ozogamicin	Mylotarg	gemtuzumab CMA-676	anti-CD 33 monoclonal antibody	AML,

Generic Name	Trade Name	Common Name	Description	Use
homoharringto-nine	Cephalotaxine	HHT	antitumor anti-biotic	AML, NHL
hydroxyurea	Hydrea	hydroxycarb amide	antimetabolite	CML, NHL, PV
histimine dihydrochloride	Maxamine	-	immunothera-peutic	AML orphan drug used with Interleukin 2
HuM195	investigatory	HuM195	humanized anti-CD33 monoclonal antibody	AML, PML still in clinical trials
131 I LYM-1	Oncolym	131 I LYM-1	radioactive monoclonal antibody	in clinical tri-als; more info as available.
idarubicin hydrochloride	Idamycin	4-demethoxy-daunorubicin	anthracycline antitumor anti-biotic	AML,
ifosfamide	Ifex, Mitoxana	isophospha-mide	alkylating agent	ALL, AML, NHL
lactacystin	investigatory	UCNO1	inhibitor of ubiquitin-pro-teasome-dependent pro-tein process-ing	induces CLL cells to apop-tosis; in trials
2-ME	investigatory	2-methox-yestradiol	inhibitor of superoxide dis-mutase (SOD)	can be used with anti-sense; still in trials
melphalan	Alkeran	L-PAM, L-phenylala-nine mustard	alkylating agent	CLL, NHL
mercaptopu-rine	Purinethal	6-mercaptopu-rine, 6-MP	purine antime-tabolite	ALL, AML,
mesna	Mesnex, Uromitexan	mesnum	rescue drug to prevent hemor-rhagic cystitis	ALL, AML,
methotexate	Mexate	MTX	antimetabolite	ALL, AML, MLL, NHL
mitoxantrone	Novantrone	DHAD	antitumor anti-biotic	AML, CLL, NHL
pegaspargase	Oncospar	PEG-L-aspara-ginase	enzyme	ALL, CLL, CML in lymphoid blast crisis, NHL,
pentostatin	Nipent	2'-deoxycofor-mycin	purine antime-tabolite	HCL, ALL, CLL, NHL
prednisone	Deltasone	prednisone	Corticosteroid	ALL, CLL, AML, NHL
rituximab	Rituxan	IDEC-C2B8	CD20 mono-clonal antibody	CLL, NHL

Generic Name	Trade Name	Common Name	Description	Use
STI571	Glivic	STI571	signal transduction inhibitor	PH+ CML still in clinical trials
teniposide	Vumon	VM-26	plant alkyoid (topo-somerase II inhibitor)	ALL
thioguanine	-	6'-thioguanine, 6-TG	purine antimetabolite	ALL, AML, CML, NHL
topotecan hydrochloride	Hycamptin	topotecan	camptothecan; topoisomerase 1 inhibitor	APL, MDS
Tositumomabiodine I 131	Bexxar	iodine I 131, anti-B1 antibody	CD20 antibody conjugated with radioactive iodine 131	AML, CLL, NHL still in trials
tretinoin	Vesanoid, Atragen	all-trans-retinoic acid, ATRA	retinoid (retinoic acid) derivative	APL
UCN-10	investigatory	7-hydroxystaurosporine	staurosporine analog that regulates signal transduction	CML, NHL
vinblastine sulfate	Velban, Velsar	vinblastine, VLB	plant alkaloid (tubulin inhibitor)	CML, NHL
vincristine sulfate	Oncovin	vincristine, VCR	plant alkaloid (tubulin inhibitor)	ALL, AML, CLL, NHL

Table G-3. Biological Response Modifiers

Generic Name	Trade Name	Common Name	Description	Use
epoitin alfa	Epogen, Procrit	erythropoitin	induces erythrocyte production	treatment of anemia
filgrastim	Neupogen	G-CSF	induces granulocyte production	decreases incidence of infection, neutropenia
alpha interferon-2A	Roferon	IFN-2A	glycoprotein	CML, HCL, NHL
oprelvekin	Neumega	IL-11	supports growth of platelets	decreases incidence of bleeding

Table G-3. Biological Response Modifiers

Generic Name	Trade Name	Common Name	Description	Use
sargramostim	Leukine, Prokine	GM-CSF	supports growth of granulocyte and monocyte precursers	decreases incidence of infection, neutropenia
thrombopoeitin	investigational	TPO	stimulates growth of platelets	decreases incidence of bleeding

Notes

Chapter 1: *What Leukemia Is*

1. D. Catovsky, "Current approach to the biology and treatment of chronic lymphoid malignancies other than CLL," *Hematology and Cell Therapy* 38, Supplement no. 2 (1996): S063–6.
2. Ibid.
3. Ibid.

Chapter 5: *Subtype, Staging, and Prognosis*

1. Department of Pathology, State University of New York at Stony Brook, Immunology tutorial. *http://www.path.sunysb.edu/hemepath/tutorial/immuno/immuno.htm.*
2. T. Wasil, et al, "IgV Gene Mutations and CD38 Expression are Prognostic Markers in Chronic Lymphocytic Leukemia," *Leukemia Insights Newsletter* Clinical Studies in Leukemia 3, no. 3 (1998 Winter).

Chapter 6: *Risks and Causes*

1. P. Schmiedlin-Ren, "Mechanisms of enhanced oral availability of CYP3A4 substrates by grapefruit constituents. Decreased enterocyte CYP3A4 concentration and mechanism-based inactivation by furanocoumarins," *Drug Metabolism Disposition* 25, no. 11 (November 1997):1228–33.
2. B. N. Singh, "Effects of food on clinical pharmacokinetics," *Clinical Pharmacokinet* 37, no. 3 (September 1999):213–55.
3. "Vitamins may interfere with cancer chemotherapy," *Reuters Health* 26 (July 2000).
4. Katrine Woznicki, "Vitamins May Affect Chemotherapy," *OnHealth.com News, http://www.onhealth.com/conditions/briefs/item%2C75845.asp.* (15 December 1999).
5. U. Elsasser-Beile, et al, "Cytokine production in leukocyte cultures during therapy with Echinacea extract," *Journal Clinical Laboratory Analysis,* 10, no. 6 (1996): 441–5.

Chapter 8: *Treatments for individual Leukemias*

1. David Loshak, "Treatment of patients with recurrent and primary refractory acute myelogenous leukemia using mitoxantrone and intermediate-dose cytarabine: A pharmacologically based regimen," *Cancer* (24 May 2000).
2. P. J. Zhang, "The use of arsenic trioxide (As2O3) in the treatment of acute promyelocytic leukemia," *Biol Regul Homeost Agents* 13, no. 4 (October–December 1999):195–200.

3. H. Agis, et al, "Successful treatment with arsenic trioxide of a patient with ATRA-resistant relapse of acute promyelocytic leukemia," *Annals of Hematology* 8, no. 7 (7 July 1999):329–32.

4. S. O'Brien, H. Kantarjian, and M. Talpaz, "Practical guidelines for the management of chronic myelogenous leukemia with interferon alpha," *Leukemia and Lymphoma* 23, no. 3–4 (October 1996):247–52. Review.

5. S. O'Brien, H. Kantarjian, et al, "Sequential homoharringtonine and interferon-alpha in the treatment of early chronic phase chronic myelogenous leukemia," *Blood* 93, no. 12 (15 June 1999:4149–53.

6. D. Catovsky, "Current approach to the biology and treatment of chronic lymphoid malignancies other than CLL," *Hematology and Cell Therapy*, 38, Supplement no. 2 (1996): S063–6.

Chapter 10: *Clinical Trials and Beyond*

1. John C. Byrd, Rai Kanti, et al, "Old and New therapies in chronic Lymphocytic Leukemia: Now is the Time for a Reassessment of Therapeutic Goals," *Seminars in Oncology* 25, no. 1 (February 1998):69–72.

2. Thomas J. Kipps, MD, PhD, "Chronic Lymphocytic Leukemia," *Current Opinions in Hematology* 7 (2000):223–34.

3. N. J. Donato, and M. Talpaz, "Clinical Use of Tyrosine Kinase Inhibitors: Therapy for Chronic Myelogenous Leukemia and Other Cancers," *Clinical Cancer Research* 6, no. 8 (August 2000):2965–6.

4. J. Pinilla-Ibarz, et al, "Vaccination of patients with chronic myelogenous leukemia with bcr-abl oncogene breakpoint fusion peptides generates specific immune responses," *Blood* 95, no. 5 (1 March 2000):1781–7.

5. P. Masdehors; H. Merle-Beral; H. Magdelenat; and J. Delic. "Ubiquitin-proteasome system and increased sensitivity of B-CLL lymphocytes to apoptotic death activation," *Leukemia Lymphoma* 38, no. 5–6 (August 2000):499–504.

Chapter 16: *After Treatment*

1. "Chemotherapy's Effect on the Brain," *American Cancer Society, News Today* (March 2000).

2. S. B. Schagen, et al, "Cognitive deficits after postoperative adjuvant chemotherapy for breast carcinoma," *Cancer* 85, no. 3 (1 February 1999):640–50.

3. F. S. van Dam, et al, "Impairment of cognitive function in women receiving adjuvant treatment for high-risk breast cancer," *Journal National Cancer Institute,* 90, no. 3 (4 February 1998):210–8.

4. B. R. Smoller and. R. A. Warnke, "Cutaneous infiltrate of chronic lymphocytic leukemia and relationship to primary cutaneous epithelial neoplasms," *Journal Cutaneous Pathology*, 25, no. 3 (March 1998):160–4.

5. J. K. Desch, and B.R. Smoller, "The spectrum of cutaneous disease in leukemias" *Journal Cutaneous Pathology* 20, no. 5, (October 1993):407–10.

6. M. Williams, "Gastrointestinal manifestations of graft-versus-host disease: diagnosis and management" *AACN Clinical Issues* 10, no. 4 (November 1999):500–6.

Glossary

This glossary lists only terms specific to leukemia. For a comprehensive glossary of cancer medical terminology, see *Taber's Cyclopedic Medical Dictionary* or *Steadman's Medical Dictionary*. For more general medical terms, any one of several inexpensive medical dictionaries available in bookstores and libraries should suffice.

Guides to pronunciation are included.

To start: Unusual phrases

Before we list terms you may find when reading about leukemia, we must point out that there are a few specific words and phrases that may be jarring because they mean something other in medicine than they do in everyday usage:

Anecdotal
> When used in a medical context, it does not mean a funny story. It means a single case report not yet substantiated by studies using large numbers of people.

Impressive or not impressive
> When used in a medical context, it does not mean anything derogatory. It means that, when the patient was examined, a particular feature did not strike the examiner as overwhelmingly unusual. For instance, after palpating your abdomen, the doctor may note in your medical record that your spleen was "not impressive." This means it did not feel enlarged, and that you did not report pain when she pressed on it.

Morbid or morbidity
> In a medical context, they do not mean that you have a neurotic outlook. They simply mean illness, and are somewhat the opposite of mortality. You might read, for example, that a treatment resulted in 20 percent low-level morbidity, but only 2 percent mortality. Likewise, comorbidity means the illnesses a person has in addition to cancer, such as high blood pressure or diabetes.

The patient denies
> This phrase does not mean that the doctor thinks you're lying. It's just used as the opposite of "the patient reports." For instance, your medical record might read, "The patient reports frequent morning cough, but denies the presence of phlegm."

Tolerable
> A word often used by medical staff to describe the side effects of treatment. Your idea of what is tolerable may be much lower than their definition, because medicine defines a tolerable side effect as one that can be ameliorated with supportive care and that does not result in permanent organ damage. For you, these side effects may be intolerable.

Leukemia terminology

Absolute lymphocyte count (LIM-fo-site)
 The total number of lymphocytes. in a standard unit of whole blood. For example, if a total white blood count was 60,000 and the percentage of lymphocytes was 75 percent the absolute lymphocyte count would be 45,000 (60,000 X 75% = 45,000).

Absolute lymphocytosis
 The presence of more than 15,000 lymphocytes in a cubic millimeter of blood.

Absolute neutrophil count (NEW-tro-fil), also called ANC
 The total number of neutrophils in the blood, a measure of one's ability to fight infection. Also called absolute granulocyte count or AGC. See Appendix B.

Acute Granulocytic Leukemia (gran-you-lo-SIT-ik)
 See AML.

ALL (Acute Lymphocytic Leukemia) (lim-fo-SIT-ik)
 An acute form of leukemia occurring predominantly in children, characterized by the unrestrained production of immature lymphoblasts (a type of white cell) in the blood forming tissues, particularly the bone marrow, spleen, and lymph nodes.

AML (Acute Myeloid Leukemia) (MY-loyd) also known as Acute Myelogenous Leukemia (MY-loj- uhn- us)
 An acute form of leukemia characterized by a massive proliferation of mature and immature abnormal granulocytes (a type of white cell).

ANLL (Acute Nonlymphocytic Leukemia) (non-lim-fo-SIT-ik)
 See Acute Myeloid Leukemia.

APL (Acute Promyelocytic Leukemia) (PRO-my-lo-SIT-ik)
 A form of AML characterized by the presence in the blood of large mononuclear cells called promyelocytes.

Allogeneic transplant (al-lo-jeh-NAY-ic)
 Marrow or stem cell transplant using donor stem cells of the same species that are immunologically different from the patient's.

Anemia (an-NEE-me-uh)
 A lack of adequate numbers of oxygen-carrying red blood cells.

Anesthesia (an-es-THEE-zee-uh)
 Partial or total loss of sensation, with or without loss of consciousness, induced by the administration of a drug.

Anorexia (an-o-REK-see-uh)
 Loss of appetite.

Antibody (AN-ti-bah-di)
 A protein produced by certain white blood cells in order to kill foreign substances (antigens). Each antibody can bind to only one specific antigen.

Antigen (AN-ti-jehn)
 Any substance that the body regards as foreign. When introduced into the body, an antigen causes the immune system to produce a corresponding antibody to fight it.

Apheresis (AF-er-EE-sis)

The channeling of blood out of the body and through specialized single-use tubing and equipment in order to extract various blood cell types, such as platelets or stem cells, from the bloodstream. After these cells are extracted, the remaining blood is returned to the body. Also called hemapheresis, or leukapheresis for the extraction of white blood cells.

Apoptosis (app-uh-TOE-sis or A-pop-TOE-sis)

Normal genetically programmed cell death. Some chemotherapy drugs induce apoptosis; others cause cell lysis (bursting).

Aspirate (AS-pir-ate, second meaning AS-pir-it)

To remove material from a body cavity, by suction, through a needle. Also used to describe that material.

Asymptomatic (A-sim-toe-MAH-tik)

Without symptoms.

ATL (Adult T-cell leukemia))

A chronic lymphocytic leukemia that affects the T-Cells. ATL appears later in life with frequent rashes, skin involvement, and lymph node and spleen enlargement. There are four subtypes: acute or prototypic ATL, lymphoma type ATL, chronic ATL, and smoldering ATL.

AIHA (Autoimmune Hemolytic Anemia)

A form of anemia characterized by autoantibodies that react with red blood cells. It often follows chemotherapy treatments for leukemia.

Autologous transplant (aw-TAHL-uh-gus)

A marrow or stem cell transplant using the patient's own blood products.

B cells

White blood cells found in the bone marrow that have not traveled to the thymus (see T-Cell). B cells are responsible for many immune functions, such as producing proteins called antibodies that tag invaders for destruction.

Basophil (BAY-so-fil)

Type of granulocyte (white cell) which plays a special role in allergic reactions and helps in the healing of inflammations.

Biological response modifier (BRM)

A substance, like inteferon and the interleukins, that boosts, directs, or restores the body's normal immune system for defense. BRMs are produced in the body naturally and may also be produced in the laboratory.

Biological therapy

A therapy which uses protein or cells that are involved in the body's natural defense mechanism. Often the cells used are man-made clones of human cells.

Biopsy

A biopsy refers to a procedure that involves obtaining a tissue specimen for microscopic analysis to establish a precise diagnosis. Biopsies can be accomplished with a biopsy needle passed through the skin into the organ in question. With leukemia, the biopsy may be done to get material from the bone marrow, or from an enlarged lymph node.

Blast Cell

An undifferentiated normal cell in an early stage of development; also means a leukemic cell of indeterminable type.

Blood-Brain Barrier

A network of blood vessels located around the central nervous system with very closely spaced cells that make it difficult for potentially toxic substances— including anticancer drugs—to enter the brain and spinal cord.

Blood Type

Identification of the proteins in a person's blood cells so that transfusions can be given with compatible blood products. Examples of blood types are A+, A-, B+, B-, AB+, AB-, O+, O-.

BMT

See Bone Marrow Transplant.

Bone marrow

The soft, spongy matrix of all bones that produce blood cells. As we age, some marrow is replaced by fat cells or fibers.

Bone Marrow Aspiration

Process in which a sample of fluid and cells is withdrawn from the bone marrow using a hollow needle.

Bulky Disease

A cancer-specific phrase found often in the literature on leukemias. Bulky disease is any cancerous lymph node or extranodal tissue that measures greater than ten centimeters in any dimension.

Cancer

A term for diseases in which abnormal cells divide without control.

Carcinogen (kar-SIN-o-jen)

A substance or agent that produces cancer.

CBC (Complete Blood Count)

Measurement of the numbers of white cells, red cells, and platelets in a cubic millimeter of blood.

Cerebrospinal Fluid (CSF) (suh-REE-broh-SPY-nuhl)

Fluid which surrounds and bathes the brain and spinal cord and provides a cushion from shocks.

Chemotherapy (KE-moh–theh-ruh-pee)

Treatment of disease with drugs. The term usually refers to cytotoxic drugs given to treat cancer.

Chromosome (KROH-moh-zohm)

A structure in the nucleus of a cell that contains genetic material. Normally, 46 chromosomes are inside each human cell.

Clinical Trial

A carefully designed and executed investigation of a drug, drug dosage, combination of drugs, or other method of treating disease. Each trial is designed to answer one or more scientific questions and to find better ways to prevent or treat disease.

CLL (Chronic Lymphocytic Leukemia)
A disease of the lymphocytes which progresses slowly and is characterized by increased longevity of the lymphocytes in the bone marrow .

Cluster of Differentiation (CD)
The immunoglobulin markers found on lymphocytes that are used to tell the function of the cell. Numbers, such as CD20, are used to label antigens and their respective antibodies. Clusters of differentiation are measured and labeled to tell apart white blood cells with different properties and functions. Each cell has only one kind of antigen, that's why they are called clusters of differentiation.

CML (Chronic Myelogenous Leukemia) or (Chronic Myeloid Leukemia)
A disease which progresses slowly and is characterized by increased production of granulocytes in the bone marrow. It is usually associated with a specific chromosomal abnormality called the Philadelphia chromosome.

CNS (Central Nervous System)
The brain, spinal cord, and nerves.

Colony Stimulating Factors (CSFs)
Proteins that stimulate the development of cells in the bone marrow.

Complete Remission (CR)
A term used to describe the patient when certain blood sample and physical criteria are met. Complete remission criteria is different for each type of leukemia.

Consolidation Therapy
Chemotherapy or radiotherapy intended to destroy all remaining cancer cells. Consolidation therapy frequently follows induction therapy.

Corticosteriods (KOR-ti-ko-STEER-oydz)
Complex chemical compounds produced naturally in the outer layer of the adrenal gland, near the kidney. They regulate body chemistry. Like prednisone, they can also be produced in the laboratory.

Cytogenetics (sigh-toh-GEN-eh-tikz)
The study of the structure of chromosomes. Cytogenetic tests are carried out on samples of blood and bone marrow taken from leukemia patients to detect any chromosomal abnormalities associated with the disease. These help in the diagnosis and selection of optimal treatment. For example, clinical cytogenetic studies might be done to determine whether an adult with possible CLL has the chromosome abnormality, Trisomy 12.

Cytokines (SIGH-toh-kinz)
Hormones or growth factors produced by cells that help regulate cell processes.

Cytomegalovirus or CMV (sigh-toe-MEG-uh-low-virus)
One of a group of herpes viruses that can cause serious or fatal infection among the immune-suppressed.

Cytoplasm
The fluid or liquid part of a cell surrounding the nucleus.

-cytosis (sigh-TOE-sis)
A suffix denoting an abnormally high number of blood cells: Lymphocytosis, erythrocytosis, or thrombocytosis. See also -penia.

Cytotoxic (sigh-toe-TOX-ic)
A term for anything that kills cells. Many chemotherapy and radiotherapy regimens are cytotoxic to both healthy and cancerous cells.

Differentiation (DIF-er-en-she-A-shun)
The term used to describe cells maturing and developing for a particular task. For leukemias, differentiation generally refers to white blood cells. In general, the less differentiated a cancer cell, the younger and more aggressive it is.

Enzyme
A protein molecule produced by living organisms that is a catalyst for chemical reactions of other substances without itself being destroyed or altered when the reactions are complete. They are divided into six main groups, oxidoreductases, transferases, hydrolases, lyases, isomerases and ligases.

Eosinophil (EOS) (EE-oh-sin-uh-fil)
A type of white cell which responds to allergic reactions as well as foreign bacteria.

Erythrocyte (eh-REETH-ro-site)
A red blood cell. Red blood cells are responsible for carrying oxygen to body tissues.

External Catheter
Indwelling catheter in which one end of the tubing is in the heart and the other end of the tubing sticks out through the skin, for example, a Hickman catheter.

Flow Cytometry
A method of testing the blood by tagging cancer cells and counting them as they pass through a stream of light, or by examining them for specific features.

Graft
Tissue taken from one person (donor) and transferred to another person (recipient or host).

Graft-versus-host disease or GVHD
The phenomenon of donor marrow attacking the patient's body. GVHD can be mild, moderate, severe, or fatal.

Graft-versus-leukemia effect or GVL
The phenomenon of donor marrow attacking the leukemia cells in the patient's body. Controlled GVL is desired during transplant.

Granulocytes (GRAN-you-lo-sites)
Types of white blood cells that attack bacteria by engulfing them. Eosinophils, neutrophils, basophils, and mast cells are types of granulocytes.

HCL (Hairy-Cell Leukemia)
A form of leukemia characterized by abnormal cells with a single nucleus and with irregular cytoplasmic projections.

Hepatitis (heh-PUH-tie-tuhs)
Inflammation of the liver by virus or toxic origin. Fever and jaundice are usually present, and sometimes the liver is enlarged.

Hematocrit or HCT (he-MAH-to-crit)
Describes the percentage by volume of red blood cells in whole blood drawn for a CBC.

Hematologist
> Physician who specializes in the diagnosis and treatment of disorders of blood and blood forming tissues.

Hematopoiesis (he-mah-TOE-puh-ee-sis)
> The formation and development of blood cells.

Hemorrhagic Cystitis (he-moh-RAH-jik SIS-tie-tis)
> Bleeding from the bladder, which can be a side effect of the drug cytoxan.

Hickman Catheter
> An indwelling catheter that has one end of the tubing in the heart and the other end outside the body.

Histology
> The study of the microscopic structure of tissue (cells).

Host
> In bone marrow transplantation, the person who receives the marrow.

Hemaglobin (HE-muh-glow-bin)
> The iron-containing protein found in the center of a red blood cell that can bind to and transport oxygen.

Human Leukocyte Antigens or HLAs
> The proteins on the surfaces of white blood cells that characterize white blood cells from different individuals.

Induction therapy
> Chemotherapy or radiotherapy intended to induce a remission.

Infusion Pump
> A small, computerized device which allows drugs to be given at home through an IV or indwelling catheter.

Immune Response
> The activity of the immune system to kill off foreign substances in the blood.

Immune System
> Complex system by which the body is able to protect itself from foreign invaders.

Immunoglobulin
> Protein produced by B cells to act against a substance the body has identified as an invader. An antibody on the surface of a lymphocyte.

Immunophenotyping (Im-mun-NO-fee-no-typ-ing)
> Process of classifying cells of the immune system based on structural and functional differences. The process is commonly used to analyze and sort lymphocytes into subsets based on CD antigens by the technique of flow cytometry. This technique is used by pathologists to determine the type of leukemia seen in a blood sample.

Immunosuppression
> When the immune system is unable to react to foreign substances, leaving the body susceptible to infection.

Induction
> The first part of the chemotherapy protocol for treating some types of leukemia in which several powerful chemotherapy drugs are given to kill as many cancer cells as possible.

Institutional Review Board (IRB)
    Group made up of scientists, clergy, doctors, and citizens from the community which approves and reviews all research, taking place at an institution.

Intrathecal (In-tra-THE-kuhl)
    Injecting drugs into the cerebrospinal fluid during a spinal tap or treatment for CNS involvement.

Intravenous-access Line (IV)
    A hollow metal or plastic tube which is inserted into a vein and attached to tubing, allowing various solutions or medicines to be directly infused into the blood.

Karyotype (KAH-ree-uh-type)
    A karyotype is a display of chromosomes from largest to smallest. It provides a reference tool for understanding the chromosomal characteristics of a cell, including abnormalities and transpositions.

Kidneys
    Two glands situated in the rear of the upper abdominal cavity, one on either side of the spine. Their function is to filter the blood and control the level of some chemicals in the blood such as hydrogen, sodium, potassium, and phosphate. They eliminate waste in the form of urine.

Leukemia (lu-KEE-mee-uh)
    The uncontrolled growth of white bloods cells in bone marrow, often overflowing to the circulating blood. (Spelled leukaemia in Great Britain.)

Leukocyte (LU-ko-site)
    A general term for all white blood cells.

Leukapharesis (lu-kah-FAR-ee-sis)
    A blood filtering process to reduce the number of lymphocytes in the blood.

Leukopenia (LU-ko-PEA-nee-uh)
    The condition of having abnormally low numbers of white blood cells. See also -penia.

Lidocaine (LIE-doh-kayn)
    Drug most commonly used for local anesthesia.

Lumbar Puncture (Spinal Tap)
    Procedure in which a needle is inserted between the vertebrae of the back to obtain a sample of cerebrospinal fluid and/or inject medication.

Lymph (LIMF)
    A clear, colorless fluid found in lymph vessels throughout the body, which carries cells to fight infection.

Lymph Nodes
    Rounded bodies of lymphatic tissues found in lymph vessels.

Lymph System
    A system of vessels and nodes throughout the body which helps filter out bacteria as well as performs numerous other functions.

Lymphocytes (LIM-foe-sites)
    A subtype of white blood cells that have migrated to the lymph nodes or other lymphoid organs to await the signal to fight infection.

Lymphocytopenia (lim-FOE-sigh-toe-PEE-ne-uh)
The condition of having abnormally low numbers of certain white blood cells called lymphocytes. See also -penia.

Lymphocytosis (lim-FOE-sigh-TOE-sis)
The condition of having abnormally high numbers of certain white blood cells called lymphocytes. See also -cytosis.

Lymphomas (lim-FO-muh)
Cancers of the white blood cells and the lymph system. Lymphomas differ in important ways from leukemias, and are classified according to the microscopic appearance of the cancer cells. It is sometimes difficult to distinguish among lymphomas and leukemias.

Maintenance Therapy
Part of a leukemia protocol for treating ALL. It follows the intensive induction and consolidation phases and helps to destroy any remaining cancer cells.

Malignant
Tending to become progressively worse, ending in death.

Mean
The numerical value that is the same as an average.

Median
The midpoint. If eighty-one patients were treated with drug XYZ, and the time for white blood cell counts to recover following this treatment ranged from two to sixty days, after you rank the patients by the number of days required for their white blood cells to recover, the median is the number of days that it took patient number forty-one's white blood cells to recover.

Monoclonal Antibodies (MOABs or MABs)
Antibodies that react with a single antigen. Antibodies that react with specific cancer cells can be used to target treatments and can be produced in large quantities in the laboratory.

Monocytes (MO-no-sites)
Type of white blood cell. The largest of the white blood cells, monocytes engulf and destroy invading bacteria and fungi. Monocytes are also known as macrophages.

Morphology (mor-FOL-uh-gee)
The science of the structure and form of organisms without regard to function.

Myelodysplastic Syndromes (my-lo-dis-PLAS-tik)
A group of disorders characterized by low white blood cell counts, low platelet counts, and, in some cases, increased monocytes. The primary problem is in the cells of the bone marrow, which shows qualitative and quantitative changes suggestive of a preleukemic process. However, the disorders have a chronic course that does not necessarily terminate as acute leukemia.

Myeloproliferative Disorders (my-lo-pro-LIF-er-uh-tiv)
A group of disease states which primarily involve the bone marrow and the production of blood cells. Examples include polycythemia vera, chronic myeloid leukemia, myelofibrosis and primary thrombocytopenia.

Neoplasm
A new and abnormal form of tissue growth that serves no normal function, but grows at the expense of healthy cells.

Neurotoxic (nu-row-TOX-ik)
   Substance which is poisonous to the brain, spinal cord, and/or nerve cells.

Neutropenia (nu-trow-PEA-nee-uh)
   The condition of having abnormally low numbers of one type of white blood cell called neutrophils.

Neutrophils (NOO-truh-filz)
   The most numerous of the granulocytic white cells, they migrate through the bloodstream to the site of infection, where they ingest and destroy bacteria.

NK (Natural Killer) Lymphocyte
   Specialized white blood cells which can kill tumor cells without having been previously exposed to the cell and without the tumor cell having antigens most other white cells require to attack.

Nutritionist
   A professional who analyzes nutritional requirements and gives advice on what may be an appropriate diet for any condition.

Oncologist (Ahn-KAH-luh-jist)
   Doctor who specializes in the treatment of cancer.

Oncology
   Study of cancer.

Overall Survival
   The total amount of time that a patient survives following treatment, including relapses that were successfully retreated. See Event-free survival.

Palliative Care
   Comfort care given to the patient after all active treatment ends.

Pancreas
   A gland situated behind the stomach which has two vital functions: It secretes enzymes into the intestines which aid in the digestion of food and it produces and secretes insulin, a hormone essential for regulating carbohydrate metabolism by controlling blood sugar levels.

Pancreatitis
   Inflammation of the pancreas which can cause extreme pain, vomiting, hiccoughing, constipation, and collapse.

Partial Remission
   The reduction of leukemia cells in the body to a point where the disease has stabilized but has not reached the criteria for complete remission.

Pathologist
   Doctor who specializes in examining tissue and diagnosing disease.

-penia
   A suffix denoting abnormally low numbers of blood cells: leukopenia, erythropenia, or thrombocytopenia. See also -cytosis.

Peripheral blood (pe-RIF-er-al)
   Blood circulating in the body as opposed to bone marrow. Peripheral blood usually is withdrawn from an arm vein or central catheter.

Petechiae (pe-TEA-key-ah)
   Small red or brown spots on the skin which are actually tiny hemorrhages. They may indicate abnormally low numbers of platelets or (thrombocytes).

Philadelphia Chromosome
   A chromosome abnormality found in 90 percent of patients with CML and in some having ALL. It is caused by a translocation of the bottom of chromosome 22 on to chromosome 9 creating a gene called brc/abl. Patients with this abnormality are referred to as Ph+ (positive).

Plasma
   The liquid part of the lymph and the blood.

Platelet
   A blood cell called a thrombocyte, important in the blood clotting process.

Port-a-cath or Port
   Indwelling catheter which has a small portal under the skin of the chest attached to tubing, which goes into the heart.

Prognosis (prog-NO-sis)
   The expected or probable outcome of a treatment or disease. The chance of recovery.

PLL (Prolymphocytic Leukemia) (PRO-lim-fo-SIT-ik)
   A form of CLL characterized by the presence in the blood of large mononuclear cells called prolymphocytes.

Preleukemic Condition
   Disease of the blood that is not yet cancer, but that may become leukemia in the future.

Prophylaxis
   An attempt to prevent disease.

Protein
   A compound of substances that is part of plants and animals.

Protocol
   The "recipe" for a cancer treatment. Outlines the drugs that will be taken, when they will be taken, and in what dosages. Also includes the dates for procedures (e.g., bone marrow aspiration schedule).

Purging
   Removing leukemic cells from the patient's bone marrow cells before autologous transplantation.

Radiation
   High-energy rays which are used to kill or damage cancer cells.

Radiologist
   Doctor who specializes in using radiation and radioactive isotopes to diagnose and treat disease.

Randomized
   Chosen at random. In a randomized research project, a computer chooses which patients receive the experimental treatment(s), and which patients receive the standard treatment.

Refractory
Not responding favorably to a particular treatment.

Relapse
A return of the cancer after its apparently complete disappearance.

Remission
A period in which there is no evidence of disease in the blood and marrow by microscopic determination of a biopsy or blood sample. Remissions may be complete or partial, with subsections of each, and the definition of remission differs according to type.

Side Effect
Unintentional or undesirable secondary effect of treatment.

SLVL (Splenic lymphoma with villous lymphocytes)
A lymphoma similar to chronic lymphocytic leukemia characterized by abnormal cells with a single nucleus and with irregular cytoplasmic projections, always characterized by an enlarged spleen. (See the entry for villous.)

Spleen
An organ that produces lymphocytes, filters the blood, stores blood cells and destroys those that are aging. It is located on the left side of the abdomen near the stomach. It is always a concern with lymphocytic leukemias.

Splenectomy (splee-NEK-toe-me)
A surgical operation resulting in the removal of the spleen.

Stable disease
Blood work shows little variation from month to month. Stable disease for months or years is common among low-grade chronic leukemias. Also known as smoldering disease.

Stem cells
Young blood cells from which all blood cells develop. Also known as peripheral blood stem cells.

Subcutaneous Port
Type of catheter comprised of a portal under the skin of the chest attached to tubing leading into the heart.

Substrate
The substance acted upon and changed by an enzyme; the substance considered to be attacked in a chemical reaction.

Systemic
Affecting the body as a whole.

T- cells
Type of lymphocyte (white cell), derived from the thymus, that attacks infected cells, foreign tissue, and cancer cells.

Thrombocyte (THROM-bow-site)
A blood cell commonly called a platelet.

Thymus
A small gland located in the top of the chest, behind the breastbone, and between the lungs. It is the source of T-cells.

Veno-occlusive Disease

The closure of veins in the liver following high-dose therapy that may or may not accompany transplantation.

Vital Signs

Term which describes a patient's pulse, rate of breathing, and blood pressure.

Villous (VIL-us)

Immature, shaggy, covered with fine long hairs of cytoplasm, but the hairs are not matted.

White Blood Cells

Cells that help the body fight infection and disease.

X-ray

High-energy electromagnetic radiation used in low doses to diagnose disease or injury and in high doses to treat cancer.

Index

family and friends
     after treatment, 363–365
     effect of illness on marriages, 384
     emotional responses to diagnosis,
          45–49
     feelings about end-of-life issues,
          398–399
     impact of guilt on relationships, 47
     interactions with, as stress reducer,
          296–298
     presence at doctors' office visits,
          252–253
     relationships with doctors, 35,
          38–39
     responses/gestures of during
          recurrence, 385–386
     role at time of diagnosis, 42–43
     as support during treatments, 126
     whether to tell about diagnosis,
          336–337
     See also support
Family and Medical Leave Act (FMLA),
     351–352
fatigue
     as complication of radiation, 211
     as late effect of treatments, 370
     as side effect of treatments,
          269–270
     as symptom of leukemias, 23, 26,
          29, 31
fear, 45–46, 285–286, 386–387
fee-for-service (indemnity) policies, 344
fertility, 120–122, 374–375
fever, 26, 31, 270
filgrastim, 118, 132, 146
financial issues
     air travel, 355, 451–453
     bankruptcy, 347–348
     debt consolidation, 347
     disability income, 348–351
     at end of life, 392–393
     estate planning, 347
     fears concerning, 45–46
     fundraising, 347, 386
     funeral costs, 405
     home mortgage refinancing, 347
     lodging when traveling for care,
          355, 453

     need for professional help with,
          338
     Patient Aid Program, 335
     payment for clinical trials, 232–233
     suggestions for coping with, 347
     Supplemental Security Income (SSI)
          eligibility, 347
     traveling for care, 354–355
     See also health insurance
finding doctors, 35, 37–39
fine-needle aspiration, 76–78
FISH (fluorescence in situ
          hybridization), 60, 61, 72
flavopiridol, 241
flow cytometry, 60, 61, 72
fludarabine, 113
Foundation for Accreditation of
          Hematopoietic Cell
          Therapy, 186
free treatments, 233, 451
French-American-British classification
          scheme (FAB), 83–84,
          462–463
friends. See family and friends
fundraising, 347, 386
funerals, 404–405
fungal infections, 202–203
fungal pneumonias, 277
future treatment directions, 234

G

gallbladder dysfunction, 272
gallium scan (gallium scintigram),
          72–74
gated blood pool scan, 76
gender, leukemia rates and, 99
gene therapy, 240
genetic predisposing conditions, 19
glossary, 477–489
graft-versus-host disease, 142, 203,
          208–209, 370
graft-versus-leukemia effect, 142
"GrannyBarb and Art's Leukemia Links,"
          xv, 414
granulocyte colony-stimulating factor
          (G-CSF), 118, 132, 146

granulocyte-macrophage colony-stimulating factor (GM-CSF), 118, 132, 146
granulocytes, 5
grapefruit juice, 107
Gribben, John
    importance of information and resources, xi–xii
grief, 383
guilt, 47
GW506U78, 241

H

H-LL2 (epratuzumab), 235–236
hair loss/growth, 133, 270–271, 371
hairy cell leukemia (HCL)
    cell (CD) markers, 97
    chemotherapy, 165–166
    diagnosis, 43–45
    email discussion list, 329
    generally, 13
    no staging system for, 97
    splenectomy, 165
    symptoms, 32–33
haplotyping, 173
harvest of bone marrow, 195–196
harvest of peripheral stem cells, 196–198
harvesting, generally, 195
headaches, 31
health insurance, 338-346
    approval/denial of transplantation, 189–190
    catastrophic insurance policies, 345
    denial of insurance coverage, 189–190
    at end-of-life, 391–392
    fears concerning, 45–46
    fee-for-service (indemnity) policies, 344
    hospital indemnity policies, 346
    laws
        COBRA (Consolidated Omnibus Budget Reconciliation Act of 1985), 340
        Employee Retirement Income Security Act (ERISA), 340
        Health Insurance Portability and Accountability Act of 1996 (HIPPA), 340
    for long-term care, 345–346
    losing coverage, 340
    managed care plans (HMOs)
        as for-profit companies, 340–341
        Point of Service (POS) plans, 341
        Preferred Physicians Organization (PPO) plans, 341
        questions to ask about, 341–342
    medical savings accounts, 344–345
    Medicare/Medicaid
        advocacy/patient service organizations, 343
        enrollment, 343
        limitations on payments, 343–344
        resources about, 342
        suggestions for older survivors, 343–344
        various options within, 342
    overview of US system, 338–339
    payment
        for acupuncture, 295
        for biofeedback treatments, 295
        for clinical trials, 232–233
        for counseling, 295
    resources, 450–451
Health Insurance Portability and Accountability Act of 1996 (HIPPA), 340
healthcare powers of attorney, 250, 393–394
healthy denial, 301
heart damage, 271, 371
hematologists. See doctors
Hemlock Society, 404
hemorrhagic cystitis, 280
hemorrhoids, 273–274
herbal medicines, 386
herpes viruses/herpes zoster, 156, 280–281, 370, 375

LMB-2, 235–236
lodging when traveling for care, 355, 453
long-term care insurance, 345–346
losing health insurance coverage, 340
loss of trust in medical system, 383
low blood counts, 371–372
lung damage, 272, 372
lymph nodes, swelling of, 23, 29, 41
lymphocytes (lymphs), 5
lymphoid cells, 86
lymphoma type adult T-cell leukemia, 17
    See also adult T-cell leukemia (ATL)

M

magnetic resonance imaging (MRI), 74–75
managed care plans (HMOs), 340–342
marriage, 384
massage therapy, 299–300
Maxamine, 146
mechlorethamine (nitrogen mustard), 112
medical case managers, 254–255
medical dictionaries, 410, 430
medical journals, 414–415
medical libraries, 417–418
medical powers of attorney, 250, 393–394
medical records, 39, 51, 53, 253, 352–354
medical savings accounts, 344–345
medical textbooks, 419
Medicare/Medicaid, 342–344
meditation, 300–301
MEDLINE, 415–417
melatonin, 107–108
memorial ceremonies, 404–405
memory problems, 368–369
meningeal CML, 154
menopause, 211
mental confusion, 202
mercaptopurine, 113
mesna, 115
metabolic imbalances, 273

meters squared method of dosage calculation, 137, 423, 459–461
methods for tests and procedures. See specific names of tests and procedures
methotrexate, 113
methylprednisone, 114
military (VA) disability income, 351
mind-body exercise, 109, 296
mini-transplantation, 179–180
mini-vacations, 301
misdiagnoses possible, 41
mitomycin, 114
mitoxantrone (Novantrone), 114
MoAbs/Mabs, 115–117, 149, 235–238
molecular genetic analysis, 85
monoclonal antibodies (MoAbs or Mabs), 115–117, 149, 235–238
monocytes (monos), 5
mouth pain/problems, 273, 372
MRI, 74–75
mucositis, 273
MUGA scan (multiple gated acquisition scan), 76
multiple myeloma (MM), 20
muscle cramps, 274
music, 301–302
myeloproliferative disorders (MPDs), 20–22
myelosuppression, 141, 146
Mylotarg, 117, 149

N

National Cancer Institute, 413, 420
natural-killer cells, 86, 115
nausea, 23, 126–127, 274–275
needle biopsy, 76–78
Neumega, 118
Neupogen, 118
neutropenia, 272
neutrophils (polys/segs), 6
night sweats, 23, 29
nitrogen mustard (mechlorethamine), 112
node biopsy, 78–79

signs and symptoms (*continued*)
in common with other conditions, 23
ensuring credence of, 24–25
of hairy cell leukemia, 32–33
honoring instincts about, 25
not always present, 24
similar in many leukemias, 23
See also specific types and names of leukemias
singing, 301–302
skeletal damage, 375
skin problems, 279, 375–376
sleep, 134, 269–270, 304, 307–308
small lymphocytic lymphoma, 12, 158
smoking, 104
smoldering adult T-cell leukemia, 17
See also adult T-cell leukemia (ATL)
Social Security Disability Income (SSDI), 348–350
sonogram (sonography), 79–80
Southern blot assay, 62
speculative causes of leukemia, 101–105
spirituality, 304–305, 383, 387, 399
spleen, swelling of, 23, 26, 32
splenectomy, 152, 159–160, 165, 167
splenic lymphoma w/villous lymphocytes (SLVL), 13–15, 90, 166–167
staging. *See* subtype and staging
stem cell transplantation. *See* bone marrow transplantation
stem cells, 2, 169, 466–468
See also bone marrow transplantation
sterility, 207–208
STI-571, 153, 241
stigmatization, 46
stomach distress, 376
storage of specimens, 50–51
stress, 282–308
as adaptation to interaction of immune system and central nervous system, 283
associations, or lack of, with cancer, 282–283
and cancer, 109, 290–291
effect on immune system
the "cancer personality," 292
effect on cancer unclear, 290–291
medications
antianxiety drugs (anxiolytics), 307
antidepressants, 307–308
sleep medications, 307–308
reduction techniques, 293–306
acupuncture, 294–295
biofeedback, 295
counseling, 296
dance, 301–302
exercise, 296
family interaction/support, 296–297
friends interaction/support, 297–298
healthy denial and escapism, 301
hobbies, 298
hugging, 305–306
humor/laughter, 299
learning about cancer, 298–299, 407–409
massage therapy, 299–300
as means of dealing with illness, 292–294
meditation, 300–301
mind-body exercise, 109, 296
mini-vacations, 301
music, 301–302
nutrition, 302–303
pets, 303
positive thinking, 303
reading, 304
relaxation training, 304
religious beliefs, 304–305
singing, 301–302
sleep, 304
spirituality, 304–305
support groups, 305
touching, 305–306
visualization, 303
volunteer work, 298
water/swimming/bathing, 306
writing, 306

About the Author

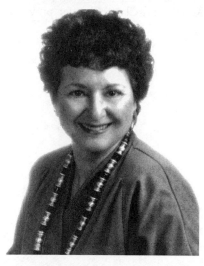

Barbara B. Lackritz is a retired educator, speech/language pathologist, and four-term alderwoman and member of the Planning and Zoning Commission for the City of Town and Country, Missouri.

Barb received her undergraduate degree from the University of Michigan in 1959 and her master's degree from Columbia University Teachers College in 1962. She has accumulated about 50 post-master's degree credits.

A leukemia survivor and cancer patient advocate, Barb manages 30 cancer support lists for the Association of Cancer Online Resources (ACOR), and is webmaster, with AML survivor Arthur Flatau, PhD, of the award-winning GrannyBarb and Art's Leukemia Links. Barb's own leukemia story is on the Web and is used by doctors at the NCI for training new doctors. She deals daily with requests for information and support from patients who have found her web site or joined her hematological cancer lists.

In addition, Barb is currently President of the American Association of University Women-Missouri (AAUW-MO) and is a member of the National Institutes of Health Director's Council of Public Representatives. She sits on the Board of Directors of ACOR and of the Chronic Lymphocytic Leukemia (CLL) Foundation.

Colophon

Patient-Centered Guides are about the experience of illness. They contain personal stories as well as a mixture of practical and medical information. The faces on the covers of our Guides reflect the human side of the information we offer.

The cover of *Adult Leukemia: A Comprehensive Guide for Patients and Families* was designed by Terri Driscoll using Adobe Photoshop 5.5 and QuarkXPress 4.1 with Onyx BT and Berkeley fonts from Bitstream. The cover photo is from Digital Stock, and is used by permission.

The interior layout for the book was designed by Melanie Wang, based on a series design by Edie Freedman and Alicia Cech. The interior fonts are Berkeley and Franklin Gothic. Anne-Maire Vaduva implemented the design using FrameMaker 5.5.6. Illustrations were created by Robert Romano and Jessamyn Read using Adobe Photoshop 5.5 and Macromedia FreeHand 8.0.

Sarah Jane Shangraw was the production editor and copyeditor for *Adult Leukemia: A Comprehensive Guide for Patients and Families*. Matt Hutchinson proofread the text and worked on page composition. Catherine Morris and Claire Cloutier provided quality control. Kate Wilkinson wrote the index.

Patient-Centered Guides™

Questions Answered
Experiences Shared

We are committed to empowering individuals to evolve into informed consumers armed with the latest information and heartfelt support for their journey.

When your life is turned upside down, your need for information is great. You have to make critical medical decisions, often with information that seems little to go on. Plus you have to break the news to family, quiet your own fears, cope with symptoms or treatment side effects, figure out how you're going to pay for things, and sometimes still get to work or get dinner on the table.

Patient-Centered Guides provide authoritative information for intelligent information seekers who want to become advocates for their own health. The books cover the whole impact of illness on your life. In each book, there's a mix of:

- **Medical background for treatment decisions**
  We can give you information that can help you to work with your doctor to come to a decision. We start from the viewpoint that modern medicine has much to offer and we discuss complementary treatments. Where there are treatment controversies, we present differing points of view.

- **Practical information**
  Once you've decided what to do about your illness, you still have to deal with treatments and changes to your life. We cover day-to-day practicalities, such as those you'd hear from a good nurse or a knowledgeable support group.

- **Emotional support**
  It's normal to have strong reactions to a condition that threatens your life or that changes how you live. It's normal that the whole family is affected. We cover issues such as the shock of diagnosis, living with uncertainty, and communicating with loved ones.

Each book also contains stories from both patients and doctors—medical "frequent flyers" who share, in their own words, the lessons and strategies they have learned while maneuvering through the often complicated maze of medical information that's available.

We provide information online, including updated listings of the resources that appear in this book. This is freely available for you to print out and copy to share with others, as long as you retain the copyright notice on the printouts.

www.patientcenters.com

Other Books in the Series

Cancer

Advanced Breast Cancer
A Guide to Living with Metastatic Disease, Second Edition
By Musa Mayer
ISBN 1-56592-522-X, Paperback, 6" x 9", 544 pages, $24.95 US, $36.95 CAN

"An excellent book...if knowledge is power, this book will be good medicine."
—*David Spiegel, MD, Stanford University, Author,* Living Beyond Limits

Cancer Clinical Trials
Experimental Treatments and How They Can Help You
By Robert Finn
ISBN 1-56592-566-1, Paperback, 5" x 8", 232 pages, $14.95 US, $21.95 CAN

"I highly recommend this book as a first step in what will be for many a difficult, but crucially important, part of their struggle to beat their cancer."
—*From the* Foreword *by Robert Bazell, Chief Science Correspondent for NBC News Author,* Her-2: The Making of Herceptin, a Revolutionary Treatment for Breast Cancer

Colon & Rectal Cancer
A Comprehensive Guide for Patients & Families
By Lorraine Johnston
ISBN 1-56592-633-1, Paperback, 6" x 9", 556 pages, $24.95 US, $36.95 CAN

"I sure wish [this book] had been available when I was first diagnosed. I wouldn't change a thing: informative, down-to-earth, easily understandable, and very touching."
—*Pati Lanning, colon cancer survivor*

Non-Hodgkin's Lymphomas
Making Sense of Diagnosis, Treatment & Options
By Lorraine Johnston
ISBN 1-56592-444-4, Paperback, 6" x 9", 584 pages, $24.95 US, $36.95 CAN

"When I gave this book to one of our patients, there was an instant, electric connection. A sense of enlightenment came over her while she absorbed the information. It was thrilling to see her so sparked with new energy and focus."
—*Susan Weisberg, LCSW, Clinical Social Worker, Stanford University Medical Center*

0065

Patient-Centered Guides
Published by O'Reilly & Associates, Inc.
Our products are available at a bookstore near you.
For information: 800-998-9938 • 707-829-0515 • info@oreilly.com
101 Morris Street • Sebastopol • CA • 95472-9902
www.patientcenters.com